Handboo...
MECHANICAL VE...

Handbook of
MECHANICAL VENTILATION

SECOND EDITION

B Umesh Kumar BRCT MD (AM)
Department of Respiratory Medicine
Hamad General Hospital—HMC
Doha, Qatar

Foreword
Jose Chacko

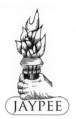

JAYPEE *The Health Sciences Publisher*

New Delhi | London | Philadelphia | Panama

Jaypee Brothers Medical Publishers (P) Ltd

Headquarters

Jaypee Brothers Medical Publishers (P) Ltd
4838/24, Ansari Road, Daryaganj
New Delhi 110 002, India
Phone: +91-11-43574357
Fax: +91-11-43574314
Email: jaypee@jaypeebrothers.com

Overseas Offices

J.P. Medical Ltd
83, Victoria Street, London
SW1H 0HW (UK)
Phone: +44 20 3170 8910
Fax: +44 (0)20 3008 6180
Email: info@jpmedpub.com

Jaypee-Highlights Medical Publishers Inc.
City of Knowledge, Bld. 237, Clayton
Panama City, Panama
Phone: +1 507-301-0496
Fax: +1 507-301-0499
Email: cservice@jphmedical.com

Jaypee Medical Inc
325 Chestnut Street
Suite 412, Philadelphia, PA 19106, USA
Phone: +1 267-519-9789
Email: jpmed.us@gmail.com

Jaypee Brothers Medical Publishers (P) Ltd
17/1-B Babar Road, Block-B, Shaymali
Mohammadpur, Dhaka-1207
Bangladesh
Mobile: +08801912003485
Email: jaypeedhaka@gmail.com

Jaypee Brothers Medical Publishers (P) Ltd
Bhotahity, Kathmandu, Nepal
Phone: +977-9741283608
Email: kathmandu@jaypeebrothers.com

Website: www.jaypeebrothers.com
Website: www.jaypeedigital.com

Handbook of Mechanical Ventilation

First Edition: 2011
Second Edition: **2016**
ISBN 978-93-5152-921-7
Printed at Sanat Printers

Dedicated to

Dr Ashwini Murthy, Consultant and Head, Apollo Hospitals, Bengaluru,
who motivated me to go on and publish this book to medical professionals,
who will achieve knowledge about mechanical ventilation and its purpose

Foreword

The intensive care unit can often be a daunting experience, especially to the uninitiated. Mechanical ventilation has come a long way since its first use during the polio epidemic of Copenhagen in the 1950s. Modern intensive care units are able to offer mechanical ventilatory support for prolonged periods of time often running into many weeks while giving the underlying disease process a chance to recover. The machines, we use today, have also evolved over time, capable of supporting patients in respiratory failure in a more efficient and versatile fashion. Much has been written on ventilatory support; however, a short handbook with access to basic information that can be carried to the bedside would always be welcome.

Umesh Kumar has compiled this bedside manual with respiratory therapists, nurses and trainee doctors in mind. He has made use of several years of experience and expertise to construct this practical guide. Written in a clear and lucid style without getting bogged down in trivia that might put off most readers, it covers the basics of mechanical ventilation in a refreshingly readable manner.

I would unhesitatingly recommend this book to all healthcare professionals involved in the care of sick patients in the intensive care unit. In particular, it will be of benefit to respiratory therapists preparing for their examinations as it covers much of their syllabus. A candidate familiar with the contents of this short book and taking note of the tips offered will be at an advantage while facing the examination. I can confidently say that Umesh Kumar's work would go a long way in making a complex topic more amenable to those who seek a better understanding of ventilating the sick patient.

Jose Chacko MD DNB EDIC
Director and Head
Department of Critical Care Medicine
Narayana Multispecialty Hospital
Whitefield, Bengaluru, Karnataka, India

Preface to the Second Edition

This *Handbook of Mechanical Ventilation* provides an opportunity to the medical and paramedical professionals like doctors, respiratory therapists, physiotherapists, nurses and other paramedical staff, who require a clear, concise yet-comprehensive guide to mechanical ventilation, airway management procedures and also to denote their skills, knowledge and competencies required during treating a patient on mechanical ventilation. This is designed to be effective for use in hospital as well as in domiciliary setting.

The successful completion of this book was a unique experience for me because by treating many different types of cases on mechanical ventilation and interacting with many medical professionals, I achieved knowledge about mechanical ventilation. The experience which I gained by doing this book was an essential point of my career.

B Umesh Kumar

Preface to the First Edition

This *Handbook of Mechanical Ventilation* is intended for use by doctors, respiratory therapists, physiotherapists, nurses and paramedical staff, who require a clear, concise yet-comprehensive guide to mechanical ventilation and procedures. This is designed to be effective for use in hospital as well as in domiciliary setting. The basic understanding of pulmonary anatomy, physiology and pathophysiology are clearly explained in the book in simple words.

B Umesh Kumar

Acknowledgments

I would like to express my gratitude to all my consultants of critical care medicine, who helped and supported me a lot in writing and giving a shape to this book. My most sincere gratitude and love, for without them, this book could not have been completed.

I would like to express my heartfelt gratitude to Dr Jose Chacko, Dr Somnath Chattrerje, Dr Ullas Gopala Krishna, Dr Padmakumar, Dr Sunil Karanth, Dr Rajesh Shetty, Dr Ashok, and Dr Ashwini Murthy, who trained and helped me gain a lot of knowledge in the field of intensive care.

Finally, to all my students who, with all their questions, can only make me a better trainer and educator, my deepest thanks.

Contents

Chapter 1: **Basic Principles of Mechanical Ventilation**   1
- *Airway Resistance   1*
- *What is the Plateau Pressure   5*
- *Lung Compliance   6*
- *Dead Space Ventilation   8*
- *Ventilation-Perfusion Ratio   10*

Chapter 2: **Pulmonary Anatomy and Physiology**   17
- *Lungs   17*
- *Breathing   20*
- *Blood Pressure   22*
- *Respiratory Physiology   22*
- *Gas Exchange in Humans and Mammals   32*
- *Pulmonary Vascular Resistance   39*

Chapter 3: **Respiratory Pathophysiology**   40
- *Pulmonary Insufficiency   40*
- *Anxiety Assessment Findings   40*
- *Respiratory Breathing Patterns   41*
- *Diagnostic Approach to Patient with Dyspnea   41*
- *Locations for Placement of the Stethoscope   44*
- *Classification of Dyspnea   45*
- *Examination of the Trachea   45*
- *Sputum Observation   46*
- *Chest X-rays   46*
- *Findings and Physical Examination   50*
- *Respiratory Diseases   52*
- *Pulmonary Hypertension   73*

Chapter 4: **Arterial Blood Gas Analysis**   77
- *Arterial Puncture   77*
- *Etiology and Clinical Manifestations   81*
- *Rules for Respiratory Acid-Base Disorders   84*
- *Rules for Metabolic Acid-Base Disorders   86*
- *Further Analysis in Cases of Metabolic Acidosis   86*

Chapter 5: **Indication for Mechanical Ventilation**   92
- *Hypoxemia   92*
- *Oxyhemoglobin Dissociation Curve   99*
- *Respiratory Failure   107*
- *Classification of Respiratory Failure   110*
- *Pathophysiology   113*
- *Treatment   114*

Chapter 6: Modes of Ventilation   **116**
- *Negative Pressure Ventilation   117*
- *Positive Pressure Ventilation   118*
- *Indication for Use   118*
- *Spontaneous Mode   119*
- *Positive End-expiratory Pressure   119*
- *Continuous Positive Airway Pressure (CPAP)   120*
- *Controlled Mandatory Ventilation (CMV)   121*
- *Pressure Controlled Ventilation   122*
- *Pressure-Assist Ventilation   123*
- *Assist Control   123*
- *Intermittent Mandatory Ventilation   124*
- *Synchronized Intermittent Mandatory Ventilation   124*
- *Pressure Regulated Volume Control (PRVC)   125*
- *How the Ventilator Achieves PRVC Mode   126*
- *Airway Pressure Release Ventilation   126*
- *Complications   126*
- *Other Supportive Modes   127*
- *Closed Loop Control   127*
- *Ventilator Settings   127*
- *High Frequency Ventilation   130*
- *High Frequency Oscillatory Ventilation   131*
- *Basic Principles   133*

Chapter 7: Initiation and Monitoring during Ventilation   **137**
- *Initial Ventilator Settings   137*
- *Tidal Volume and Inspiratory Pressure Limit   137*
- *Respiratory Rate   138*
- *Initial FiO_2 138*
- *Sighs   139*
- *Inspiratory Plateau or Hold   140*
- *Variable and Waveform Control   141*
- *Phase Variables   141*
- *Goals   142*
- *Patient Assessment   144*
- *Ventilator Settings and Alarms   144*
- *Patient-Ventilator Dyssynchrony   147*
- *Monitoring   153*
- *Contraindications   155*
- *Hazards/Complications   156*
- *Limitations of Procedure/Validation of Results   156*
- *Assessment of Need   156*
- *Assessment of Outcome   156*
- *ARDS/ALI Ventilator Protocol   156*

Chapter 8: Hemodynamic Waveform Analysis   **161**
- *Arterial Catheter   161*
- *Central Venous Catheter   165*

- *Pathologic CVP Waveforms   166*
- *Pulmonary Artery Catheter   168*
- *Pulse Oximetry   171*
- *Capnography   173*
- *Cardiac Output   175*
- *Fick Principle   176*

Chapter 9: **Weaning from Mechanical Ventilation**   178
- *Weaning Success   178*
- *Weaning Failure   178*
- *Weaning Criteria   179*
- *Method of Weaning   181*
- *Rapid Weaning   182*
- *Approach to Difficult Weaning   183*
- *When to Stop   184*
- *Procedure   186*

Chapter 10: **Ventilator Graphics**   190
- *General Concepts   190*
- *Analysis of Scalar Graphics   192*

Chapter 11: **Airway Management**   212
- *Manual Methods   212*
- *Adjuncts to Airway Management   213*
- *Laryngeal Mask Airway   213*
- *Endotracheal Tube   214*
- *Intubation   214*
- *Approach to the Airway in Trauma Patients   218*
- *Oropharyngeal Airway   222*
- *Nasopharyngeal Airway   223*
- *Esophageal Obturator Airway   229*
- *Esophageal Gastric Tube Airway   230*
- *Cricothyroidotomy   231*
- *Percutaneous Tracheostomy   239*

Chapter 12: **Noninvasive Ventilation and High Flow Therapy**   248
- *Noninvasive Ventilation   248*
- *High Flow Therapy   258*
- *Contraindications   260*

Chapter 13: **Pulmonary Rehabilitation**   263
- *Who Benefits from Pulmonary Rehabilitation   263*
- *Therapy Programs   264*
- *Flexibility and Stretching   266*
- *Balance   269*
- *Inspiratory Muscle Training   269*
- *Home Training   269*
- *Nutritional Guidance   270*
- *What to Expect after Treatment   270*
- *Why it is Done   270*
- *How Well it Works   270*
- *Risks   270*
- *What to Think About   271*

Chapter 14: Chest Physiotherapy   272
- *Goals of Chest Physiotherapy 272*
- *Techniques Promoting Bronchial Hygiene 273*
- *Lung Segments 275*
- *Techniques Improving Breathing Efficiency 280*
- *Chest Physiotherapy Positions for Infants and Children 281*

Index   *285*

Abbreviations

ABP	:	Arterial blood pressure
AC	:	Assist control ventilation
ALI	:	Acute lung injury
APRV	:	Airway pressure release ventilation
ARDS	:	Acute respiratory distress syndrome
AVM	:	Arteriovenous malformation
BIPAP	:	Bi-level positive airway pressure
BPG	:	Biphosphoglycerate
CCHS	:	Congenital central hypoventilation syndrome
CMV	:	Controlled mandatory ventilation
CO	:	Cardiac output
COPD	:	Chronic obstructive pulmonary disease
CPAP	:	Continuous positive airway pressure
CVP	:	Central venous pressure
DP	:	Diastolic pressure
DPPC	:	Dipalmitoyl phosphatidylcholine
EDRVP	:	End diastolic right ventricular pressure
EOA	:	Esophageal obturator airway
EPAP	:	Expiratory pressure
ERA	:	Endothelin receptor antagonist
ERV	:	Expiratory reserve volume
ESRVP	:	End systolic right ventricular pressure
FiO_2	:	Inspired fraction of oxygen
FRC	:	Functional residual capacity
FVC	:	Forced vital capacity
HbO_2	:	Oxyhemoglobin
HCO_3	:	Sodium bicarbonate
HFOV	:	High frequency oscillatory ventilation
HFT	:	High flow therapy
HHb	:	Hydrohemoglobin
HHT	:	Hereditary hemorrhagic telangiectasia
IMV	:	Intermittent mandatory ventilation
IPAP	:	Inspiratory pressure
IPPB	:	Intermittent positive pressure breathing
IRV	:	Inspiratory reserve volume
MAP	:	Mean arterial pressure
MAS	:	Meconium aspiration syndrome
NAVA	:	Neurally adjusted ventilatory assist
NIV	:	Noninvasive ventilation

NPA	:	Nasopharyngeal airway
OPA	:	Oropharyngeal airway
P	:	Pressure change
$PaCO_2$	:	Partial pressure of carbon dioxide
PaO_2	:	Partial pressure of oxygen
PAP	:	Pulmonary artery pressure
PAV	:	Pressure-assist ventilation
PC	:	Pressure control ventilation
PCOP	:	Pulmonary capillary occlusion pressure
PCWP	:	Pulmonary capillary wedge pressure
PDEI	:	Phosphodiesterase-5 inhibitors
PEEP	:	Positive end expiratory pressure
PEFR	:	Peak expiratory flow rate
PEP	:	Positive expiratory pressure
PIFR	:	Peak inspiratory flow rate
PIP	:	Peak inspiratory pressure
PPHN	:	Persistent pulmonary hypertension
PRVC	:	Pressure regulated volume control
PS	:	Pressure support
PVR	:	Pulmonary vascular resistance
RACE	:	Repetitive alveolar collapse-expansion
RAW	:	Airway resistance
RQ	:	Respiratory quotient
RSBI	:	Rapid shallow breathing index
RV	:	Residual volume
SBT	:	Spontaneous breathing trail
SIMV	:	Synchronized intermittent mandatory ventilation
SP	:	Systolic pressure
SVR	:	Systemic vascular resistance
Te	:	Expiratory time
Ti	:	Inspiratory time
TLC	:	Total lung capacity
V/Q	:	Ventilation/perfusion
V	:	Inspiratory flow
VD	:	Dead space volume
VE	:	Minute ventilation
VILI	:	Ventilator-induced lung injury
VMT	:	Ventilatory muscle training
Vt	:	Tidal volume

Introduction

Mechanical ventilation was first described in the 16th century by Vesalius, who used bellows to ventilate a donkey. Advances in mechanical ventilation were encouraged by the 1952 polio epidemic in Copenhagen during which, Lassen organized relays of medical students to ventilate hundreds of patients by hand, for many weeks.

Mechanical ventilation is used when natural (spontaneous) breathing is absent (apnea) or is insufficient. This may be so in cases of intoxication, cardiac arrest, neurological disease or head trauma, paralysis of the breathing muscles due to spinal cord injury, or the effect of anesthetic or muscle relaxant drugs. Various pulmonary diseases or chest trauma, cardiac disease, such as congestive heart failure, sepsis and shock may also necessitate ventilation.

Depending on the situation, mechanical ventilation may be continued for a few minutes or many hours to weeks to, in some rare cases years. While returning to spontaneous breathing is rarely a problem in routine anesthesia, weaning an intensive care patient from prolonged mechanical ventilation can take weeks or even months. Some patients never adequately regain the ability to breathe and require permanent mechanical ventilation. This is often the case with severe brain injury, spinal cord injury, or neurological disease.

Plate 1

Hemoglobin

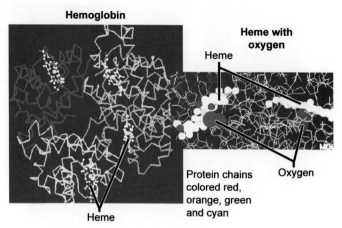

Figs 2.6: Oxygen transportation through blood

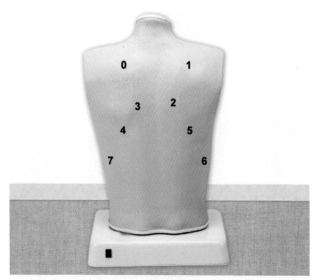

Fig. 3.1: Stethoscope placement: Dorsal. Note that the locations for placement of the stethoscope are the same general locations for percussion

Plate 2

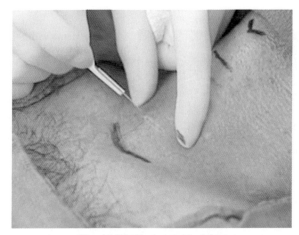

Fig. 11.21: Horizontal incision

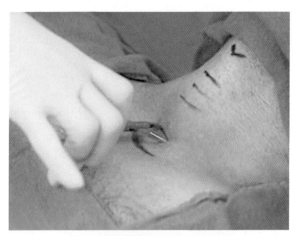

Fig. 11.22: Dilatation with forceps

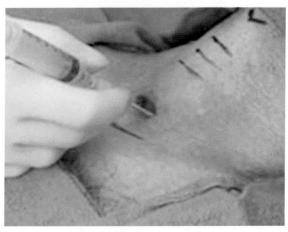

Fig. 11.23: Needle insertion

Plate 3

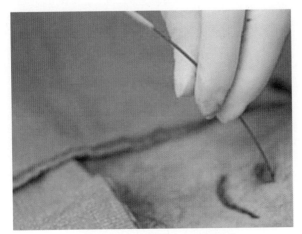

Fig. 11.25: Guidewire insertion

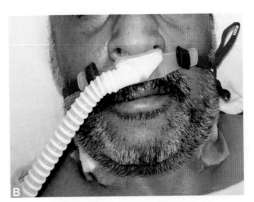

Fig. 12.3B: Nasal high flow

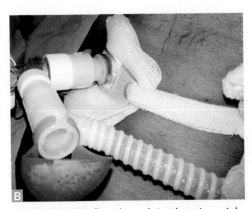

Fig. 12.4B: High flow through tracheostomy tube

BASIC PRINCIPLES OF MECHANICAL VENTILATION

■ AIRWAY RESISTANCE

Airway resistance is defined by the pressure difference between the beginning and end of a tube and the flow of gas volume per unit time. In case of pulmonary airways, it would be the difference between atmospheric pressure at the mouth and the alveolar pressure. In mechanical ventilation, the degree of airway resistance is primarily affected by the length, size and patency of the airway, endotracheal tube and ventilator circuit.

Normal Airway Resistance

Newborn	: 30–40 mbar/L/sec
Infant	: 20–30 mbar/L/sec
Small children	: 10–20 mbar/L/sec
Adult	: 2–4 mbar/L/sec
Intubated patient	: 4–6 mbar/L/sec
Raw	: Airway resistance
ΔP	: Pressure change
Pressure change	: Peak pressure—Plateau pressure
V	: Inspiratory flow

$$Raw = \frac{\Delta P}{V}$$

Alveoli—Site of Gas Exchange

An alveolus has a single layer of thin exchange epithelium and is the site of gas exchange.

There are three types of cells in alveoli:

1. Type I alveolar cells: Very thin, allowing gas exchange.
2. Type II alveolar cells: Thicker, secrete surfactant to ease lung expansion.
3. Alveolar macrophages: Protect and defend.

Alveoli do not contain muscle fibers and cannot contract. There are elastin fibers between alveoli and these do contribute to elastic recoil when lung tissue is stretched. Capillaries cover 80–90% of alveolar surface forming an almost continuous blood-air contact. Gas exchange occurs by simple diffusion. The single endothelial cell of the capillary and the single squamous epithelium of the alveoli have a fused basement membrane in between them, this arrangement allows for a rapid diffusion of gases.

300 million alveoli in lungs—0.3 mm in diameter, total surface area of lungs is about 75 m^2 (size of tennis court).

Collateral ventilation: Airflow between adjacent alveoli.

Pleurisy: Inflammation of pleural sac (painful "friction rub").

Atmospheric pressure = 760 mm Hg at sea level, decreases as altitude increases.

Intra-alveolar pressure (intrapulmonary pressure) will equilibrate with atmospheric pressure.

Intrapleural pressure (intrathoracic pressure) = 756 mm Hg – vacuum [called minus four (–4)] closed cavity.

Negative intra-alveolar, intrapleural pressures provide driving force for inhaling/exhaling.

Transmural pressure – pressure across surface of lungs = $P_{alveolus} - P_{pleural\,space}$

Two forces hold thoracic walls and lungs in close apposition:

(Cannot expand thorax without expanding lungs):

1. Intrapleural fluid's cohesiveness (like water between two slides).
2. Transmural pressure gradient (most important).

Intra-alveolar pressure = 760 mm Hg, pushes out against intrapleural pressure of 756 mm Hg.

Atmospheric pressure = 760 mm Hg, pushes in against intrapleural pressure of 756 mm Hg.

Neither chest wall nor lungs are in their resting position (both are actively pushing against space).

Pleural space has slightly negative pressure because chest is pulling out, lungs are pulling in, and there's no extra fluid to fill expanded space.

Pneumothorax: Air enters pleural cavity, pressure equalizes with atmospheric pressure, transmural pressure gradient is gone → lungs collapse, thoracic wall springs out.

Before inspiration: Respiratory muscles are relaxed, no air is flowing, intra-alveolar pressure = Atmospheric pressure.

Major inspiratory muscles (diaphragm, external intercostals) contract → thoracic cavity enlarges.

[Diaphragm is innervated by phrenic nerve; dome-shaped at rest, contracts and pulls down. Responsible for 75% of enlargement of thoracic cavity during inspiration. Contraction of external intercostals enlarges cavity in lateral and AP dimensions (elevate ribs when contracting)].

As lungs expand, pressure decreases (to 759 mm Hg) → air flows in (alveolar pressure is negative during inhalation, positive during exhalation). Intrapleural pressure drops to 754 mm Hg (ensures that lungs will be fully expanded).

Lung expansion is not caused by movement of air into lungs.

With deeper contractions, contract diaphragm and external intercostals more forcefully and contract accessory inspiratory muscles (SCM, scalenes, alae nasi, small muscles of neck/head) to raise sternum and first 2 ribs.

At end of inspiration: Inspiratory muscles relax, diaphragm is dome-shaped again, rib cage falls because of gravity once external intercostals relax, chest walls and stretched lungs recoil → volume decreases, pressure increases (to 761 mm Hg) → air flows out.

During quiet breathing, expiration is passive (due to elastic recoil of lungs, there is no muscular/energy expenditure), whereas inspiration is always active.

During heavy breathing – active expiration – contract abdominal muscles (increase intra-abdominal pressure → pushes diaphragm up → increases intrathoracic pressure), internal intercostal muscles (pull ribs downward, inward) → lungs are emptied more forcefully.

During forceful expiration, intrapleural pressure exceeds atmospheric pressure, but lungs do not collapse because intra-alveolar pressure increases, too (4 mm Hg pressure gradient stays same).

Paralysis of intercostal muscles does not affect breathing much, but in paralysis of diaphragm, one cannot breathe. Phrenic nerve is C3–C5, so patients with paralysis from neck down can still breathe.

Airflow $V = \Delta P/R$

Flow

ΔP = pressure gradient between atmosphere and alveoli.

R is primarily determined by radius.

Resistance of total airways circuit depends on length, cross-sectional area of conducting airways. Each terminal bronchiole has greater resistance to flow than trachea, but because of vast cross-sectional area, their overall contribution to total R is less than that of central airways (since bronchioles are arranged in parallel).

In healthy patient, overall respiratory system has extremely low R.

Laminar vs Turbulent Flow

Flow can be laminar (low flow rate) or turbulent (fast flow rate).

In small airways, flow is usually laminar.

For laminar flow, $R = \dfrac{8\eta l}{\pi r^4}$ (Poiseuille's Law) where, η = viscosity, l = Length

Turbulent flow has different properties, where driving pressure is proportional to square of flow (V^2).

Turbulence is most likely to occur with high velocity and large diameter.

Volume of inflation of lung has important effect on airway resistance.

Pressure = (Volume/Compliance) + Flow × Resistance; P = pressure required to breathe.

Partial pressures = P_{atm} × Percentage of gas in atmosphere. Partial pressures vary with amount of water vapor.

For example, air is a mixture of gases.

$$N_2 \quad = \quad 79\%$$
$$O_2 \quad = \quad 21\%$$
$$CO_2 \quad = \quad 0.03\%$$

If atmospheric pressure of air at sea level is 760 mm Hg (a standard value, See calculating partial pressures of gases in air at sea level) and air is a mixture of the above gases (N_2, O_2 and CO_2), then we can calculate the partial pressure exerted by each gas in this mixture. The partial pressure of N_2 is symbolized by PN_2 and partial pressure of O_2 is PO_2, etc.

Calculating partial pressures of gases in air at sea level:

1. P_{N_2} =   760 mm Hg × Percentage of gas in mixture (79% = 0.79)
             =   760 mm Hg × 0.79
             =   600 mm Hg

2. P_{O_2} =   760 mm Hg × Percentage of gas in mixture (21% = 0.21)
             =   760 mm Hg × 0.21
             =   160 mm Hg

3. P_{CO_2} =   760 mm Hg × Percentage of gas in mixture (0.03% = 0.0003)
             =   760 mm Hg × 0.0003
             =   0.24 mm Hg (which is negligible)

Factors Affecting Airway Resistance

Airway resistance causes obstruction to airflow in the airways. It is increased when the patency of the airways is reduced. That is,

- Inside the airway. For example, retained secretion.
- In the wall of the airway. For example, neoplasm of the bronchial muscle structure.
- Outside the airway. For example, tumor surrounding and compressing the airway.

When one of these conditions occurs, the radius of the airway decreases and airway resistance increases (Table 1.1).

- Increased airway resistance occurs with:
  - Bronchoconstrictors
    - Parasympathetic nervous system (acetylcholine)
    - Cholinergic agonists
    - Histamine (released from mast cells, e.g. in asthma)
    - Smoke, pollutants
    - Bronchitis (inflammation of the bronchi)

Table 1.1: Conditions that increase airway resistance

Type	Clinical conditions
COPD	Emphysema Chronic bronchitis Bronchiectasis Asthma
Mechanical	Post-intubation obstruction
Obstruction	Foreign body aspiration Endotracheal tube obstruction Condensation in ventilator circuit
Infection	Larygotracheobronchitis Bronchiolitis Epiglottitis

- Compression of airways
- Particles in the airways
- Low lung volumes: Less traction on airways and, hence, increased resistance
- Increased air density, as in a deep-sea dive.
- Decreased airway resistance occurs with:
  - Bronchodilation → decreased resistance
    - Sympathetic nervous system (norepinephrine)
    - β-adrenergic agonists
  - High lung volumes: Greater traction and decreased airway resistance
    - Breathing at higher volumes is a good way to decrease resistance in patients with asthma (or other diseases that lead to increased resistance).
  - Breathing in air with decreased density, as in breathing in helium.

Effects on Ventilation and Oxygenation

The work of breathing is increased when there is increased airway resistance. This affects on the patient's ventilatory and oxygenation status. If high airway resistance is sustained over a long time, fatigue of the respiratory muscle may occur, leading to ventilatory and oxygenation failure. Oxygen failure usually follows when the pulmonary system cannot provide adequate oxygen needed for metabolism. Ventilatory failure occurs when the patient's minute ventilation cannot keep up with carbon dioxide production.

■ WHAT IS THE PLATEAU PRESSURE

The plateau pressure is the pressure applied (in positive pressure ventilation) to the small airways and alveoli. It is believed that control of the plateau pressure is important, as excessive stretch of alveoli has been implicated as the cause of ventilator-induced lung injury. The peak pressure is the pressure measured by the ventilator in the major airways, and it strongly reflects airways resistance. For example, in acute severe asthma, there is a large gradient between the peak pressure (high) and the plateau pressure (normal).

Increased PIP and P$_{plat}$

- Increased tidal volume
- Decreased pulmonary compliance
- Pulmonary edema
- Pleural effusion
- Peritoneal gas insufflation
- Tension pneumothorax
- Trendelenburg
- Ascites
- Abdominal packing
- Endobronchial intubation.

Increased PIP and unchanged P$_{plat}$

- Increased inspiratory gas flow rate
- Increased airway resistance
- Kinked ET tube
- Secretions
- Foreign body aspiration
- Bronchospasm
- Airway compression
- ET tube cuff herniation.

■ LUNG COMPLIANCE

Lung compliance is volume change (Lung expansion) per unit pressure change (work of breathing). Abnormally low or high lung compliance impairs the patient's ability to maintain efficient gas exchange. Low lung compliance makes lung expansion difficult and high lung compliance induces incomplete exhalation and carbon dioxide elimination.

There are two types of compliance:

1. Static compliance
2. Dynamic compliance.

Static compliance: Static compliance is measured when there is no air flow (using plateau pressure – PEEP). When air flow is absent, airway resistance is not a determining factor. Thus static compliance reflects the elastic resistance of the lung and chest wall.

Dynamic comliance: Dynamic compliance is measured when air flow is present (using the peak pressure-PEEP). Here airway resistance becomes a critical factor. This, therefore, reflects the condition of airway (non-elastic resistance) as well as the elastic properties of the lung and chest wall (elastic resistance).

Static compliance:	Corrected tidal volume
	Plateau pressure—PEEP
Dynamic compliance:	Corrected tidal volume
	Peak pressure—PEEP
Normal values:	Static compliance: 40–60 cm H$_2$O
	Dynamic compliance: 30–40 cm H$_2$O

Elastic Forces

- Due to tendency of tissue to resume its original position after an applied force has been removed
  Note: The chest wall is naturally larger than the lungs, but the chest wall and lungs cannot assume their natural positions because (normally) no air can enter the intrapleural space
- At the resting (muscles relaxed) volume (FRC), the tendency of the isolated lungs is to collapse and the tendency of the isolated chest wall is to expand. Relaxed intrapleural pressure (Ppl) is negative, about × 5 cmH$_2$O
  Note: Negative intrapleural pressure helps keep airways open
- Rest or relaxed position: Position in which the lung and chest wall elastic forces just balance with no active muscle contraction (that is, the forces are balanced because the force developed by the tendency of the lungs to collapse is equal in magnitude and opposite in direction to the force developed by the tendency of the chest wall to expand). (Question: Volume in the lungs at the rest/relaxed position?) If expanded from this position, the system will tend to collapse; if compressed, the lung-chest wall system will tend to expand when the force is removed. Thus, force is necessary to maintain any position other than the relaxed position. The volume change per unit force (pressure) is termed as the compliance (C). The inverse of compliance is stiffness.

Basis of Compliance (or Stiffness)

- Total system stiffness (S$_t$) is the sum of the lung stiffness (S$_L$) and chest wall stiffness (S$_{cw}$)

$$S_t = S_L + S_{cw}$$

  Note: If either the lung tissue or the chest wall is more stiff than normal, total compliance will be less than normal.
- Chest wall stiffness: Due to elasticity of tissue; normally responsible for one-half of the total system stiffness.
- Lung stiffness: Contributing factors.
  - Elasticity of lung tissue
  - Surface tension.
    - Due to air-liquid interface in the alveoli (alveoli are lined with a monomolecular layer of liquid because of high permeability).
    - Important because of large alveolar surface area.
      - High stiffness (low compliance).
      - Alveolar instability, with small alveoli emptying into large alveoli; can cause atelectasis—alveolar collapse.
      - Movement of interstitial fluid into the alveoli (life-threatening).
- Effects greatly reduced by the pulmonary surfactant dipalmitoyl phosphatidylcholine (DPPC) secreted by lung type 2 alveolar cells.

Table 1.2: Conditions that decrease compliance

Compliance	Clinical condition
Static compliance	Atelectasis Tension pneumothorax ARDS Retained secretion Obesity
Dynamic compliance	Airway obstruction Kinking of ET tube/circuit Bronchospasm

- Role of surfactant
    - Lower surface tension to about 1/3rd of plasma (increase lung compliance).
    - Lower surface tension more in small alveoli (increase alveolar stability).
    - Helps keep alveoli "dry."

Note: Structures surrounding the alveoli tend to support them and so help counteract the action of surface tension in causing alveolar collapse.

Note: Even though pulmonary surfactant lowers surface tension, some alveoli will still collapse unless the lungs are periodically inflated to a larger volume.

■ DEAD SPACE VENTILATION

The portion of the respiratory system, in which no significant gas exchange occurs is referred to as dead space ventilation. There are three types of dead space:

Anatomic dead space: The volume in the conducting airways is called anatomic dead space. It includes nasopharynx, trachea, bronchi and the bronchiolds. Its air filling volume is referred as dead space volume. The anatomical dead space volume (VD) is about 2 mL/kg of body weight.

$$\frac{V_d}{V_t} = \frac{P_{aCO_2} - P_{eCO_2}}{P_{aCO_2}}$$

Where V_d is the dead space volume and V_t is the tidal volume.

P_{aCO2} is the partial pressure of carbon dioxide in the arterial blood.

P_{eCO2} is the partial pressure of carbon dioxide in the expired (exhaled) air.

Alveolar dead space: The inhaled air reaching the alveoli is not utilized due to insufficient perfusion of the relevant alveoli and this is called as alveolar dead space.

$$\frac{V_{alveolar\ dead\ space}}{V_t} = \frac{P_{aCO_2} - P_{end\ tidal\ CO_2}}{P_{aCO_2}}$$

Physiological dead space: It is the sum of anatomical and alveolar dead space volume (Table 1.3).

Normally, dead space ventilation involves 30% of the tidal volume and alveolar ventilation involves about 70%. Any increase in dead space ventilation can be compensated for by increasing the tidal volume. The dead space quotient V_D/V_t is 0.3.

$$\frac{V_{\text{physiologic dead space}}}{V_t} = \frac{P_{aCO_2} - P_{\text{mixed expired } CO_2}}{P_{aCO_2}}$$

How gas gets to the alveoli: Ventilation, which can be spontaneous (as in breathing) or artificial (as in mechanical ventilation) is the movement of air (Air is a mixture of gases. According to Dalton's law, the total pressure of a mixture of gases is the sum of the pressures of the individual gases. In dry air, at an atmospheric pressure of 760 mm Hg, 78% of the total pressure is due to nitrogen molecules and 21% is due to oxygen) between the environment and the alveoli. It is measured as the frequency of breathing multiplied by the volume of each breath. Ventilation maintains normal concentrations of oxygen and carbon dioxide in the alveolar gas and, through the process of diffusion, also maintains normal partial pressures of oxygen and carbon dioxide in the blood flowing from the capillaries.

Minute ventilation, the volume of gas ventilated in one minute, is expressed as
Minute ventilation = Tidal Volume × Breaths/Minute

Alveolar ventilation, the volume of gas available to the alveolar surface per minute, is expressed as:
Alveolar Ventilation = Tidal Volume – Dead Space) × Breaths/Minute

Ventilation-perfusion relationships: Ventilation and perfusion are normally matched in the lungs so that gas exchange (ventilation) nearly matches pulmonary arterial blood flow (perfusion). If mismatched, impairment of oxygen and carbon dioxide transfer results.

The concentration of oxygen (PO_2) in any lung unit is measured by the ratio of ventilation to blood flow:

Concentration of oxygen (PO_2) in any lung unit = Ventilation/Perfusion
or V/Q

Table 1.3: Clinical conditions that increase physiological dead space

Type of change	Clinical condition
Decrease in TV	Relative increase in V_D/V_t ratio (Drug over dose, neuromuscular disease)
Increase in alveolar dead space	Decreased cardiac output (Congestive heart failure, blood loss) Obstruction of pulmonary vessels (Pulmonary vasoconstriction, pulmonary embolism)

This relationship also applies to carbon dioxide, nitrogen and any other gas present.

The ventilation-perfusion relationship can be measured by calculating difference between the alveolar (a) and arterial (A) pO_2. PaO_2 can be calculated using the equation:

$$PaO_2 = FiO_2 (P_{atm} - pH_2O) - (PaCO_2/R)$$

At sea level, $FiO_2 = 0.21$, $pH_2O = 47$, $P_{breath} = 760$, $PaCO_2$ measured by laboratory analysis, $R = 0.8$.

$$PAO_2 = 150 - (PaCO_2/0.8)$$

PaO_2 is measured by laboratory analysis.

Normal $PAO_2 - PaO_2$ gradient $= 10$, increasing by 5–6 per decade over 50.

■ VENTILATION-PERFUSION RATIO

Ideally, each alveolus in the lungs would receive the same amount of ventilation and pulmonary capillary blood flow (perfusion). In reality, ventilation and perfusion differ depending on the region of the lung.
- On an average, the alveolar ventilation is about 4 L/min.
- Normal pulmonary capillary blood flow is about 5 L/min.
- Thus, the ventilation-perfusion ratio 0.8.

In the upright lung, the ventilation-perfusion ratio progressively decreases from the apex to the base.
- The alveoli in the upper lung portions receive moderate ventilation and little blood flow.
- The resulting ventilation-perfusion ratio is higher than 0.8 (ventilation > perfusion).
- In lower regions of the lung, the alveolar ventilation is moderately increased and the blood flow is greatly increased (since blood flow is gravity dependent). Thus, the ventilation-perfusion ratio is lower than 0.8 (perfusion > ventilation).

Two key relationships to remember are:
- When the ventilation-perfusion ratio increases, ventilation > perfusion.
- When the ventilation-perfusion ratio decreases, perfusion > ventilation.

How the ventilation-perfusion ratio affects the alveolar gases
- The ventilation-perfusion ratio profoundly affects the oxygen pressure (PaO_2) and carbon dioxide pressure ($PaCO_2$) in the alveoli:
  - The normal average PaO_2 of 100 mm Hg is determined by:
    - The amount of oxygen entering the alveoli.
    - The removal of oxygen by the capillary blood flow.
  - The normal average $PaCO_2$ of 40 mm Hg is determined by:
    - The amount of carbon dioxide that diffuses into the alveoli from the capillary blood.
    - The removal of carbon dioxide from the alveoli by means of ventilation.

   – Changing ventilation-perfusion ratios alters the PaO_2 and $PaCO_2$ in the following ways:

Increased ventilation-perfusion ratio
- The PaO_2 increases because the oxygen does not diffuse into the blood as fast as it enters the alveoli.
- The $PaCO_2$ falls, allowing the PaO_2 to move closer to the partial pressure of the atmospheric oxygen (approx 159 mm Hg).
- The $PaCO_2$ decreases because the CO_2 is washed out of the alveoli faster than it is replaced by venous blood.
- This ventilation-perfusion relationship is present in the upper segments of the upright lung.

Decreased ventilation-perfusion ratio
- The PaO_2 decreases because the O_2 moves out of the alveoli and into the pulmonary capillary blood faster than it is replenished by ventilation.
- The $PaCO_2$ increases because the CO_2 moves out of the capillary blood and into the alveoli faster than it is washed out of the alveoli by breathing.
- This ventilation-perfusion relationship is present in the lower segments of the upright lung.

How the ventilation-perfusion ratio affects the end-capillary gases
- In end capillary blood, the oxygen pressure (PcO_2) and the carbon dioxide pressure ($PcCO_2$) mirror changes in the PaO_2 and $PaCO_2$.
- As the ventilation-perfusion ratio decreases from the top to the bottom of the upright lung:
   – The PaO_2 increases and the $PaCO_2$ decreases.
   – The PcO_2 increases and the $PcCO_2$ decreases.
- Distal to the pulmonary capillary bed, in the pulmonary veins, the different
- PcO_2 and $PcCO_2$ are mixed, producing an oxygen pressure of about 100 mm Hg and a carbon dioxide pressure of about 40 mm Hg.
- This PcO_2 $PcCO_2$ mixture that occurs in the pulmonary veins is reflected downstream in the PaO_2 and $PaCO_2$ of an arterial blood gas sample. As $PaCO_2$ decreases from the bottom of the lung to the top, the reduced CO_2 levels in the end-capillary blood result in a relative respiratory alkalosis in these regions. Once mixing occurs, the overall pH in the pulmonary veins, and subsequent in the arterial blood is about 7.35 to 7.45.

Respiratory Quotient
- Internal respiration is the gas exchange between the systemic capillaries and the tissue cells.
- The ratio between the volume of oxygen consumed and the volume of carbon dioxide produced is called the respiratory quotient (RQ).
- Normally, the tissues consume about 250 mL of oxygen each minute and produce about 200 mL of carbon dioxide.

- Calculation
    - RQ = CO_2/O_2
    - RQ = 200 mL CO_2/min/250 mL O_2/min.
    - RQ = 200/250 = 0.8
- Normal value is 0.8.

Respiratory Exchange Ratio

- External respiration is the gas exchange between the pulmonary capillaries and the alveoli.
    - The gas exchange is between the body and the external environment.
- The quantity of oxygen and carbon dioxide exchanged during 1 minute is called the respiratory exchange ratio (RR).
- Calculation is the same as for the RQ:
    - RR = CO_2/O_2
    - RQ = 200 mL CO_2/min/250 mL O_2/min.
- RQ = 200/250 = 0.8
- Normal value is 0.8
- Under normal conditions, the RR equals the RQ.

Respiratory Physiology Equations

Gas velocity:

$$V = \frac{F}{A}$$

V = velocity, F = flow, A = cross-sectional area

Compliance (the "give" of the lung):

$$C = \frac{V}{P}$$

C = compliance, V = volume, P = pressure

Specific compliance:

$$S = \frac{C}{TLC}$$

C = compliance, S = specific compliance, TLC = total lung compliance

Elastance (the "stiffness" of the lung):

$$E = \frac{1}{C}$$

E = elastance, C = compliance

Ohm's law:

$$R = \frac{\Delta P}{F}$$

R = resistance, ΔP = change in pressure, F = flow

Respiratory system resistance:

$$R_{RS} = R_L + R_{CW}$$

R_{RS} = respiratory system resistance
R_L = lung resistance
R_{CW} = chest wall resistance

Pulmonary resistance:

$$R_L = R_{air} + R_{tis}$$

R_L = lung resistance
R_{air} = airway resistance
R_{tis} = tissue resistance

Laminar resistance:

$$R = \frac{8\eta l}{\pi r^4}$$

R = resistance, η = viscosity, r = radius, l = tube length

Turbulent resistance:

$$Re = \frac{2rvd}{\eta}$$

Re = Reynold's number (over 2000 = turbulent flow), r = radius, d = density, v = velocity, η = viscosity

Specific resistance:

$$SR = (R)(LV)$$

SR = specific resistance
R = resistance
LV = lung volume

Conductance (ability to flow through the airways):

$$C = \frac{1}{R}$$

C = conductance, R = resistance

Specific conductance:

$$SC = \frac{C}{LV}$$

SC = specific conductance, C = conductance, LV = lung volume

Respiratory pressures:

$$P_{tot} = (V)(E) + (F)(R)$$

P_{tot} = total pressure
F = flow
V = volume
R = resistance
E = elastance

Minute ventilation:

$$MV = (RR)(TV)$$

MV = minute ventilation
RR = respiratory rate
TV = tidal volume

Ideal gas law:

$$PV = nRT$$

P = pressure
R = ideal gas constant
V = volume
T = temperature
n = moles of gas

Oxygen uptake:

$$V'O_2 = (V'I)(FiO_2) - (V'E)(FEO_2)$$

$V'O_2$ = oxygen uptake/min
$V'I$ = inspired minute ventilation
FiO_2 = $[O_2]$ in inspired air
$V'E$ = expired minute ventilation
FEO_2 = $[O_2]$ in expired air

Carbon dioxide elimination:

$$V'CO_2 = (V'E)(FECO_2)$$

$V'CO_2$ = carbon dioxide eliminated/min
$V'E$ = expired minute ventilation
$FECO_2$ = $[CO_2]$ in expired air

Respiratory quotient:

$$R = \frac{CO_{2made}}{O_{2taken}}$$

R = respiratory quotient, CO_{2made} = CO_2 production, O_{2taken} = O_2 consumption

Respiratory exchange ratio:

$$R = \frac{V'CO_2}{V'O_2}$$

R = respiratory exchange ratio, $V'CO_2$ = CO_2 output, $V'O_2$ = O_2 uptake

Physiologic dead space (in a tidal volume):

$$V_T = V_A + V_D$$

V_T = tidal volume
V_A = alveolar volume
V_D = physiologic dead space

Physiologic dead space (Bohr method):

$$V_D = V_T \frac{PaCO_2 - PECO_2}{PaCO_2}$$

V_D = physiologic dead space, V_T = tidal volume, $PaCO_2$ = partial arterial pressure of CO_2, $PECO_2$ = partial expired pressure of CO_2

Alveolar dead space

$$V_D/V_T = (PaCO_2 - PEtCO_2)/PaCO_2$$

Normal ranges from 20 to 30%

Alveolar gas equation:

PaO_2 = alveolar partial pressure of O_2
FiO_2 = $[O_2]$ in inspired air

$$PaO_2 = FiO_2(BP - WVP) - (PaCO_2/R)$$

PaCO$_2$ = arterial partial pressure of CO$_2$
R = respiratory quotient
BP = barometric pressure (normally 760 mm Hg)
WVP = water vapor pressure (normally 47 mm Hg)

Diffusion rate:

$$R \propto \frac{1}{\rho^{0.5}}$$

R = diffusion rate, ρ = density

Diffusion capacity:

$$D_L = \frac{F}{\Delta P}$$

D$_L$ = diffusion capacity, F = flow, ΔP = pressure change

Diffusion capacity using CO:

$$D_L CO = \frac{V'CO}{PaCO}$$

D$_L$CO = diffusion capacity, V'CO = flow of CO, PACO = partial alveolar pressure of CO

Starling equation:

$$F = K[(P_c - P_i) - \sigma(\pi_c - \pi_i)]$$

F = fluid flow
K = filtration coefficient
P$_c$ = capillary hydrostatic pressure
P$_i$ = interstitial hydrostatic pressure
σ = reflection coefficient
π_c = capillary oncotic pressure
π_i = interstitial oncotic pressure

Ventilation/perfusion matching:

$$\frac{V'}{Q'} = R \frac{PaO_2 - PvO_2}{PaCO_2}$$

V' = ventilation, Q' = perfusion, R = respiratory exchange ratio, PaO$_2$ = alveolar pressure of oxygen, PvO$_2$ = mixed venous pressure of oxygen, PaCO$_2$ = alveolar pressure of carbon dioxide.

Shunt equation:

$$\%S = \frac{CcO_2 - CaO_2}{CcO_2 - CvO_2}$$

%S = shunt fraction, CcO$_2$ = pulmonary capillary oxygen content, CaO$_2$ = systemic arterial oxygen content, CvO$_2$ = mixed venous oxygen content.

Alveolar-arterial gradient

A-a Gradient $= P_AO_2 - P_aO_2$

Where, $P_AO_2 =$ Alveolar PO_2, $P_aO_2 =$ Arterial PO_2

$$P_AO_2 = F_iO_2\,(P_{atm} - P_{H_2O}) - \frac{P_aCO_2}{0.8}$$

- A normal A-a gradient for a young adult non-smoker breathing air, is between 5–10 mm Hg.
- A-a increases 5 to 7 mm Hg for every 10% increase in F_iO_2
- However, the A-a gradient increases with age, i.e. [age/4] + 4

Shunt equation:

$$\%S = \frac{CcO_2 - CaO_2}{CcO_2 - CvO_2}$$

Where, %S(Qs/Qt) = shunt fraction, $CcO_2 =$ pulmonary capillary oxygen content, $CaO_2 =$ systemic arterial oxygen content, $CvO_2 =$ mixed venous oxygen content.

Normal shunt fraction (QS/QT) is less than 0.05 (<5%)

$CcO_2 = 1.39 \times Hb + 0.003 \times PAO_2$

$CaO_2 = Hb \times SaO_2 \times 1.39 + 0.003 \times PaO_2$

$CvO_2 = Hb \times SvO_2 \times 1.39 + 0.003 \times PvO_2$

Before we can calculate the CcO_2, we must calculate the PAO_2:

Example:

$P_AO_2 = P_IO_2 - (P_aCO_2 \times 1.25)$, or

$P_AO_2 = (760 - 47) \times F_iO_2 - P_aCO_2/0.8$ (or 1)

$P_IO_2 = F_iO_2 \times (PB - 47)$

$P_IO_2 = 0.4 \times 713 = 285.2''$ mm Hg

$P_AO_2 = 285.2 - (45 \times 1.25)$

$P_AO_2 = 285.2 - 56.25 = 228.95$ mm Hg

■ BIBLIOGRAPHY

1. Briscoe WA, Dubois AB. The relationship between airway resistance, airway conductance and lung volume in subjects of different age and body size. J Clin Invest. 1958;37(9):1279-85.
2. Dubois AB, Botelho SY, Bedell GN, Marshall R, Comroe JH. A rapid plethysmographic method for measuring thoracic gas volume: A comparison with a nitrogen washout method for measuring functional residual capacity in normal subjects. J Clin Invest. 1956;35(3):322-6.
3. Dubois AB, Botelho SY, Comroe JH. A new method for measuring airway resistance in man using a body plethysmograph: values in normal subjects and in patients with respiratory disease. J Clin Invest. 1956;35(3):327-35.
4. Marino PL, Byrd RP. The ICU Book. 2nd edition. Mechanical ventilation. Medicine, 1998.
5. Moon, Richard and Enrico Camporesi "Respiratory Monitoring". Miller's Anesthesia, Sixth edition, Ronald Miller (Ed), Elsevier, New York, 2005.pp.1466.
6. Morgan, Edward G, Mikhail M and Murry M. Clinical Anesthesiology, Fourth edition. McGraw Hill, Philadelphia, 2006. pp.82.
7. Sena MJ, et al. Mechanical Ventilation. ACS Surgery: Principles and Practice. 2005. pp. 1-16.

PULMONARY ANATOMY AND PHYSIOLOGY

Clinical medicine is predicated on the basic sciences of anatomy, pharmacology, physiology, and biochemistry. The following is an overview of the functional anatomy and physiology of the pulmonary system. It is not a definitive treatise, but rather a useful and up-to-date presentation of anatomy and function as related to respiratory care.

■ LUNGS

The **lungs** flank the heart and great vessels in the chest cavity. Air enters and leaves the lungs via a conduit of cartilaginuous passageways—the bronchi and bronchioles. In Figure 2.1, lung tissue has been dissected away to reveal the bronchioles.

The **lung** is the essential respiration organ in air-breathing vertebrates. Its principal function is to transport oxygen from the atmosphere into the bloodstream, and to excrete carbon dioxide from the bloodstream into the atmosphere. This exchange of gases is accomplished in the mosaic of specialized cells that form millions of tiny, exceptionally thin-walled air sacs called alveoli. The lungs also have nonrespiratory functions.

Medical terms related to the lung often begin with *pulmo-*, from the Latin *pulmonarius* ("of the lungs"), or with *pneumo-* (from Greek *pnévmonas* "lung").

Respiratory Function

Energy production from aerobic respiration requires oxygen and produces carbon dioxide as a byproduct, creating a need for an efficient means of oxygen delivery to cells and excretion of carbon dioxide from cells.

In air-breathing vertebrates, respiration occurs in a series of steps. Air is brought into the animal via the airways—this consists of the nose, the pharynx; the larynx, the trachea (also called the wind pipe), the bronchi and bronchioles; and the terminal branches of the respiratory tree. The lungs are a rich lattice of alveoli, which provide an enormous surface area for gas exchange. A network of fine capillaries allows transport of blood over the surface of alveoli. Oxygen

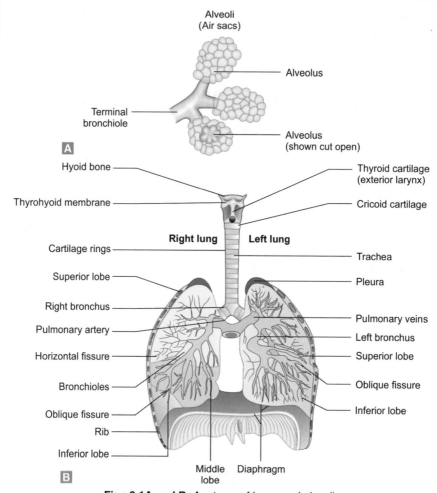

Figs 2.1A and B: Anatomy of lungs and alveoli

from the air inside the alveoli diffuses into the bloodstream, and carbon dioxide diffuses from the blood to the alveoli, both across thin alveolar membranes. The drawing and expulsion of air is driven by muscular action; a complicated musculoskeletal system is used. A large muscle, the diaphragm (in addition to the internal intercostal muscles), drive ventilation by periodically altering the intrathoracic volume and pressure; by increasing volume and thus decreasing pressure, air flows into the airways down a pressure gradient, and by reducing volume and increasing pressure, the reverse occurs. During normal breathing, expiration is passive and no muscles are contracted (the diaphragm relaxes).

Another name for this inspiration and expulsion of air is ventilation.

The lungs of mammals have a spongy texture and are honey-combed with epithelium having a much larger surface area in total than the outer surface area of the lung itself.

Breathing is largely driven by the muscular diaphragm at the bottom of the thorax. Contraction of the diaphragm pulls the bottom of the cavity, in which the lung is enclosed, downward. Air enters through the oral and nasal cavities; it flows through the larynx and into the trachea, which branches out into bronchi. Relaxation of the diaphragm has the opposite effect, passively recoiling during normal breathing. During exercise, the diaphragm contracts, forcing the air out more quickly and forcefully. The rib cage itself is also able to expand and contract to some degree, through the action of other respiratory and accessory respiratory muscles. As a result, air is sucked into or expelled out of the lungs, always moving down its pressure gradient. This type of lung is known as a **bellows lung** as it resembles a blacksmith's bellows.

Anatomy

In humans, it is the two main bronchi (produced by the bifurcation of the trachea) that enter the roots of the lungs. The bronchi continue to divide within the lung, and after multiple divisions, give rise to bronchioles. The bronchial tree continues branching until it reaches the level of terminal bronchioles, which lead to alveolar sacs. Alveolar sacs are made up of clusters of alveoli, like individual grapes within a bunch. The individual alveoli are tightly wrapped in blood vessels, and it is here that gas exchange actually occurs. Deoxygenated blood from the heart is pumped through the pulmonary artery to the lungs, where oxygen diffuses into blood and is exchanged for carbon dioxide in the hemoglobin of the erythrocytes (red blood cells). The oxygen-rich blood returns to the heart via the pulmonary veins to be pumped back into systemic circulation.

Human lungs are located in two cavities on either side of the heart. Though similar in appearance, the two are not identical. Both are separated into lobes, with three lobes on the right and two on the left. The lobes are further divided into lobules, hexagonal divisions of the lungs that are the smallest subdivision visible to the naked eye. The connective tissue that divides lobules is often blackened in smokers and city dwellers. The medial border of the right lung is nearly vertical, while the left lung contains a cardiac notch. The cardiac notch is a concave impression molded to accommodate the shape of the heart (Fig. 2.2A).

Lungs are to a certain extent 'overbuilt' and have a tremendous reserve volume as compared to the oxygen exchange requirements when at rest. This is the reason that individuals can smoke for years without having a noticeable decrease in lung function while still or moving slowly; in situations like these, only a small portion of the lungs are actually perfused with blood for gas exchange. As oxygen requirements increase due to exercise, a greater volume of the lungs is perfused, allowing the body to match its CO_2/O_2 exchange requirements (Fig. 2.2B).

The environment of the lung is very moist, which makes it hospitable for bacteria. Many respiratory illnesses are the result of bacterial or viral infection of the lungs.

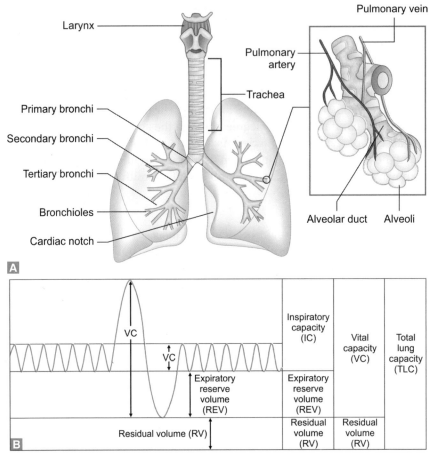

Figs 2.2A and B: (A) Bronchi, bronchial tree and lungs; (B) Different lung capacities and volumes

Vital Capacity

Vital capacity (VC) is the maximum volume of air that a person can exhale after maximum inhalation.

A person's vital capacity can be measured by a spirometer which can be a wet or regular spirometer (Spirometry). In combination with other physiological measurements, the vital capacity can help make a diagnosis of underlying lung disease.

Vital capacity is the maximum amount of air a person can expel from the lungs after first filling the lungs to their maximum extent and then expiring to the maximum extent (about 4600 milliliters). It equals the inspiratory reserve volume plus the tidal volume plus the expiratory reserve volume (Fig. 2.2B).

■ BREATHING

Breathing transports oxygen into the body and carbon dioxide out of the body. Aerobic organisms require oxygen to create energy via respiration, in the form of energy-rich molecules such as glucose. The medical term for normal relaxed breathing is eupnea.

Mechanics

Breathing in, or inhaling, is usually an active movement, with the contraction of the diaphragm muscles needed. At rest, breathing out, or exhaling, is normally a passive process powered by the elastic recoil of the chest, similar to a deflating balloon.

Gas Exchange

Breathing is only part of the process of delivering oxygen to where it is needed in the body. The process of gas exchange occurs in the alveoli by passive diffusion of gases between the alveolar gas and the blood passing by in the lung capillaries. Once in the blood, the heart powers the flow of dissolved gases around the body in the circulation.

As well as carbon dioxide, breathing also results in loss of water from the body. Exhaled air has a relative humidity of 100% because of water diffusing across the moist surface of breathing passages and alveoli.

Control of Breathing

Breathing is one of the few bodily functions which, within limits, can be controlled both consciously and unconsciously.

Unconsciously, breathing is controlled by specialized centers in the brainstem, which automatically regulate the rate and depth of breathing depending on the body's needs at any time.

When carbon dioxide levels increase in the blood, it reacts with the water in blood, producing carbonic acid. The drop in the blood's pH will then cause the medulla oblongata signaling center in brain to send nerve impulses to the diaphragm and the intercostal muscles, increasing the rate of breathing.

While exercising, the level of carbon dioxide in the blood increases due to increased cellular respiration by the muscles, and so breathing rate increases. During rest, the level of carbon dioxide is lower, so breathing rate is lower. This ensures that an appropriate amount of oxygen is delivered to the muscles and other organs. It is important to reiterate that it is the build-up of carbon dioxide making the blood acidic that elicits the desperation for a breath much more than lack of oxygen. Rarely, individuals with chronic lung disease may adapt to high CO_2 levels in their blood by regulating their breathing according to O_2 levels.

Hyperventilation causes a drop in CO_2 below normal levels, lowering blood acidity to trick the brain into thinking it has more oxygen than is actually present.

Respiratory Rate

Humans typically breathe between 12 and 20 times per minute.

Composition of Air

The air we inhale is roughly 21% oxygen (% by volume).

Not all of the oxygen breathed in is converted into carbon dioxide; around 13% of what we breathe out is still oxygen. This is what makes resuscitation possible. Also our reliance on this relatively small amount of oxygen can cause overactivity or euphoria in pure or oxygen rich environments.

Gas Exchange

The process of gas exchange occurs in the alveoli by passive diffusion of gases between the alveolar gas and the blood passing by in the lung capillaries. Once in the blood, the heart powers the flow dissolved gases around the body in the circulation.

■ BLOOD PRESSURE

Blood pressure refers to the force exerted by circulating blood on the walls of blood vessels, and constitutes one of the principal vital signs. The pressure of the circulating blood decreases as blood moves through arteries, arterioles, capillaries, and veins; the term *blood pressure* generally refers to **arterial pressure,** i.e. the pressure in the larger arteries, the blood vessels that take blood away from the heart. Arterial pressure is most commonly measured via a sphygmomanometer, which historically used the height of a column of mercury to reflect the circulating pressure (*See* Non-invasive measurement). Today blood pressure values are reported in millimeters of mercury (mm Hg), though aneroid and electronic devices do not use mercury.

The systolic arterial pressure is defined as the peak pressure in the arteries, which occurs near the beginning of the cardiac cycle when the ventricles are contracting; the diastolic arterial pressure is the lowest pressure during the resting phase of the cardiac cycle. The average pressure throughout the cardiac cycle is reported as mean arterial pressure; the pulse pressure reflects the difference between the maximum and minimum pressures measured.

Typical values for a resting, healthy adult human are approximately 120 mm Hg systolic and 80 mm Hg diastolic (written as 120/80 mm Hg, and spoken as "one twenty over eighty") with large individual variations. These measures of arterial pressure are not static, but undergo natural variations from one heart beat to another and throughout the day (in a circadian rhythm); they also change in response to stress, nutritional factors, drugs, or disease. Hypertension refers to arterial pressure being abnormally high, as opposed to hypotension, when it is abnormally low. Along with body temperature, blood pressure measurements are the most commonly measured physiological parameters.

■ RESPIRATORY PHYSIOLOGY

Respiratory physiology is the branch of human physiology focusing upon respiration.

Volumes

Lung volumes refer to physical differences in lung volume, while lung capacities represent different combinations of lung volumes, usually in relation to inhalation and exhalation.

The average pair of human lungs can hold about 6 liters of air, but only a small amount of this capacity is used during normal breathing.

Breathing mechanism in mammals is called "tidal breathing". Tidal breathing means that air goes into the lungs the same way that it comes out.

Several factors affect lung volumes, some that can be controlled and some that cannot. Lung volumes can be measured using the terms given in Table 2.1.

A person who is born and lives at sea level will develop a slightly smaller lung capacity than a person who spends their life at a high altitude. This is because the atmosphere is less dense at higher altitude, and therefore, the same volume of air contains fewer molecules of all gases, including oxygen. In response to higher altitude, the body's diffusing capacity increases in order to be able to process more air.

When someone living at or near sea level travels to locations at high altitudes, she/he can develop a condition called altitude sickness because their lungs cannot respirate sufficiently in the thinner air.

These values vary with the age and height of the person; the values that follow in Table 2.2 are for a 70 kg (154 lb), average-sized adult male.

The *tidal volume, vital capacity, inspiratory capacity* and *expiratory reserve volume* can be measured directly with a spirometer. Determination of the *residual volume* can be done by radiographic planimetry, body plethysmography, closed circuit dilution and nitrogen washout.

These are the basic elements of a ventilatory *pulmonary function test*. The results (in particular FEV1/FVC and FRC) can be used to distinguish between restrictive and obstructive pulmonary diseases (Table 2.3).

Vital capacity is the maximum volume of air that a person can exhale after maximum inhalation. It can also be the maximum volume of air that a person can inhale after maximum exhalation.

A person's vital capacity can be measured by a spirometer which can be a wet or regular spirometer. In combination with other physiological measurements, the vital capacity can help make a diagnosis of underlying lung disease.

Table 2.1: Terms used to measure lung volume

Larger volumes	Smaller volumes
Males	Females
Taller people	Shorter people
Non-smokers	Smokers
Athletes	Non-athletes
People living at high altitudes	People living at low altitudes

Table 2.2: Different lung capacities and volumes

Measurement	Value	Calculation	Description
Total lung capacity (TLC)	6.0 L	IRV + TV + ERV + RV	The volume of gas contained in the lung at the end of maximal inspiration. The total volume of the lung (i.e. the volume of air in the lungs after maximum inspiration)
Vital capacity (VC)	4.6 L	IRV + TV + ERV	The amount of air that can be forced out of the lungs after a maximal inspiration. Emphasis on completeness of expiration. The maximum volume of air that can be voluntarily moved in and out of the respiratory system
Forced vital capacity (FVC)	4.8 L	Measured	The amount of air that can be maximally forced out of the lungs after a maximal inspiration. Emphasis on speed
Tidal volume (TV)	500 mL	Measured	The amount of air breathed in or out during normal respiration. The volume of air an individual is normally breathing in and out
Residual volume (RV)	1.2 L	Measured	The amount of air left in the lungs after a maximal exhalation. The amount of air that is always in the lungs and can never be expired (i.e. the amount of air that stays in the lungs after maximum expiration)
Expiratory reserve volume (ERV)	1.2 L	Measured	The amount of additional air that can be breathed out after the end expiratory level of normal breathing. (At the end of a normal breath, the lungs contain the residual volume plus the expiratory reserve volume, or around 2.4 liters. If one then goes on and exhales as much as possible, only the residual volume of 1.2 liters remains).
Inspiratory reserve volume (IRV)	3.6 L	Measured IRV = VC − (TV + ERV)	The additional air that can be inhaled after a normal tidal breath in. The maximum volume of air that can be inspired in addition to the tidal volume
Functional residual capacity (FRC)	2.4 L	ERV + RV	The amount of air left in the lungs after a tidal breath out. The amount of air that stays in the lungs during normal breathing
Inspiratory capacity (IC)	4.1 L	TV + IRV	The volume that can be inhaled after a tidal breathe-out
Anatomical dead space	150 mL	Measured	The volume of the conducting airways. Measured with Fowler method
Physiologic dead volume	155 mL		The anatomic dead space plus the alveolar dead space

Table 2.3: Difference between restrictive and obstructive diseases

Type	Examples	Description	FEV1/FVC
Restrictive diseases	Pulmonary fibrosis	Volumes are decreased	Often in a normal range (0.8–1.0)
Obstructive diseases	Asthma or COPD	Volumes are essentially normal but flow rates are impeded	Often low (Asthma can reduce the ratio to 0.6. Emphysema can reduce the ratio to 0.3–0.4)

Vital capacity is the maximum amount of air a person can expel from the lungs after first filling the lungs to their maximum extent and then expiring to the maximum extent (about 4600 milliliters). It equals the inspiratory reserve volume plus the tidal volume plus the expiratory reserve volume.

Functional residual capacity (FRC) is the volume of air present in the lungs at the end of passive expiration. At FRC, the elastic recoil forces of the lungs and chest wall are equal but opposite and there is no exertion by the diaphragm or other respiratory muscles.

FRC is the sum of expiratory reserve volume (ERV) and residual volume (RV) and measures approximately 2400 mL in a 70 kg, average-sized male. It can be estimated through spirometry, but in order to measure it more precisely, one would need to perform a test that directly measures RV such as nitrogen washout, helium dilution or body plethysmography.

A lowered or elevated FRC is often an indication of some form of respiratory disease. For instance, in emphysema, the lungs are more compliant and therefore are more susceptible to the outward recoil forces of the chest wall. Emphysema patients often have noticeably broader chests because they are breathing at larger volumes.

Body plethysmography is a very sensitive lung measurement used to detect lung pathology that might be missed with conventional pulmonary function tests. This method of obtaining the absolute volume of air within one's lungs may also be used in situations where several repeated trials are required or where the patient is unable to perform the multibreath tests. The technique requires moderately complex coaching and instruction for the subject. In the USA, such tests are usually performed by certified or registered pulmonary function technologists (CPFT or RPFT) who are credentialed by the National Board for Respiratory Care.

More specifically, the test is done by enclosing the subject in an airtight chamber often referred to as a body box; a pneumotachometer is used to measure airflow while a mouth pressure transducer with a shutter measures the alveolar pressure. The most common measurements made using body plethysmographs are thoracic gas volume (VTG) and airway resistance (R_{AW}). This test is used mainly in the Pulmonary Function Testing Laboratories.

Using body plethysmography, doctors can examine the lungs' resistance to airflow, distinguish between restrictive and obstructive lung diseases, determine the response to bronchodilators, and determine bronchial hyperreactivity in response to methacholine, histamine, or isocapnic hyperventilation.

Flow and pressure plethysmographs: There are two types of plethysmographs: flow and pressure. In flow plethysmography, airway resistance is measured by two maneuvers. The patient first pants while the mouth shutter is open to allow flow changes to be measured. Then, the mouth shutter closes at the patient's end expiratory or FRC level and the patient continues panting while maintaining an open glottis. This provides a measure of the driving pressure used to move air into the lungs.

Pressure plethysmographs are usually measured at the end-expiratory level and are then equal to FRC. The patient sits in the box, which has the pressure transducer in the wall of the device, and breathes through a mouth-piece connected to a device that contains an electronic shutter and a differential pressure pneumotachometer. The mouth pressure and box pressure changes that are measured during tidal breathing and panting maneuvers, which are performed during the test by the patient at the end of expiration are sent to a microprocessor unit that calculates thoracic gas volume.

A **peak flow meter** is a small, hand-held device used to manage asthma by monitoring airflow through the bronchi and thus the degree of obstruction in the airways.

Function

The peak flow meter measures the patient's maximum ability to exhale, or **peak expiratory flow rate** (PEFR or PEF). Peak flow readings are higher when patients are well and lower when the airways are constricted. From changes in recorded values, patients and doctors may determine lung functionality, severity of asthma symptoms, and treatment options.

The measurement of peak expiratory flow was pioneered by Dr Martin Wright, who produced the first meter specifically designed to measure this index of lung function. Since the original design of instrument was introduced in the late 1950s, and the subsequent development of a more portable, lower cost version (the 'Mini-Wright' peak flow meter) (Fig. 2.3), other designs and copies have become available across the world.

Measurement of PEFR requires training to correctly use a meter and the normal expected value depends on a patient's sex, age and height. It is classically reduced in obstructive lung disorders such as asthma.

Mechanics: Breathing in, or inhaling, is usually an active movement. The contraction of the diaphragm muscles causes a pressure variation, which is equal to the pressures caused by elastic, resistive and inertial components of the respiratory system.

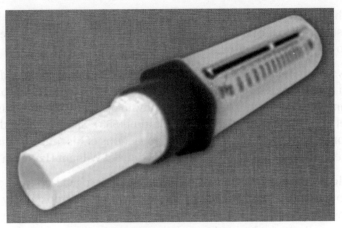

Fig. 2.3: Mini-Wright Peak flow meter

$$P = P_{el} + P_{re} + P_{in}$$
$$P = EV + RV + IV$$

Where P_{el} equals the product of elastance E (inverse of compliance) and volume of the system V, P_{re} equals the product of flow resistance R and time derivate of volume V (which is equivalent to the flow), P_{in} equals the product of iterance I and second time derivate of V. R and I are sometimes referred to as Rohrer's constants.

Circulation, ventilation, and perfusion: Pulmonary circulation is the portion of the cardiovascular system which carries oxygen-depleted blood away from the heart, to the lungs, and returns oxygenated blood back to the heart. The term is contrasted with systemic circulation.

Course: In the pulmonary circulation, deoxygenated blood exits the heart through the pulmonary arteries, enters the lungs and oxygenated blood comes back through pulmonary veins. The blood moves from right ventricle of the heart to the lungs back to the left atrium.

Right heart: Oxygen-depleted blood from the body leaves the systemic circulation when it enters the right heart, more specifically the right atrium through the superior vena cava. The blood is then pumped through the tricuspid valve (or right atrioventricular valve), into the right ventricle. From the right ventricle, blood is pumped through the pulmonary semilunar valve into the pulmonary artery. This blood enters the two pulmonary arteries (one for each lung) and travels through the lungs.

Lungs: The pulmonary arteries carry blood to the lungs, where red blood cells release carbon dioxide and pick up oxygen during respiration. Exchanges carbon dioxide for oxygen in the lungs.

Veins: The oxygenated blood then leaves the lungs through pulmonary veins, which return it to the left heart, completing the pulmonary cycle. This blood then enters the left atrium, which pumps it through the bicuspid valve, also called the mitral or left atrioventricular valve, into the left ventricle. The blood is then distributed to the body through the systemic circulation before returning again to the pulmonary circulation.

History: Pulmonary circulation was first discovered and published by Ibn Nafis in his Commentary on Anatomy in Avicenna's Canon (1242), for which he is considered the father of circulatory physiology. It was later published by Michael Servetus in Christianismi Restitutio (1553). Since it was a theology work condemned by most of the Christian factions of his time, the discovery remained mostly unknown until the dissections of William Harvey in 1616.

Hypoxic pulmonary vasoconstriction is a physiological phenomenon in which pulmonary arteries constrict in the presence of hypoxia (low oxygen levels) without hypercapnia (high carbon dioxide levels), redirecting blood flow to alveoli with higher oxygen tension.

The process might at first seem illogical, as low oxygen levels should theoretically lead to increased blood flow to the lungs to receive increased gaseous exchange. However, it is explained by the fact that constriction leads to increased blood flow to better-aerated areas of the lung, which increases the total area involved in gaseous exchange.

Several factors inhibit this process including increased cardiac output, hypocarbia, hypothermia, acidosis/alkalosis, increased pulmonary vascular resistance, inhaled anesthetics, calcium channel blockers, PEEP, HFV, isoproterenol, nitrous oxide and vasodilators.

Perfusion: Perfusion is the process of nutritive delivery of arterial blood to a capillary bed in the biological tissue. The word is derived from the French verb "perfuser" meaning to "pour over or through."

Tests of adequate perfusion are a part of patient triage performed by medical or emergency personnel in a mass casualty incident.

Calculation: Perfusion ('F') can be measured with the following formula, Where PA is mean arterial pressure, PV is mean venous pressure, and R is vascular resistance:

$$F = PA - PV/R$$

The term 'PA – PV' is sometimes presented as 'ΔP', for the change in pressure.

The terms 'perfusion' and 'perfusion pressure' are sometimes used interchangeably, but the equation should make clear that resistance can have an effect on the perfusion, but not on the perfusion pressure.

Overperfusion and underperfusion: The terms 'overperfusion' and 'underperfusion' are measured relative to the average level of perfusion across all tissues in an individual body, and the terms should not be confused with hypoperfusion and 'hyperperfusion', which measure the perfusion level to the tissue's current need.

Tissues like the skin are considered overperfused and receive more blood than would be expected to meet the metabolic needs of the tissue. In the case of the skin, extra blood flow is used for thermoregulation. In addition to delivering oxygen, the blood helps dissipate heat by redirecting warm blood close to the surface where it can cool the body through the sweating and thermal radiation. Ventilation/perfusion ratio: In respiratory physiology, the ventilation/perfusion ratio (or V/Q ratio) is a measurement used to assess the efficiency and adequacy of the matching of two variables:

- 'V' - ventilation—the air which reaches the lungs
- 'Q' - perfusion—the blood which reaches the lungs

These two variables constitute the main determinants of the blood oxygen concentration. In fact since V determines the quantity of oxygen mass reaching the alveoli per minute (g/min) and Q expresses the flow of blood in the lungs (v/min), the V/Q ratio refers to a concentration (g/L).

$$V = \frac{g}{min} ; Q = \frac{L}{min} \Rightarrow \frac{V}{Q} = \frac{\frac{g}{min}}{\frac{L}{min}} = \frac{g}{L}$$

However, actually the V/Q ratio is an adimensional measure since V is expressed as a flow too.

Physiology: Ideally, the oxygen provided via ventilation would be just enough to saturate the blood fully. In the typical adult, 1 liter of blood can hold about 200 mL of oxygen. Coincidentally, 1 liter of dry air has about 210 mL of oxygen. Therefore, under these conditions, the ideal ventilation perfusion ratio would be about 0.95. If one were to consider humidified air (with less oxygen), then the ideal V/Q ratio would be in the vicinity of 1.0.

The actual values in the lung vary depending on the position within the lung. If taken as a whole, the typical value is approximately 0.8.

Because the lung is centered vertically around the heart, one part of the lung is superior to the heart, and other part is inferior. This has a major impact on the V/Q ratio:

- Apex of lung—higher
- Base of lung—lower.

In a subject standing in orthostatic position, the apex of the lung shows higher V/Q ratio, while at the base of the lung the ratio is lower but nearer to the optimal value for reaching adequate blood oxygen concentrations. The main reason for lower V/Q ratios at the base is that both ventilation and perfusion increase when going from the apex to the base, but Q does it more strongly, thus lowering the V/Q ratio. The principal factor involved in the genesis of V/Q dishomogeneity between the apex and the base of the lung is gravity (this is why V/Q ratios change in positions other than the orthostatic one).

Ventilation: Gravity and lung's weight act on ventilation by increasing pleural pressure at the base (making it less negative) and thus reducing the alveolar volume. However, at these smaller volumes, the alveoli are more compliant (more distensible) and so capable of wider oxygen exchanges with the external environment. On the other side the apex, though showing a higher oxygen partial pressure, ventilates less efficiently since its compliance is lower and so smaller volumes are exchanged.

Perfusion: The impact of gravity on pulmonary perfusion expresses itself as the hydrostatic pressure of the blood passing through the branches of the pulmonary artery in order to reach the apical and basal district of the lung, acting respectively against or synergistically with the pressure developed by the right ventricle. Thus at the apex of the lung, the resulting pressure can be insufficient for developing a flow (which can be sustained only by the negative pressure generated by venous flow towards the left atrium) or even for preventing the collapse of the vascular structures surrounding the alveoli, while the base of the lung shows an intense flow due to the higher resulting pressure.

A ventilation/perfusion lung scan, also called a V/Q lung scan, is a type of medical imaging used to evaluate the circulation of air and blood within a patient's lungs. The ventilation part of the test looks at the ability of air to reach all parts of the lungs, while the perfusion part evaluates how well the blood circulates within the lungs. This test is most commonly done in order to check for the presence of a blood clot or abnormal blood flow inside the lungs (pulmonary embolism or PE), although computed tomography with radiocontrast is now more commonly used for this purpose. A V/Q lung scan may also be performed in the case of serious lung disorders such as COPD or pneumonia as well as a lung performance quantification tool pre- and post-lung lobectomy surgery.

Procedure: The ventilation and perfusion phases of a V/Q lung scan are performed together and may include a chest X-ray for comparison or to look for other causes of lung disease. A defect in the perfusion images requires a mismatched ventilation defect to be indicative of pulmonary embolism.

In the ventilation phase of the test, a gaseous radionuclide xenon or technetium DTPA in an aerosol form is inhaled by the patient through a mouthpiece or mask that covers the nose and mouth. The perfusion phase of the test involves the intravenous injection of radioactive technetium macro aggregated albumin (Tc99m-MAA). A gamma camera acquires the images for both phases of the study.

Gas Exchange/Transport (Primarily Oxygen and Carbon Dioxide)

Gas exchange or respiration takes place at a respiratory surface—a boundary between the external environment and the interior of the body (Figs 2.4A and B).

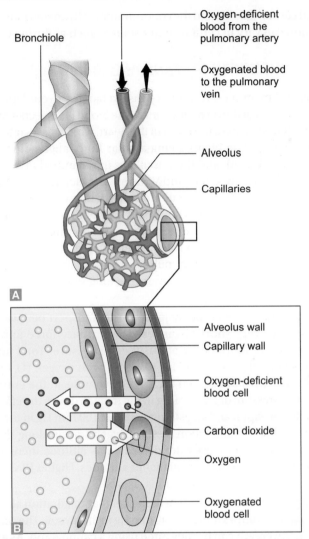

Figs 2.4A and B: Process of gas exchange at a respiratory surface

For unicellular organisms, the respiratory surface is only the cell membrane. From Fick's law, we can predict that respiratory surfaces must have:

- A large surface area
- A thin permeable surface
- A moist exchange surface.

Many also have a mechanism to maximize the diffusion gradient by replenishing the source and/or sink.

Control of respiration is due to rhythmical breathing generated by the phrenic nerve to stimulate contraction and relaxation of the diaphragm during inspiration and expiration. Ventilation is controlled by partial pressures of oxygen and carbon dioxide and the concentration of hydrogen ions. The control of respiration can vary in certain circumstances such as during exercise.

■ GAS EXCHANGE IN HUMANS AND MAMMALS

In humans and mammals, respiratory gas exchange or ventilation is carried out by mechanisms of the heart and lungs. The blood is subjected to a transient electric field (QRS waves of the EKG) in the heart, which dissociates molecules of different charge. The blood, being a polar fluid, aligns dipoles with the electric field, is released, and then oscillates in a damped driven oscillation to form J or Osborn waves, T, U, and V waves. The electric field exposure and subsequent damped driven oscillation dissociate gas from hemoglobin, primarily CO_2, but more importantly BPG, which has a higher affinity for hemoglobin than does oxygen, due in part to its opposite charge. Completely dissociated hemoglobin (which will even effervesce if the electric field is too strong—the reason defibrillation joules are limited, to avoid bubble emboli that may clog vessels in the lung) enters the lung in red blood cells ready to be oxygenated.

Convection occurs over the majority of the transport pathway. Diffusion occurs only over very short distances. The primary force applied in the respiratory tract is supplied by atmospheric pressure. Total atmospheric pressure at sea level is 760 mm Hg (101 kPa), with oxygen (O_2) providing a partial pressure (pO_2) of 160 mm Hg, 21% by volume, at the entrance of the nares, a partial pressure of 150 mm Hg in the trachea due to the effect of partial pressure of water vapor, and an estimated pO_2 of 100 mm Hg in the alveoli sac, pressure drop due to conduction loss as oxygen travels along the transport passageway. Atmospheric pressure decreases as altitude increases making effective breathing more difficult at higher altitudes. Higher BPG levels in the blood are also seen at higher elevations, as well.

Similarly CO_2 which is a result of tissue cellular respiration also exchange. The pCO_2 changes from 45 mm Hg to 40 mm Hg in the alveoli. The concentration of this gas in the breath can be measured using a capnograph. As a secondary measurement, respiration rate can be derived from a CO_2 breath waveform.

Gas exchange occurs only at pulmonary and systemic capillary beds, but anyone can perform simple experiments with electrodes in blood on the bench-top to observe electric field stimulated effervescence.

Trace gases present in breath at levels lower than a part per million are ammonia, acetone and isoprene. These can be measured using selected ion flow tube mass spectrometry.

Diffusion

Blood carries oxygen, carbon dioxide and hydrogen ions between tissues and the lungs.

The majority (70%) of CO_2 transported in the blood is dissolved in plasma (primarily as dissolved bicarbonate; 60%). A smaller fraction (30%) is transported in red blood cells combined with the globin portion of hemoglobin as carbaminohemoglobin.

As CO_2 diffuses into the blood stream, 93% goes into red blood cells and 7% is dissolved in plasma. 70% is converted into H_2CO_3 by carbonic anhydrase. The H_2CO_3 dissociates into H^+ and HCO_3^-. The HCO_3^- moves out of the red blood cells in exchange for Cl^- (chloride shift). The hydrogen is removed by buffers in the blood (Hb).

Oxygen Transport

General Cell Metabolism

Cell metabolism is based on the same general principle as the combustion of any fuel, whether it be in the automobile, power plant, or a home furnace. The general combustion reaction is:

$$CH_2O \text{ (fuel)} + O_2 \Rightarrow CO_2 + HOH$$

The same reaction occurs in the cells. The 'fuel' comes from food in the form of carbohydrates, fats, and proteins.

The important principle to remember is that oxygen is needed by the cell and that carbon dioxide is produced as a waste product of the cell. Carbon dioxide must be expelled from the cells and the body.

The lungs serve to exchange the two gases in the blood. Oxygen enters the blood from the lungs and carbon dioxide is expelled out of the blood into the lungs. The blood serves to transport both gases. Oxygen is carried to the cells. Carbon dioxide is carried away from the cells (Fig. 2.5).

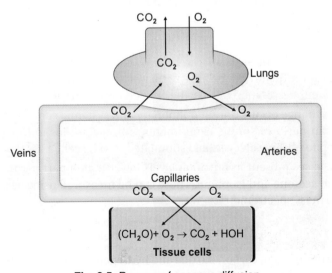

Fig. 2.5: Process of gaseous diffusion

Gaseous Diffusion

Partial pressures are used to designate the concentrations of gases. Dalton's law of partial pressures states that the total pressure of all gases is equal to the sum of the partial pressures of each gas. For example, the total atmospheric pressure of air is 760 mm Hg. In equation form:

$$P\ (total\ air) = P(O_2) + P(N_2) + P(CO_2) + P(HOH)$$

The movement or exchange of gases between the lungs, blood, and tissue cells is controlled by a diffusion process. The gas diffusion principle is: A gas diffuses from an area of higher partial pressure to an area of lower partial pressure.

In the lungs, oxygen diffuses from alveolar air into the blood because the venous blood has a lower partial pressure. The oxygen dissolves in the blood. Only a small amount is carried as a physical solution (0.31 mL per 100 mL). The remainder of the oxygen is carried in chemical combination with the hemoglobin in red blood cells (erythrocytes) (Fig. 2.6).

Hemoglobin (molecular weight of 68,000) is made from 4 hemes, a porphyrin ring containing iron and globin, a 4 protein chains. Oxygen is bound to the iron for the transport process. Hydrohemoglobin (HHb) behaves as a weak acid ($K = 1.4 \times 10^{-8}$; pKa = 7.85). Oxyhemoglobin (HbO_2) also behaves as a weak acid ($K = 2.5 \times 10^{-7}$; pKa = 6.6).

Because both forms of hemoglobin are weak acids, and a relationship of the numerical values of the equilibrium constants, the net reaction for the interaction of oxygen with hemoglobin results in the following equilibrium:

$$HHb + O_2 \Leftrightarrow HbO_2 + H^+$$

If O_2 is increased in the blood at the lungs, the equilibrium shifts to the right and H^+ ions increase.

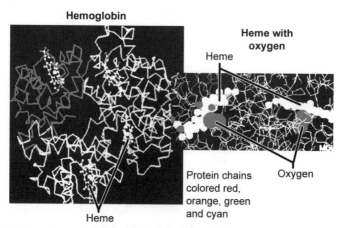

Fig. 2.6: Oxygen transportation through blood (*For color version, see Plate 1*)

Oxyhemoglobin can be caused to release oxygen by the addition of H^+ ions at the cells. The difference in pH (7.44) of arterial blood and venous blood (pH = 7.35) is sufficient to cause release of oxygen from hemoglobin at the tissue cells.

Carbon Dioxide Transport

Bicarbonate Buffer

Carbon dioxide produced in the tissue cells diffuses into the blood plasma. The largest fraction of carbon dioxide diffuses into the red blood cells. The carbon dioxide in the red blood cells is transported as: dissolved CO_2, combined with hemoglobin, or as bicarbonate (largest fraction).

The formation of bicarbonate ions, (HCO_3^-) takes place by the following reactions:

Hydration of CO_2: $CO_2 + HOH = H_2CO_3$

Dissociation of H_2CO_3: $H_2CO_3 = H^+ + HCO_3^-$

The H_2CO_3/HCO_3^- combination acts as the primary buffer of the blood. The hydration of carbon dioxide is a slow process but occurs rapidly in the red blood cells because a high concentration of the enzyme carbonic anhydrase catalyzes the reaction.

Bicarbonate diffuses out of the red blood cells into the plasma in venous blood and visa versa in arterial blood. Chloride ion always diffuses in an opposite direction of bicarbonate ion in order to maintain a charge balance. This is referred to as the 'chloride shift'.

The changes in concentration of CO_2 or HCO_3^- ion can influence slight pH changes in the blood even though it is buffered. At the same time, the concentration of H^+ ions will influence the concentrations of CO_2 and HCO_3^- ions.

Combined Oxygen and Carbon Dioxide Transport

The reactions for both oxygen and carbon dioxide are coupled together and work in cooperation with each other. The main reason for this 'coupled' effect is that both systems are influenced by hydrogen ions and equilibrium principles.

At the lungs, the diffusion of oxygen into the blood triggers the reactions. The oxygen reacts with and attaches to hemoglobin. This oxygenation reaction with hemoglobin produces excess H^+ ions which react with HCO_3^- to produce H_2CO_3. The carbonic acid decomposes to CO_2, which diffuses out of the blood.

Equilibrium at the Tissue Cells

Example: Use equilibrium principles to explain the reactions occurring at the tissue cells.

Solution: Two equilibrium equations are needed:

Reaction 1: Carbon dioxide $\leftrightarrow$ Carbonic Acid $\leftrightarrow$ Bicarbonate Buffer reaction

$$CO_2 + HOH \Leftrightarrow H_2CO_3 \Leftrightarrow H^+ + HCO_3^-:$$

Reaction 2: Hemoglobin/oxygenation and deoxygenation reaction

$$HHb + O_2 \Leftrightarrow HbO_2 + H^+$$

At cells CO_2 diffuses out of the tissue cells and causes an increase of CO_2 in the blood. Reaction 1 shifts right (all the way). H_2CO_3 increases and H^+ increases. The increase of H^+ causes Reaction 2 to shift left which causes O_2 to be released to the blood and can then diffuse into the tissue cells.

pH Changes in the Blood

The changes in concentration of CO_2 or $H^+ + HCO_3^-$ ion can influence slight pH changes in the blood even though it is buffered. At the same time, the concentration of H^+ ions will influence the concentrations of CO_2 and $H^+ + HCO_3^-$ ions.

Example:
Predict the change in pH in venous blood caused by the diffusion of CO_2 from tissue cells using equilibrium principles.

Solution:
Always write the blood buffer equations first:

Reaction 3: $CO_2 + HOH = H_2CO_3 = H^+ + H^+ + HCO_3^-$

Increased carbon dioxide causes reaction (1) to shift right causing H_2CO_3 to increase. The increased H_2CO_3 causes reaction (2) to shift right causing H^+ to increase and finally causing pH to decrease. Using reaction (3), increased carbon dioxide causes a shift in equilibrium all the way to the right with consequent H^+ increase, which causes the pH to decrease in the venous blood.

Pulmonary Blood Flow and Metabolism (Fig. 2.7)

The pulmonary artery arises from the right ventricle and transports deoxygenated blood (oxygen-poor) to the lungs, where the blood becomes oxygenated again. The four pulmonary veins return the oxygenated blood (oxygen-rich) to the left atrium of the heart. The pulmonary circulation is also referred to as the lesser circulation. The summary of the pulmonary circulation is thus: Right ventricle $\rightarrow$ pulmonary artery $\rightarrow$ lungs $\rightarrow$ pulmonary veins $\rightarrow$ left atrium $\rightarrow$ left ventricle.

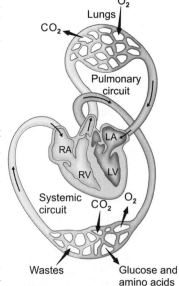

Fig. 2.7: Pulmonary blood flow

Systemic Circulation

Oxygenated blood is pumped from the left ventricle into the aorta. Branches of the aorta convey blood to all the tissues and organs of the body (except the lungs). The tissue cells are oxygenated and deoxygenated blood returned to the heart via the superior and inferior vena cava. The blood then flows via the tricuspid valve into the right ventricle, from where it joins the pulmonary circulation. The systemic circulation is also referred to as the greater circulation. The summary of the systemic circulation is thus:

> Left ventricle → aorta → organs → vena cava → right atrium → left ventricle.

Hepatic Portal System of Circulation

This system serves the intestines, spleen, pancreas and gall bladder. The liver receives blood from two main sources. The main sources are the hepatic artery, which as a branch of the aorta, supplies oxygenated blood to the liver and the hepatic portal vein, which is formed by the union of veins from the spleen, the stomach, pancreas, duodenum and the colon. The hepatic portal vein transports, inter alia, the following blood to the liver:

- Absorbed nutrients from the duodenum
- White blood cells (added to the circulation) from the spleen
- Poisonous substances, such as alcohol which are absorbed in the intestines
- Waste products, such as carbon dioxide from the spleen, pancreas, stomach and duodenum.

The hepatic artery and hepatic portal vein open into the liver sinuses, where the blood is in direct contact with the liver cells. The deoxygenated blood, which still retains some dissolved nutrients, eventually flows into the inferior vena cava via the hepatic veins.

Coronary Circulation

This circulation supplies the heart muscle itself with oxygen and nutrients and conveys carbon dioxide and other waste products away from the heart. Two coronary arteries lead from the aorta to the heart wall, where they branch off and enter the heart muscle. The blood is returned from the heart muscle to the right atrium through the coronary vein, which enters the right atrium through the coronary sinus.

Pressures within Pulmonary Circulation

The right ventricle (RV) pumps blood to the lungs via main pulmonary artery trunk, which divides into left and right pulmonary arteries. Pulmonary arteries continue into arterioles and capillaries which surround the alveoli, where oxygen exchange occurs. Once this occurs, oxygenated blood moves forward via pulmonary veins coming from both right and left lungs, to the left atrium (LA) which then continues to enter the left ventricle (LV) and to the body.

An increase in the pulmonary pressures will eventually affect the heart, initially and predominantly the right ventricle (RV). RV failure secondary to pulmonary hypertension is known as cor pulmonale.

Normal Pulmonary Artery Pressures (PAP)

Systolic pressure	15–25 mm Hg
Diastolic pressure	8–15 mm Hg
Mean pressure	9–18 mm Hg
Capillary wedge pressure	6–12 mm Hg

During rest (diastole), right RV pressure are very low, close to zero, between 1–6 mm Hg, known as end diastolic right ventricular pressure (EDRVP) and end systolic pressure range between 15 and 25 mm Hg (ESRVP). The systolic pressure is same as the pulmonary pressure because when pulmonary valve opens, these pressures equalize.

There is an important thing to remember that pulmonary artery carry deoxygenated blood which is not totally true because under the normal circumstances, the body utilizes approximately 25% of oxygen delivered, while 60 – 75% of this oxygen in our blood goes unused, still available in venous blood. This is known as mixed venous blood saturation (SvO_2).

Pulmonary capillary wedge pressure (PCWP) provides an indirect estimate of left atrial pressure (LAP). Although left ventricular pressure can be directly measured by placing a catheter within the left ventricle, it is not feasible to advance this catheter back into the left atrium. LAP can be measured by placing a special catheter into the right atrium then punching through the interatrial septum.

PCWP is measured by inserting balloon-tipped, multi-lumen catheter (Swan-Ganz catheter) into a peripheral vein, then advancing the catheter into the right atrium, right ventricle, pulmonary artery, and then into a branch of the pulmonary artery. Just behind the tip of the catheter is a small balloon that can be inflated with air (~1 cc). The catheter has one opening (port) at the tip (distal to the balloon) and a second port several centimeters proximal to the balloon. These ports are connected to pressure transducers. When properly positioned in a branch of the pulmonary artery, the distal port measures pulmonary artery pressure (~25/10 mm Hg; systolic/diastolic pressure) and the proximal port measures right atrial pressure (~0–3 mm Hg). The balloon is then inflated, which occludes the branch of the pulmonary artery. When this occurs, the pressure in the distal port rapidly falls, and after several seconds, reaches a stable lower value that is very similar to left atrial pressure (normally about 8–10 mm Hg). The balloon is then deflated. The same catheter can be used to measure cardiac output by the thermodilution technique.

The pressure recorded during balloon inflation is similar to left atrial pressure because the occluded vessel and its distal branches that eventually form the pulmonary veins act as a long catheter that measures the blood pressures within the pulmonary veins and left atrium.

■ PULMONARY VASCULAR RESISTANCE

Pulmonary vascular resistance (PVR) is the resistance to flow that must be overcome to push blood through the circulatory system. The total pressure drop from pulmonary artery to left atrium in the pulmonary circulation is only some 10 mm Hg, against about 100 mm Hg for the systemic circulation. Because the blood flows through the two circulations is virtually identical, it follows that the pulmonary vascular resistance is only one-tenth that of the systemic circulation. The pulmonary vascular resistance is normally ranges from 20 to 130 dyn·s/cm^5. The high resistance of the systemic circulation is largely caused by very muscular arterioles that allow the regulation of blood flow to various organs of the body. The pulmonary circulation has no such vessels and appears to have as low a resistance as is compatible with distributing the blood in a thin film over a vast area in the alveolar walls.

■ BIBLIOGRAPHY

1. Bepler G. Lung Cancer epidemiology and genetics. J Thorac Imaging. 1999;14:228-34.
2. Boffetta P, Pershagen G, Jockel KH, et al. Cigar and pipe smoking and lung cancer risk: a multicentre study from Europe. Journal of the National Cancer Institute. 1999;91(8):697-701.
3. Fuster V, Alexander RW, O'Rourke RA. Hurst's the heart, book 1. 11th Edition, McGraw-Hill Professional, Medical Pub. Division, 2004.
4. Goers TA. Washington University School of Medicine Department of Surgery; Klingensmith, Mary E; Li Ern Chen; Sean C Glasgow, 2008.
5. Iribarren C, Tekawa IS, Sidney S, et al. Effect of cigar smoking on the risk of cardiovascular disease, chronic obstructive pulmonary disease, and cancer in men. New England Journal of Medicine. 1999;340(23):1773-80.
6. Reis LA, Kosary CL, Hankey BF, et al. SEER Cancer Statistics Review. 1973-1996. Bethesda, Md: National Cancer Institute, 1998.
7. Roth JA, Ruckdeschel JC, Weisenburger TH. Thoracic Oncology, 2nd ed. Philadelphia, Pa: WB Saunders Co, 1995.
8. University of Virginia Health System. "The Physiology: Pulmonary Artery Catheters."

RESPIRATORY PATHOPHYSIOLOGY

■ PULMONARY INSUFFICIENCY

Degree of respiratory failure that may occur when the exchange of respiratory gases between the circulating blood and the ambient atmosphere is impaired. This impairment can be caused by disease or trauma that to some degree anatomically alters the lung and chest wall.

Clinical information may be gained by inspecting the chest. The majority of this information should be gathered without the patient's knowledge. This is done by listening and by observation of the patient.

Things to look for: Is the patient short of breath while talking, note the use of accessory muscle and retractions. Note the patient's posture, respiratory rate and pattern, pursed-lip breathing, grunting or nasal flaring. Also note symmetry of the chest, skin color, nail beds, digital clubbing, type of cough (dry, hacking, loose, wet). Is the cough productive, and if it is, how much? When is the cough present (morning, night, all the time)? What time of the year is the cough present? Note the color of the sputum, audible wheezing or rhonchi, evidence of edema or dehydration.

This information is the basis for proper treatment of the patient with respiratory problems.

■ ANXIETY ASSESSMENT FINDINGS

The patient's fear of being in a hospital or physician's office or just the fear of the unknown can affect your physical findings of the patient. The appearance, conversation, behavior, and vital signs may dramatically increase when anxiety is present. A thorough patient interview and physical examination are necessary for prompt and proper treatment. Help reduces the amount of anxiety by asking open-ended questions. When needed, obtain additional information from the patient's family, if possible.

The following are things to look for in patients with anxiety:

Appearance: Muscular tension, pale clammy skin, fatigue, and restlessness.

Conversation: Does the patient frequently ask questions? Shifts topic of conversation, describes fears with a sense of helplessness, and avoids focusing on his own feelings?

"Though most of the symptoms listed may be caused by factors other than anxiety, a thorough physical examination with proper lab work can give you a good overall clinical picture.

Behavior: Does the patient have a shortened attention span? Does the patient have an inability to follow directions?

Physiologic signs: Increased heart rate, respiratory rate, blood pressure, and perspiration.

■ RESPIRATORY BREATHING PATTERNS

Eupnea: Normal respiratory rate and rhythm with occasional deep breath.

Tachypnea: Increased respiratory rate as seen in patients with fever, pneumonia, respiratory insufficiency, lesions of the brain's respiratory control center.

Bradypnea: Slower respiratory rate but regular, affected by narcotics, tumors, alcohol, and during normal sleep.

Apnea: Absence of breathing, which may be periodic.

Hyperpnea: Deeper than normal breaths but with a normal rate.

Cheyne-Stokes: Slower respiratory rate that gets faster and deeper than normal, with periods of apnea of 20 to 60 seconds. Causes are increased intracranial pressure, severe congestive heart failure, meningitis, and drug overdose.

Blot's: Faster and deeper respiratory rate with abrupt pauses between breaths. Each breath has the same depth. Causes are spinal meningitis or other central nervous system conditions.

Kussmaul's: Faster and deeper than normal respiratory rate without pauses. Breathing sounds are labored, with deep breaths that resemble sighs. Causes may be renal failure or diabetic ketoacidosis.

Apneustic: Prolonged gasping inspiration, followed by short, inefficient expiration. It can be caused by lesions in the respiratory control center.

■ DIAGNOSTIC APPROACH TO PATIENT WITH DYSPNEA
Causes
Cardiac
- Left ventricular failure
- Mitral valve disease
- Cardiomyopathy
- Pericardial effusion or constriction.

Non-cardiorespiratory

- Psychogenic
- Anemia
- Hemorrhage
- Acidosis
- Hypophthalmic lesions.

Respiratory

- Airways disease:
  - Chronic bronchiolitis and emphysema
  - Asthma
  - Bronchiectasis and cystic fibrosis
  - Laryngeal or pharyngeal tumor
  - Bilateral lord palsy
  - Cricoarytenoid rheumatoid
  - Tracheal obstruction
  - Tracheomalacia
  - Amyloid of airways.
- Parenchymal disease:
  - Allergic alveolitis
  - Sarcoidosis
  - Fibroses + diffuse alveolitis
  - Obliterative bronchiolitis
  - Pneumonias + toxic pneumonitis
  - Diffuse infections
  - Respiratory distress syndrome
  - Infiltrative + metastatic tumor
  - Pneumothorax.
- Pulmonary circulation
  - Pulmonary embolism + hypertension
  - Pulmonary arteritis + thrombosis.
- Chest wall and pleura
  - Effusion or pleural fibrosis
  - Fractured ribs
  - Ankylosing spondylitis
- Kyphoscoliosis
- Neuromuscular, bilateral diaphragm paralysis
- Hematologic
- Psychiatric
- Renal
- Skeletal, endocrine, rheumatologic.

A comprehensive history and physical examination are required for diagnosis of dyspnea.

History
- Onset/intermittent/progressive
- Nocturnal
- Relation to exercise/provoking factors
- Aggrevating + relieving factors
- Orthopnea/PND, etc.

Physical Examination
- Respiratory rate
- Body habitus
- Posture
- Use of pursed lips
- Accessory muscles
- Clubbing
- Emotional state
- Chest expansion
- Intensity of breath sounds
- Pedal edema?
- CCF
- Thromboembolic diseases
- Signs of pulmonary arterial hypertension or right
- Ventricular failure.

Laboratory Evaluation
Hemoglobin
- Anemic bleeding
- Polycythmia chronic hypoxia
- Renal, metabolic, thyroid
- CXR, spirometry, ECG.

Special Test
- Pulmonary function testing
- ABG.

Cardiopulmonary exercise testing
- Pulmonary or CVS System
- Unrelated.

Spiral CT
- Ventilation perfusion scan (Pulmonary embolism)
- Gallium—*Pneumocystis carinii* infection
- HRCT—Interstitial lung disease.

Cardiac Cause
- ECG, Radionucleide scan
- Cardiac catheterization
- Rule out psychiatric cause (anxiety).

LOCATIONS FOR PLACEMENT OF THE STETHOSCOPE

Figures 3.1 and 3.2 shows the dorsal and frontal placement of the stethoscope.

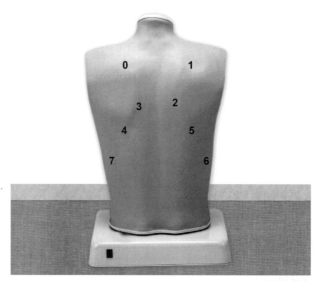

Fig. 3.1: Stethoscope placement: Dorsal. Note that the locations for placement of the stethoscope are the same general locations for percussion (*For color version, see Plate 1*)

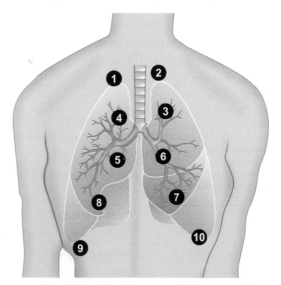

Fig. 3.2: Stethoscope placement: Frontal

Breath Sounds
Abnormal

The results of a movement by pulmonary physicians five years ago to change terms, such as rates, sibilant, musical and so on to more descriptive terms have made breath sounds easier to describe and easier to explain (Table 3.1).

Normal

Vesicular breath sounds are heard over most of the chest, except over major airways. The pitch is low in tone. The inspiratory-to-expiratory ratio is 1:2. The sound is said to be breezy.

Tracheal breath sounds are heard over the trachea. The pitch is very high in tone. The inspiratory-to-expiratory ratio is 5:6. The sound is said to be loud, harsh, and tubular.

Bronchial breath sounds are heard over the major central airways. They are high in pitch, with an inspiratory-to-expiratory ratio of 2:3, and are described as hollow or tubular in sound.

Bronchial-vesicular breath sounds are heard over the major central airways. The pitch is of medium tone, with an inspiratory-to-expiratory ratio of 1:1, and the sound is breezy.

■ CLASSIFICATION OF DYSPNEA

- Class I: Dyspnea only on severe exertion (appropriate).
- Class II: Can keep pace with persons of the same age and body size on level surface without breathlessness, but not on hills or stairs.
- Class III: Can walk a mile at own pace without dyspnea but cannot keep pace on level surface with a normal person.
- Class IV: Dyspnea present after walking about 100 yards on a level surface with a normal person or on climbing one flight of stairs.
- Class V: Dyspnea on even less activity or even at rest.

■ EXAMINATION OF THE TRACHEA

With certain pulmonary conditions, the trachea may shift toward or away from the affected lung. Some causes that would pull the trachea toward the affected

Table 3.1: Terms used now and before 1982 for abnormal breath sounds

Recommended Terms	Terms Used Before 1982
Crackles	Rales or crepitation
Wheezes	Sibilant rales, musical rales, and
	Sibilant rhonchus
Rhonchi	Low-pitched wheeze and sonorous rales
Stridor	Stridor (no change).

side are pulmonary atelectasis, pulmonary fibrosis, pneumonectomy, and diaphragmatic paralysis. When the trachea is pushed to the unaffected side, the possible causes are neck tumors, thyroid enlargement, mediastinal mass, massive pleural effusion, tension pneumothorax, and hemothorax.

■ SPUTUM OBSERVATION

This is presented in Table 3.2.

■ CHEST X-RAYS (FIG. 3.3)

Reasons for Obtaining

There are five major reasons for obtaining a chest X-ray:
1. Detect changes in the lung caused by pathologic processes.
2. Determine appropriate therapy.
3. Evaluate effectiveness of treatment.
4. Determine proper tube and catheter placement.
5. Provide a way of trending the progression or decline of lung disease and tumors.

Standard View

The standard views of the chest are the posteroanterior (PA). The PA view is preferred because, since the heart is in the anterior half of the chest, there will

Table 3.2: Sputum observation

Appearance	Possible Causes
Mucoid, clear, thin, frothy	Bronchial asthma, legionnaires disease, pulmonary tuberculosis, emphysema, early chronic bronchitis
Mucopurulent, yellow-green	All of the above and infection, pneumonia, cystic fibrosis
Purulent, yellow, thick, viscid	Bronchiectasis, advanced chronic bronchitis, *Pseudomonas pneumonia*
Apple green, thick pink, thin blood – streaked	*Haemophilus influenzae pneumonia* *Streptococcus pneumonia*
Blood-rust	*Klebsiella pneumonia*, pneumococcal pneumonia, lung abscess, bronchiectasis, anaerobic infections, aspiration
Black	Smoke, coal dust
Frothy pink	Pulmonary edema
Blood	Pulmonary emboli with infarction, tuberculosis, abscess, trauma, mitral valve disease

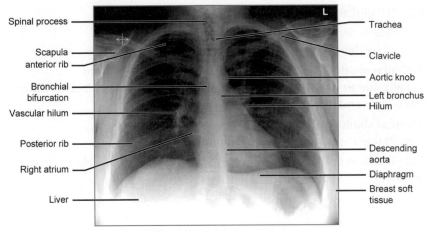

Spinal process
Scapula
anterior rib
Bronchial
bifurcation
Vascular hilum
Posterior rib
Right atrium
Liver

Trachea
Clavicle
Aortic knob
Left bronchus
Hilum
Descending
aorta
Diaphragm
Breast soft
tissue

Fig. 3.3: Normal chest X-ray

be less cardiac magnification. The left lateral view is also preferred because there is less cardiac magnification and a sharper view of the left lower lobe, which is partially obscured on the PA film.

Correlation between X-rays

Chest X-ray Interpretation

Always start with name of patient, date, and type of X-ray (AP, PA and lateral). Comment on penetration, rotation, projection and patient position.

A general rule is to start with bones, then fat, liquids/soft tissues, and finally air spaces. Other abnormalities such as metallic opacities, lines etc. should also be commented on.

- Penetration: Can individual vertebrae be identified?
- Rotation: Clavicle heads level? Trachea in line with vertebrae?
- Projection: Can the apices and lung bases be seen?
- Position: Patient lordotic/kyphotic?

Respiratory

- Trachea—should be central. Deviated towards affected side in fibrosis, collapse and pneumothorax, away from affected side in tension pneumothorax and large effusion.
- Heart—enlarged, (cor pulmonale), tall and narrow (hyperinflation).
- Hila—left usually higher than right. Pulled down by fibrosis or collapse. Enlarged by infection, carcinoma, pulmonary hypertension.
- Diaphragm—right side usually higher than left. Raised in fibrosis, phrenic nerve palsy, hepatomegaly. Low in hyperinflation.

Abnormalities in Lung Fields

- *Nodular shadowing:* Well-defined.
- May be due to neoplasia, granulomas, pneumoconiosis.

Reticular shadowing: 'Net-like'. Due to disease of interstitium.
Usually due to pulmonary interstitial edema. Other causes include fibrosis, sarcoidosis and interstitial lung diseases.

Alveolar shadows: 'Fluffy'.
Usually due to pulmonary edema or pneumonia.

Ring shadows and tram lines: Bronchiectasis. Rings also rarely due to tumor or abscess.

Typical Appearances

Asthma:	X-ray normal in between episodes. Hyperinflated during attacks (tall narrow heart, >6 anterior ribs, low flat diaphragm. May be nodular opacity if lobe collapse (mucus plugging, ABPA). Pigeon chest deformity may be seen on lateral view. No abnormalities on CT.
COPD:	X-ray often normal, may be signs of hyperinflation—tall narrow heart, >6 anterior ribs, low flat diaphragm, bullae. CT can be used to view emphysema—appears as a fine shadow.
Bronchiectasis:	X-ray shows no abnormalities unless severe disease. Ring shadows/tram lines may be seen. Complications such as collapse/infection may be apparent. CT is diagnostic. Shows dilated airways and thickened walls.
Pneumonia:	X-ray—consolidation, often lobular or segmental. May be parapneumonic effusion. May be hilar lymphadenopathy. CT not indicated unless something else is suspected (i.e carcinoma).
Tuberculosis:	X-ray—consolidation/collapse. Cavitation (granuloma). Pleural effusion/empyema, 'miliary' shadowing; diffuse, speckled. CT not indicated unless something else is suspected (i.e. carcinoma).
Bronchial carcinoma:	X-ray signs differ depending on site and size of tumor. Common findings—unilateral hilar enlargement (central tumor). Peripheral opacity; usually irregular and can be very large.

Collapse (distal to tumor); appears as a hazy shadowing.
Pleural effusion (due to invasion of pleural space or infection)
Broadening of mediastinum (paratracheal lympha-denopathy)
Enlarged cardiac shadow (Malignant pericardial effusion)
Elevated hemidiaphragm (phrenic nerve palsy)
Rib destruction (Bone mets)
Tumors that are too small to be picked up on X-ray may be obtained on CT.

Mediastinal carcinoma: May present on X-ray as broadening of the mediastinum, but CT and MRI are the investigations of choice.

Sarcoidosis: In early stages, X-rays show BHL, enlarged para-tracheal nodes, which progress to include diffuse pulmonary opacities. BHL subsides in later stages. Frank fibrosis is seen in stage 4.
Contast enhanced CT may show lymph nodes with 'rim enhancement' and central necrosis. Whatever that looks like.

CFA: X-ray shows typical firbrotic changes: Small lungs, high diaphragm, basal and peripheral opacities. Honey-combing in late stage disease.
HRCT shows characteristic changes (see Davidson's 552 old edn). Particularly useful in early disease, where X-ray may be normal.

PE: X-ray may be normal. Otherwise—opacities that may be any size or shape, can caviate. Elevated hemidiaphragm. Bilateral horizontal opacities (usually in lower zones), pleural effusion. Rarely: Wedge-shaped opacity.
CTPA investigation of choice. Pick up emboli like nobody's business.

Pneumothorax: X-ray shows reduced lung field with sharply defined edge. Will show extent of any mediastinal displacement (i.e. tension pneumothorax).
CT indicated if doubt exists between large emphy-sematous bulla and pneumothorax.

Cardiovascular

Best reviewed by PA in full inspiration.

Cardiothoracic ratio: Maximum width of cardiac silhouette/widest aspect of lung fields. Can only be accurately measured on a PA. >0.5 suggests cardiac hypertrophy/dilatation. Imp: Cardiomyopathies, pericardial effusion, heart failure, valvular disease.

Specific dilatations:
- Left atrium produces straight left heart border, double cardiac shadow to right of sternum, and widened carina
- Right atrium protrudes out into the right lung space
- Left ventricle causes prominence of the left lower heart border and widening of the cardiac silhouette
- Right ventricle displaces apex upwards and straightens left heart border.

Pulmonary edema:
- 'Ground glass' of alveolar edema
- Prominence of upper lobe vessels
- Enlarged hilar vessels
- Enlarged cardiac silhouette
- Kerley B lines (horizontal lines in lower zones).

Aortic dissection: Broadened upper mediastinum, distorted aortic knuckle. (absent in 40% cases).

▓ FINDINGS AND PHYSICAL EXAMINATION

There should be a correlation between what is seen on an X-ray and the physical examination. The following is a list of physical findings with related X-ray findings for certain disease states.

Atelectasis

Physical findings: Elevated diaphragm on the affected side on palpation of the lower chest. Decreased or absent breath sounds on the affected side by auscultation. Shift of the trachea to the affected side only if a large area of the lung is affected (Fig. 3.4).

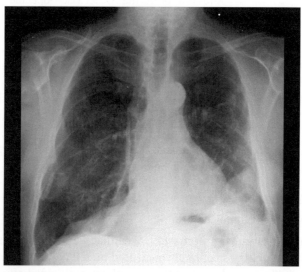

Fig. 3.4: X-Ray findings: Shift of the fissure lines and hilar structures toward the affected area and overall loss of volume with elevation of the hemidiaphragm

Consolidation

Physical findings: Dullness on percussion over affected areas. Auscultation reveals crackles over the affected area. Whispered voice sounds are usually louder than normal (Fig. 3.5).

Congestive Heart Failure

Physical findings: Increased heart rate with either a regular or irregular rhythm. A third heard sound (S3) is a consistent finding. The peripheral pulse may be strong, alternating to a weak pulse every other beat. Pedal edema is usually present during the day but is somewhat relieved after a night of sleep. Patient usually complains of coughing, attacks of severe shortness of breath, fatigue, and weakness (Fig. 3.6).

Hyperinflation (COPD)

Physical findings: Barrel-chested with decreased breath sounds, wheezing, limited motion of the diaphragm, increased respiratory rate, and the use of accessory muscles to breathe (Fig. 3.7).

Interstitial Fibrosis

Physical findings: May have a dry, nonproductive cough, dyspnea on exertion, and a history of exposure to inhaled agents (Fig. 3.8).

Pleural Effusion

Physical findings: Decreased breath sounds over affected side, pain on inspiration, coughing, and shortness of breath (Fig. 3.9).

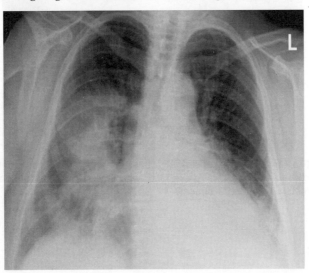

Fig. 3.5: X-ray findings: Minimal loss of volume with lobar distribution and homogeneous density (whiter area) late in the consolidation process

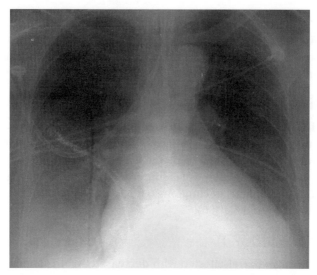

Fig. 3.6: X-ray findings: Usually shows prominent pulmonary blood vessels. Development of Kerley B lines, which are seen in the right base. These Kerley B lines are horizontal and start at the periphery; they are usually 1 mm thick and 1 to 2 cm in length

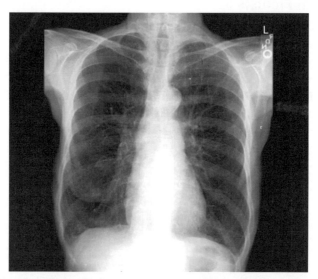

Fig. 3.7: X-ray findings: Increased AP chest dimensions and anterior air space. Depressed diaphragms, marked hyperinflation with large lung volumes, and small narrow heart with enlarged intercostal spaces

■ RESPIRATORY DISEASES

The following is the listing of possible causes, clinical findings, and treatment of common respiratory diseases.

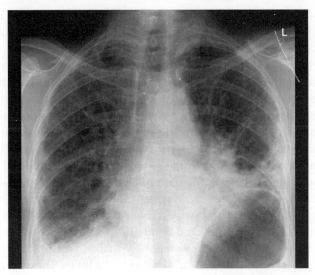

Fig. 3.8: X-ray findings: Peripheral markings are enlarged and white in color. The air-filled airways are seen as clear with dark straight shadows. The peripheral white markings are said to have the appearance of ground glass, representing affected alveolar spaces

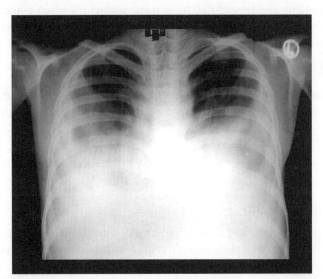

Fig. 3.9: X-ray findings: Large volumes of complete "white out" on the affected side completely obscuring the hemi-diaphragm. With small-volume effusion, only partial 'white-out' on the affected side is seen, with only partial obstruction of the hemi-diaphragm

Chronic Bronchitis
Structural Changes

Chronic inflammation and swelling of the peripheral air was excessive mucus production and accumulation bronchial.

In the early stages of chronic bronchitis, a cough usually occurs in the morning. As the disease progresses, coughing persists throughout the day. This chronic cough is commonly referred to as 'smoker's cough.'

Also in the early stages of chronic bronchitis, only the larger airways are affected, but eventually all airways are involved. Over time the patient experiences abnormal ventilation-perfusion, insufficient oxygenation of blood (hypoxemia), labored breathing (hypoventilation) and right-sided heart failure (cor pulmonale). Compared with acute bronchitis, which may respond quickly to medications, such as antibiotics, chronic bronchitis can be difficult to treat because many patients with chronic bronchitis are susceptible to recurring bacterial infections. Excessive mucous production in the lungs provides a good environment for infection, which also causes inflammation and swelling of the bronchial tubes and a reduction in the amount of airflow in and out of the lungs.

In the later stages of chronic bronchitis, the patient cannot clear this thick, tenacious mucus, which then causes damage to the hair-like structures (cilia) that help sweep away fluids and/or particles in the lungs. This in turn impairs the lung's defense against air-borne irritants. Cigarette smoking is the most common cause of chronic bronchitis. People who have been exposed for a long time to irritants, like chemical fumes, dust and other noxious substances, can also get chronic bronchitis. As chronic bronchitis often coincides with emphysema, it is frequently difficult for a physician to distinguish between the two. Chronic bronchitis also can have an asthmatic component.

Possible Causes

Exact causes are not known; cigarette smoking, atmospheric pollutants, and repeated infection of the respiratory tract have been linked to the disorder.

Clinical Findings

Pulmonary function tests: Decreases in FEF25-75, FEV1, MVV, PEFR, VC, IRV; increases in Vt, RV, FRC, VC and FVC (Fig. 3.10).

Respiratory Findings

Use of accessory muscles, diminished breath sounds with wheezing and/or rhonchi, chronic cough with excessive sputum production for three months per year for two or more successive years.

Arterial blood gases

Early: Decreased PaO_2 normal or decreased $PaCO_2$ normal or decreased pH.

Advanced Stage: Decreased PaO_2, increased $PaCO_2$, increased HCO_3, normal or decreased pH.

Treatment

Avoidance of smoking, inhaling of irritants, and infections, mostly people with contagious respiratory tract infections. Mobilize bronchial secretions

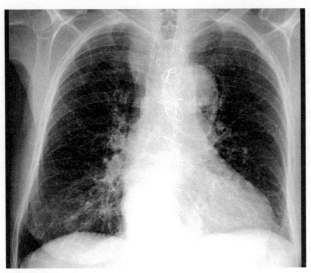

Fig. 3.10: Chest X-ray: Translucent, depressed or flattened diaphragm, spike-like projections on bronchogram, enlarged heart, pulmonary vascular engorgement, and increased anteroposterior chest diameter (barrel chest)

by nebulizer or aerosol therapy, increased fluid intake, chest physical therapy, postural drainage, deep breathing aids (incentive spirometer), and suctioning. Sympathomimetics (Bronkosol, Alupent, etc), methylxanthines (aminophylline, etc), expectorants (Robitussin, etc), antibiotics (ampicillin, tetracycline). Proper education and psychological and sociologic support.

There is no cure for chronic bronchitis. Treatment is aimed at relieving symptoms and preventing complications. Lying down at night can worsen the condition, so some people with advanced chronic bronchitis must sleep sitting up. In late, severe stages people who often have emphysema as well, are called 'blue bloaters' because lack of oxygen causes the skin to have a blue cast (cyanosis) and because the body is swollen from fluid accumulation caused by congestive heart failure.

Emphysema

Permanent enlargement and deterioration of air spaces distal to the terminal bronchioles. Destruction of pulmonary capillaries. Weakening of the distal airways, primarily the respiratory bronchioles.

Emphysema is a long-term, progressive disease of the lungs that primarily causes shortness of breath. In people with emphysema, the lung tissues necessary to support the physical shape and function of the lung are damaged. It is included in a group of diseases called chronic obstructive pulmonary disease or COPD (pulmonary refers to the lungs). Emphysema is called an obstructive lung disease because the destruction of lung tissue around smaller airways, called bronchioles, makes these airways unable to hold their shape properly when you exhale. This makes them inefficient at transferring oxygen into the blood, and in taking carbon dioxide out of the blood.

Emphysema changes the anatomy of the lung in several important ways.

Normally, the lungs are very spongy and elastic. When a breath is taken, the chest wall expands, expanding the sponge. Just as a squeezed sponge will draw water into it when released, suction draws air into the lungs when the chest wall expands. Air is brought through the trachea (windpipe) and bronchi (the main air tubes going to right and left lungs). These tubes divide into smaller and smaller tubes, finally ending in alveoli. Alveoli, the tiniest structures in the lung, are very small air sacs that are arranged like a bunch of grapes. The alveoli are at the ends of the smallest tubes called bronchioles. The alveoli and the bronchioles are very important structures for the lungs to function properly. It is these structures that are damaged by emphysema.

A sponge works to pick up water because all the tiny little holes expand at once after being squeezed. If the holes were larger, the sponge would not pick up as much water. This is because a larger hole cannot expand enough by itself to equal the action of multiple smaller ones. Thinking of the lungs as a sponge in this way, it becomes easier to see how emphysema acts to cause impaired lung function. Lungs require an elastic quality, so that they can expand and contract well. Also, as with the holes of the sponge, the lungs need many alveoli (hundreds of millions, in fact) to draw enough air into them. The fewer and the bigger the alveoli, the less effectively they perform.

Types

There are three types of emphysema:
- Centrilobular: Changes mostly in the respiratory bronchioles.
- Panlobular: Changes at the alveolar level.
- Bullous: Changes at the alveolar and respiratory bronchioles.

Possible Causes

Cigarette smoking, alpha-antitrypsin deficiency, infections of the respiratory tract during childhood and inhaled irritants (sulfur dioxide, nitrogen oxides, and ozone).

Clinical Findings

Pulmonary functions tests: Increased Vt, RV, FRC, VC decreased IRV, ERV, FVC, and FEF25-75, FEV1, MVV, PEFR (Fig. 3.11).

Respiratory Findings

Increases in respiratory infections, respiratory rate, heart rate, cardiac output, and blood pressure. The patient will show an increase in use of accessory muscles with pursed-lip breathing. Cyanosis and digital clubbing may also be seen.

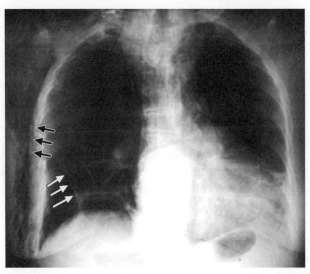

Fig. 3.11: Chest X-ray: Increased anteroposterior chest diameter (barrel chest); translucent, depressed, or flattened diaphragm; elongated cardiac silhouette, and small heart

Arterial Blood Gases

Early stages: Decreased PaO_2, normal or decreased $PaCO_2$, normal or decreased HCO_3 normal or increased pH.

Advanced stages: Decreased PaO_2, increased $PaCO_2$, increased HCO_3, normal or decreased pH.

Treatment

Avoidance of smoking, people with contagious respiratory tract infections, and inhaling irritants. Proper nutrition; meals (possible high protein) should be given in small amounts but more often, 6 to 8 a day. Mobilization of bronchial secretions by aerosol or nebulizer therapy, increase in fluids, chest physical therapy, deep breathing aids (incentive spirometer), and suctioning. Supplemental oxygen at low flow. Possible medications: Sympathomimetic agents (Bronkosol, Alupent, etc). Methylxanthines (aminophylline), expectorants (nortussin, Robitussion, etc) antibiotics, digitalis (Lanoxin, etc) for patients with ventricular heart failure with emphysema. Proper education of patient and family.

Complications of Emphysema

Recurrent chest infections, including pneumonia, the flu (influeza), cold and the common cold.

Pulmonary hypertension: Unusually high blood pressure in the arteries of the lungs.

Cor pulmonale: Enlargement and strain on the right side of the heart. This can lead to heart failure.

Asthma

Smooth muscle constriction of bronchial airways. Excessive production of thick, tenacious tracheobronchial secretions. Hyperinflation of alveoli. Thickening of subepithelial membranes.

The inflammatory reaction in bronchial asthma is brought about by four types of cells: namely the dendritic cells and macrophages, T-helper lymphocytes, mast cells and eosinophils. Dendritics cells and macrophages present antigens to T-helper cells and induce the switching of B lymphocytes to produce immunoglobulin E (IgE). These cells are influenced by corticosteroids (e.g. beclomethasone, prednisolone) though beta receptor antagonists have no influence on them.

T helper lymphocyte is the key in the pathogenesis of bronchial asthma. They induce B cells to synthesize and secrete IgE through the production of interleukin 4 (IL-4) and induce eosinophilic inflammation via interleukin 5 (IL-5). T helper cells are also influenced by corticosteroids but not by the beta receptor agonists.

Mast cells contribute to the inflammatory reaction by the production and release of histamine, tryptase, prostaglandin D_2 (PGD_2) and leukotriene C_4 (LTC_4). These cells are involved in the early phases of asthma known as the early reaction. Unlike other types of cells, mast cell membranes are stabilized by beta receptor agonists (such as salbutamol and terbutaline) and chromones (such as sodium cromoglycate).

Eosinophils are involved in the late phase reaction of bronchial asthma. They are attracted to the bronchial walls by interleukins 3 and 5 (IL-3, IL-5) and the granulocyte monocyte colony stimulating factor (GM-CSF) secreted by the T helper cells. Corticosteroids are effective in decreasing the entry of eosinophils as well as the number of eosinophils in circulation. In addition, corticosteroids prevent activation of eosinophils which have entered the bronchial walls.

Possible Causes

Extrinsic asthma (allergic reaction to pollen, house dust, feathers, etc). Hypersensitivity to common environmental allergens. Intrinsic asthma (nonallergic or nonatopic), infection, cold air, vapor, drugs (aspirin) emotional stress and exercise.

Clinical Findings

Pulmonary function tests: Decreases in FEF25-75, FEV1, MVV, PEFR, VC, IRV, ERV; increases in RV, FRC, RV/TLC ratio (Fig. 3.12).

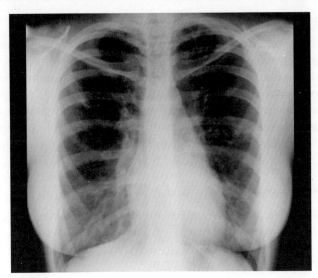

Fig. 3.12: Chest X-ray: Increased anteroposterior chest diameter, translucent, depressed, or flattened diaphragm

Respiratory Findings

Increased respiratory rate, heart rate, blood pressure, use of accessory muscles, pursed-lip breathing, cough with expectoration, decreased breath sounds with wheezing and/or rhonchi often audible without a stethoscope, and a prolonged expiratory time.

Arterial Blood Gases

Acute: Decreased PaO_2, decreased $PaCO_2$, decreased HCO_3, increased pH.
Status asthmaticus: Decreased PaO_2, increased $PaCO_2$, increased HCO_3, decreased.

Treatment

Medications: Sympathomimetic agents, methylxanthines, corticosteroids. Supplemental oxygen and possible mechanical ventilation in patients with status asthmaticus. Pneumothorax frequently develops in status asthmaticus, necessitating the need for chest tubes. Mobilization of bronchial secretions: suctioning, aerosol therapy, increased fluid intake—systemic, possible chest physical therapy. Monitoring arterial blood gases, proper education of the patient, psychological and sociologic support.

Pneumonia

Inflammation of the alveoli. Alveolar consolidation.

Pathophysiology

There are different categories of pneumonia. Two of these types are hospital-acquired and community-acquired. Common types of community-acquired pneumonia are Pneumococcal pneumonia and Mycoplasma pneumonia. In some people, particularly the elderly and those who are debilitated, pneumonia may follow influenza. Hospital-acquired pneumonia tends to be more serious because defense mechanisms against infection are often impaired. Some of the specific pneumonia-related disorders include aspiration pneumonia, pneumonia in immunocompromised host and viral pneumonia.

Possible Causes

Gram-positive, Gram-negative organisms, viral, rickettsial infection, prittacoris, varicella, rubella and aspiration.

Clinical Findings

Pulmonary function tests: Decreases in VC, RV, FRC, TLC, Vt (Fig. 3.13).

Respiratory Findings

Increases in respiratory rate, heart rate, blood pressure, cough with expectoration, chest pain with decreased chest expansion, bronchial breath sounds with rales/rhonchi/wheezing, possible pleural friction rub.

Arterial Blood Gases

Early stages: Decreased PaO_2, normal to decreased $PaCO_2$, normal to decreased HCO_3, increased pH.

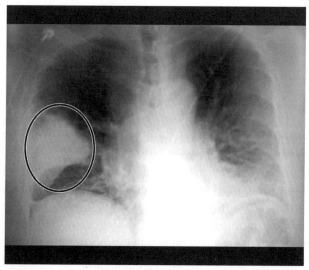

Fig. 3.13: Chest X-ray: Increased opacity (whiter in appearance), increased lung density

Advanced stages: Decreased PaO_2, increased $PaCO_2$, increased HCO_3, decreased pH.

Treatment

Medications: Antibiotic agents, sympathomimetic, non-sedative analgesic agents. Oxygen therapy (keeping the PaO_2 60 to 80 mm Hg), possible mechanical ventilation for patients with chronic lung problems and pneumonia, increases in fluid intake, deep breathing aids (IPPB, incentive spirometer), chest physical therapy, nebulizer therapy, possible thoracentesis, bronchoscope, control of fever and excess cough. Keep a close watch for complications.

Pulmonary Edema

Interstitial edema, including fluid engorgement of the perivascular and peribronchial spaces and the alveolar wall interstitium, increased surface tension, alveolar shrinkage, frothy secretions throughout the tracheobronchial tree.

Pathophysiology

Pulmonary vessels create an imbalance in the startling forces, leading to an increase in the fluid filtration into the interstitial spaces of the lungs that exceeds the lymphatic capacity to drain the fluids away. Increasing volumes of fluid leak into the alveolar space.

The lymphatic system drains excess interstitial fluid volume. Additional fluid in the pleural drains into the titer lymph nodes. In this, pathway becomes overwhelmed, however, fluid moves from the interstitial in the alveolar walls. If the alveolar epithelium is damaged, the fluid accumulates in the alveoli. Alveolar edema is a series late sighs in the progression of fluids imbalance. Hypoxemia develops when the alveolar membrane is thickened by fluid that impairs gas exchange of oxygen and CO_2. As fluid fills interstitial and alveolar space, lung compliance decreases and oxygen diffusion.

Possible Causes

Cardiogenic causes: Increases in hydrostatic pressure, arrhythmias, excessive fluid administration, left ventricle failure, mitral valve disease, myocardial infarction, pulmonary embolus, renal failure and systemic hypertension.

Noncardiogenic causes: Pulmonary edema, alveolar hypoxia, adult respiratory distress syndrome (ARDS), inhalation of toxic gas (chlorine, sulfur dioxide, ammonia), therapeutic radiation of the lungs, lymphatic insufficiency, overtransfusion or rapid transfusion, uremia, hypoproteinemia, acute nephritis, allergic reaction to drugs, aspiration, central nervous system stimulation, encephalitis and head trauma.

Clinical Findings

Pulmonary function tests: Decreases in VC, RV, FRC, TLC and Vt (Fig. 3.14).

Respiratory Findings

Increased respiratory rate, nocturnal dyspnea, cough with expectoration, cyanosis, breath sounds, rales/rhonchi/wheezing, and increase in pulmonary wedge pressure—cardiogenic only.

Arterial Blood Gases

Early: Decreased PaO_2, normal or decreased $PaCO_2$, normal or decreased HCO_3, normal to decreased pH.

Advanced stage: Decreased PaO_2, increased $PaCO_2$, increased HCO_3, decreased pH.

Pulmonary wedge pressure for cardiogenic pulmonary edema >12 mm Hg.

Treatment

Medications—morphine sulfate, diuretic agents, digitalis, sympathomimetic agents, albumin, possible inhaled ethanol; positioning patients in Fowler's position; hyperinflation and oxygen (keeping PaO_2 60–80 mm Hg) possible intubation with volume-cycled ventilator with PEEP or CPAP. Hemoglobin below 10 g should be corrected by blood transfusion and fluid management.

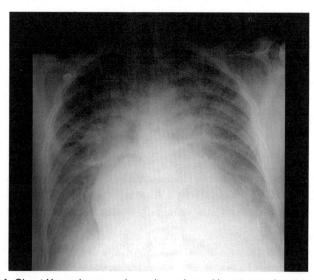

Fig. 3.14: Chest X-ray: Increased opacity, enlarged heart, prominent pulmonary vessels, and Kerley B lines

Pulmonary Embolism

Blockage of the pulmonary vascular system. Pulmonary infarction. Pulmonary tissue necrosis.

Thrombotic pulmonary embolism is not an isolated disease of the chest but a complication of venous thrombosis. Deep venous thrombosis (DVT) and pulmonary embolism are therefore parts of the same process, venous thromboembolism. Evidence of leg DVT is found in about 70% of patients who have sustained a pulmonary embolism; in most of the remainder, it is assumed that the whole thrombus has already become detached and embolized. Conversely, pulmonary embolism occurs in up to 50% of patients with proximal DVT of the legs (involving the popliteal and/or more proximal veins), and is less likely when the thrombus is confined to the calf veins. Rarely, the source of emboli are the iliac veins, renal veins, right heart, or upper extremity veins; the clinical circumstances usually point to these unusual sites.

Pathophysiology

The effects of an embolus depend on the extent to which it obstructs the pulmonary circulation, the duration over which that obstruction accumulates, and the pre-existing state of the patient, which has been defined only imprecisely. Some humoral mediators (for example, serotonin or thromboxane from activated platelets) can probably produce vasospasm in nonembolized segments of the lung. As a result, a degree of pulmonary hypertension may develop disproportionate to the amount of vasculature that is mechanically occluded. In general, a patient who has pre-existing cardiopulmonary disease or who is old, frail or debilitated will be more sensitive to the effects of pulmonary embolism than a patient who was well until the embolic event occurred. Most emboli are multiple. As both the extent and chronicity of obstruction vary so widely, pulmonary embolism can produce widely differing clinical pictures. Disregarding chronic thromboembolic pulmonary hypertension. The first and most common presentation is dyspnea with or without pleuritic pain and hemoptysis (acute minor pulmonary embolism). The second presentation is hemodynamic instability, which is associated with acute massive pulmonary embolism. The third and least common presentation mimics heart failure or indolent pneumonia, especially in the elderly (subacute massive pulmonary embolism).

Possible Causes

Prolonged bed rest and/or immobilization; prolonged sitting (car, plane, bus, etc); congestive heart failure; varicose veins; long bone fractures—trauma; injury of the soft tissues, vessels; extensive hip, abdominal, or chest surgery; oral contraceptives; obesity; pregnancy; and burns.

Clinical Findings

Physical findings: Chest pain, increased respiratory rate, cough with hemoptysis, syncope, lightheadedness, confusion, cyanosis, breath sounds-rales/rhonchi/wheezing/pleural friction rub, abnormal perfusion lung scan, pulmonary hypertension, systemic hypotension. ECG—sinus tachycardia or atrial arrhythmia or possible incomplete right bundle-branch block.

Arterial Blood Gases

Decreased PaO_2, normal to decreased $PaCO_2$, normal to decreased HCO_3, normal to increased pH.

Treatment

Heparin dicumarol, supplemental oxygen, possible embolectomy, and treat any cardiac problems that might arise.

Anticoagulants or blood thinners, decrease your blood's ability to clot. They are used to stop blood clots from getting larger and prevent clots from forming. Blood thinners do not break up blood clots that have already formed. (The body dissolves most clots with time).

Blood thinners as either a pill, an injection, or through a needle or tube inserted into a vein (called intravenous, or IV, injection). Warfarin is given as a pill. Heparin is given as an injection or through an IV tube.

Adult Respiratory Distress Syndrome (ARDS)

Interstitial and intra-alveolar edema and hemorrhage. Alveolar consolidation. Intra-alveolar hyaline membrane. Pulmonary surfactant deficiency or abnormality. Atelectasis.

Pathophysiology

- Exudative phase with alveolar edema, capillary congestion, and hyaline membrane formation.
- Proliferative phase with proliferation of type II alveolar cells and cellular infiltration.
- Fibrotic phase with fibrosis of membranes, septae, and ducts.

Two defining characteristics of ARDS are edema/infiltration and fibrosis/low compliance. Edema occurs because the membranes become permeable to protein. Oncotic gradient is lost, and protein leaks into the interstitium and alveoli. The filtration coefficient (K_f) goes way up. Capillaries also vasoconstrict due to hypoperfusion. This protein permeability and increased pressure serve to fill the interstitium and alveoli with protein and water. This edema distributes with gravity because of the weight of the lungs pressing down and closing alveoli. So if they lie on their back, posterior regions close off, and vice versa. This is in contrast to CHF edema, which is due solely to high capillary pressure and is therefore a protein-poor edema. There is also fibrosis and loss of surfactant, both of which give the lungs reduced compliance (Fig. 3.15).

ARDS is characterized by the following criteria:

- Lung injury of acute onset, within 1 week of an apparent clinical insult and with progression of respiratory symptoms
- Bilateral opacities on chest imaging not explained by other pulmonary pathology (e.g. pleural effusion, pneumothorax, or nodules)
- Respiratory failure not explained by heart failure or volume overload.

Decreased arterial PaO$_2$/FiO$_2$ ratio:

- Mild ARDS: ratio is 201–300 mm Hg ($\leq$ 39.9 kPa)
- Moderate ARDS: 101–200 mm Hg ($\leq$ 26.6 kPa)
- Severe ARDS: $\leq$100 mm Hg ($\leq$13.3 kPa)

The above characteristics are the "Berlin criteria" of 2012 by the European Society of Intensive Care Medicine, endorsed by the American Thoracic Society and the Society of Critical Care Medicine. They are a modification of the previously used criteria:

Acute onset

- Bilateral infiltrates on chest radiograph sparing costophrenic angles

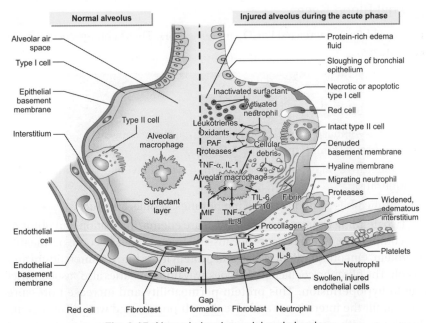

Fig. 3.15: Normal alveolus vs injured alveolus

- Pulmonary artery wedge pressure <18 mm Hg (obtained by pulmonary artery catheterization), if this information is available; if unavailable, then lack of clinical evidence of left atrial hypertension.

If PaO$_2$: FiO$_2$ <300 mm Hg (40 kPa) acute lung injury (ALI) is considered to be present.

If PaO$_2$: FiO$_2$ <200 mm Hg (26.7 kPa) acute respiratory distress syndrome (ARDS) is considered to be present.

Possible Causes

Aspiration; central nervous system disease; cardiopulmonary bypass; congestive heart failure; disseminated intravascular coagulation (DIC); drug overdose; fat or air emboli; fluid overload; infections; inhalation of chlorine, nitrogen dioxide, smoke, or ozone; immunologic reaction.

Clinical Findings

Pulmonary function tests: Decreases in VC, RV, FRC, TLC and Vt (Fig. 3.16).

Respiratory Findings

Increased respiratory rate and blood pressure, intercostal retractions, cough, nausea, vomiting, fever, decreased compliance, breath sounds, rales/rhonchi, mental disorientation.

Arterial Blood Gases

Decreased PaO$_2$ decreased PaCO$_2$, increased pH. These changes occur in the early stages.

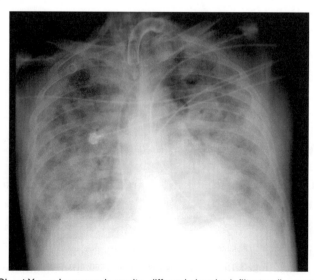

Fig. 3.16: Chest X-ray: Increased opacity, diffused alveolar infiltrates (honeycomb effect)

Treatment

Medications: Diuretic agents, corticosteroids and antibiotic, hyperinflation and oxygenation. Possible intubation with ventilation and PEEP therapy maintaining PaO_2 >60 mm Hg, possible fluid therapy, watching input and output.

Flail Chest
Structural Changes

Double fracture of multiple adjacent ribs. Rib instability. Lung restriction. Atelectasis. Lung collapse.

A flail chest occurs when a segment of the thoracic cage is separated from the rest of the chest wall. This is usually defined as at least two fractures per rib (producing a free segment), in at least two ribs. A segment of the chest wall that is flail is unable to contribute to lung expansion. Large flail segments will involve a much greater proportion of the chest wall and may extend bilaterally or involve the sternum. In these cases, the disruption of normal pulmonary mechanics may be large enough to require mechanical ventilation.

The main significance of a flail chest, however, is that it indicates the presence of an underlying pulmonary contusion. In most cases, it is the severity and extent of the lung injury that determines the clinical course and requirement for mechanical ventilation. Thus the management of flail chest consists of standard management of the rib fractures and of the pulmonary contusions underneath.

Possible Causes

Direct compression by a heavy object (automobile or industrial accident).

Clinical Findings

Pulmonary function tests: Decreases in VC, RV, FRC, TLC, Vt (Fig. 3.17).

Respiratory Findings

Increased respiratory rate, heart rate, blood pressure and paradoxical chest movement (uneven movement).

Arterial Blood Gases

Early stages: Decreased PaO_2, normal or decreased $PaCO_2$, normal or decreased HCO_3, normal or increased pH.

Advanced stages: Decreased PaO_2, increased $PaCO_2$, increased HCO_3, decreased pH.

Treatment

Deep-breathing aids (incentive spirometer), medication for pain, bronchial hygiene, stabilization of fractures, possible mechanical ventilation with PEEP. Look for possible pneumothorax.

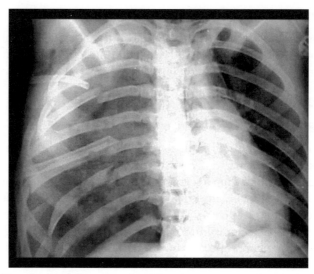

Fig. 3.17: Chest X-ray: Rib fractures involving three or more adjacent ribs, or multiple fractures of two or more ribs will increase opacity

Pneumothorax

Structural Changes

Lung collapse. Atelectasis. Compression of the great veins and decreased venous return.

In normal subjects, the pressure in the pleural space is negative with respect to the alveolar pressure during the entire respiratory cycle. The pressure gradient between the alveoli and the pleural space is the transpulmonary pressure and is the result of the inherent elastic recoil of the lung. During spontaneous breathing, the pleural pressure is also negative with respect to the atmospheric pressure. The functional residual capacity, or resting end-expiratory volume of the lung, is the volume at which the inherent outward pull of the chest wall is equal to, but opposite in direction to, the inward pull (recoil) of the lung.

A primary pneumothorax is one that occurs without an apparent cause and in the absence of significant lung disease, while a secondary pneumothorax occurs in the presence of existing lung pathology. In a minority of cases, the amount of air in the chest increases markedly when a one-way valve is formed by an area of damaged tissue, leading to a tension pneumothorax. This condition is a medical emergency that can cause steadily worsening oxygen shortage and low blood pressure. Unless reversed by effective treatment, these sequelae can progress and cause death.

A traumatic pneumothorax may result from either blunt trauma or penetrating injury to the chest wall. The most common mechanism is due to the penetration of sharp bony points at a new rib fracture, which damages lung tissue. Traumatic pneumothorax may also be observed in those exposed to blasts, even though there is no apparent injury to the chest.

Possible Causes

Traumatic pneumothorax (penetrating wounds, also called sucking chest wound). Spontaneous pneumothorax (suddenly without any obvious underlying cause). Iatrogenic pneumothorax (occurs during specific diagnostic or therapeutic procedures).

Clinical Findings

Pulmonary function tests: Decreases in VC, RV, FRC, TLC and Vt (Fig. 3.18).

Respiratory Findings

Increased difficulty in ventilating if on mechanical ventilator, vital signs will deteriorate, breath sounds will be absent on the affected side, trachea and mediastinum may shift toward unaffected side, possible pleuritic pain, and dry hacking cough.

Treatment

Decompression of the thorax by chest tube insertion or needle aspiration for pneumothorax >20%, bed rest for pneumothorax <20%, oxygen therapy, watch for atelectasis, if present deep-breathing aids (incentive spirometer). IPPB should be given only if the pneumothorax has been corrected or treated.

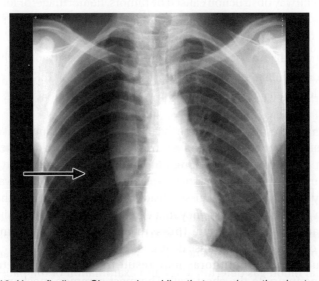

Fig. 3.18: X-ray findings: Show a pleural line that runs down the chest wall. The trachea is shifted toward the unaffected side

Respiratory Care and Surgery—Preoperative Evaluation

History: Chronic cough, shortness of breath, chest pain, smoking, edema in hands and feet, age, previous or existing heart disease, obesity, any chronic disease or muscle weakness noted.

Physical examination: State of nutrition, movement of the chest wall and abdomen, pursed-lip breathing, rib cage deformities, auscultation of the lungs.

Investigations: Chest X-ray, pulmonary function test, and arterial bloods gases.

Management: For heavy smokers, urge them to stop or at least cut down. Patients who are overweight should be placed on a diet- this only for elective surgery. Recent changes in sputum production or color – patients should be placed on antibiotics. Bronchospasm should be treated with bronchodilator drugs. Hypoxemia should be corrected if possible. Avoid excessive premeditations. If high risk for pulmonary complication, determine arterial blood gases, at least bedside pulmonary function tests, baseline ECG, and vital signs.

Acute Ventilatory Failure

Any cause that would affect ventilation.

Possible Causes

It has many etiologies. You must identify the underlying causes:

- Depression of the central drive caused by drug poisoning or craniocerebral trauma.
- Upper airway obstruction caused by tumors, hemorrhage, or foreign body.
- Lower airway and parenchymal defects caused by chronic bronchitis, emphysema asthma, or pulmonary edema.
- Chest wall disorders caused by kyphoscoliosis, obesity, or birth defects.
- Neuromuscular defects caused by myasthenia gravis, GBS, and respiratory muscle fatigue.

Physiologic Consequences

Hypoxemia, hypercapnia, academia, which are confirmed by arterial blood gases.

Clinical Findings

Tachypnea, tachycardia, hypertension or hypotension, cyanosis, confusion, coma, papilledema, asterixis, cardiac arrhythmias, and headaches.

Pulmonary function tests show decreased VC and peak inspiratory flow.

Arterial blood gas determination and examination of the patient are the best ways of determining ventilatory failure.

Treatment

Oxygen therapy, ventilatory support, correction of acid-base balance, and treatment of the underlying causes.

Caution must be taken when oxygen therapy is given to COPD patients.

Ventilatory Failure in Chronic Obstructive Pulmonary Disease (COPD)

Patients with COPD have already compromised physical and clinical features, which can hide acute ventilatory failure, up to the point of being life-threatening. Deterioration of clinical findings should alert you to impending problems.

Possible Causes

Depressed central drive caused by drugs (sedatives), excessive use of oxygen, or metabolic alkalosis. Other possible causes include acute bronchitis, pneumonia and allergies.

Clinical Findings

Decreased flow rates (pulmonary function tests), positive for overuse of sedatives, changes in sputum production, chest X-rays positive for pneumonia, positive for Gram's stain, and possible cardiovascular effects.

Treatment

Therapy should be directed for rehydration. Reduce or stop sedatives. Control oxygen percentage. Provide chest physical therapy, nebulizer or IPPB therapy, and nutritional support.

Pulmonary Arteriovenous Malformation

A pulmonary arteriovenous malformation (PAVM) is a rare vascular abnormality of the lung. Most cases tend to be simple AVM's (single feeding artery) although up to 20% of cases can have complex (2 or more) feeding vessels. They can be multiple in ~1/3 of patients.

Pathophysiology

In congenital cases, they are considered to result from a defect in the terminal capillary loops, which causes dilatation and the formation of thin-walled vascular sacs.

Anatomic shunt from pulmonary to systemic circulation:
- Shunt of material in venous system: Results in systemic embolization.
- Shunt of unoxygenated blood: Results in hypoxemia.

- Effect of exercise: Increased pulmonary blood flow (probably due to a greater than normal decrease in PVR, caused by less resistance to flow through the AVM) and decreased SVR (possibly due to underlying HHT or hypoxemic vasodilation).
- Orthodeoxia (decreased pO_2 when going from supine to erect position): occurs due to increased flow in lower lobes with erect posture—increased shunt (assuming lower lobe AVM).

Diagnosis

- ABG: Resting hypoxemia: Due to shunt (arterial pO_2 is inversely related to the size of the shunt fraction.
- Due to shape of oxygen dissociation curve, changes in arterial pO_2 are more sensitive at detecting shunt than changes in SAO_2.
- Orthodeoxia (decreased pO_2 when going from supine to erect position, as vascular dilatations are basilar-predominant): For shunts of >20%, SAO_2 decreases about 6% (as compared to 0.3% for normal).
- Exercise decrease in pO_2: Variable (pO_2 decreases 6% for shunts >30% and decreases 1–2% for shunts <12%).

100% FiO$_2$ shunt study: Assess pO_2 on 100% FiO_2 to assess degree of shunt.
- Actually measures 'physiologic shunt', which is equal to alveolar shunt (caused by V/Q mismatch) + anatomic shunt (caused by AVM). Measure arterial pO_2 and hemoglobin after breathing 100% FiO_2 × 15–20 min (deep breaths periodically to washout nitrogen).
- Normal: 5% of cardiac output.
- Calculate shunt as % of cardiac output (assuming O_2 content of 5 mL per 100 mL): This calculation may underestimate the % shunt.
- Supine and upright A-a gradient on 100% FiO_2: Only 68% sensitive in detecting a shunt from an AVM.

Exercise study: High ventilatory drive during exercise (similar to patients with congenital heart disease and right-to-left shunts) with preserved work capacity.

Swan: PVR is usually normal (with no pulmonary HTN).
CXR/Chest CT pattern: CXR is abnormal in 60–90% of cases.
- Shape: Round or oval, slightly lobulated, well-defined nodule (range from 1 to several cm).
- Maneuvers: AVM may change in size with Valsalva or Mueller maneuvers.
- Growth: AVM may increase in size during puberty, pregnancy, or in presence of pulmonary venous hypertension (due to mitral stenosis or LV dysfunction).

Helical CT: Useful to demonstrate AVM.

Chest MRI: Less sensitive than CT or pulmonary angiography, as small AVM's with rapid flow are not visualized.

Pulmonary angiogram: May demonstrate macroscopic, microscopic, or smaller diffuse AVM's.

- Allows identification of feeder vessels and assessment of rest of lungs prior to surgery.
- Transthoracic Echo with Bubble study: Best screening test for shunt from an AVM.
- Immediate appearance of bubbles in left side: Indicates intracardiac shunt.
- Delayed appearance of bubble in left side (after at least 4 cardiac cycles): indicates intrapulmonary shunt.

Clinical Presentation of AVM

- Asymptomatic (50% of cases):
- Respiratory symptoms:
  - Dyspnea (48% of cases):
  - Platypnea: Hypoxemia with upright position (as vascular dilatations are basilar-predominant)
  - Pulmonary bruit (49% of cases)
  - Clubbing (32% of cases)
  - Cyanosis (30% of cases)
  - Chest pain (14% of cases)
  - Hemoptysis (11% of cases): Due to endobronchial telangiectasia, increased risk during pregnancy
  - Hemothorax (<1% of cases): Due to pleural telangiectasia.
- Embolic phenomena: Serious neurologic events occur in 30–40% of AVM's with feeder vessels >3 mm.
  - Embolic CVA or TIA (27% of cases)
  - Brain abscess (10% of cases)
- Other symptoms
  - Anemia
  - High-output CHF: Due to intrapulmonary shunt
  - Endocarditis
  - Migraine
  - Seizures.

Treatment

Transcatheter coil embolization.

Surgery

Once successfully treated (embolotherapy, surgical resection), prognosis is generally good for an individual lesion.

▉ PULMONARY HYPERTENSION

Pulmonary hypertension is raised blood pressure within the pulmonary arteries, which are the blood vessels that supply the lungs.

Pulmonary arteries carry blood from your heart to the lungs, where it picks up oxygen to be delivered throughout your body. In PAH, the pulmonary arteries constrict abnormally. This forces your heart to work faster and causes blood pressure within the lungs to rise.

There are several types of PAH. It can be caused by or occur at the same time as a variety of other medical problems. PAH also can be the result of taking certain medicines. The cause of some cases of PAH is unknown.

PAH worsens over time and is life-threatening because the pressure in a patient's pulmonary arteries rises to dangerously high levels, putting a strain on the heart. There is no cure for PAH, but several medications are available to treat symptoms.

Possible Causes

- Congestive heart failure.
- Venous thromboembolic disease (blood clots in the lungs).
- Human immunodeficiency virus infection.
- Illegal drug use (cocaine, methamphetamine).
- Cirrhosis of the liver.
- Appetite suppressant medications (fenfluramine, dexfenfluramine, diethylpropion.
- Autoimmune diseases (lupus, scleroderma, and rheumatoid arthritis).
- Heart shunts (abnormal blood flow between heart chambers).
- Chronic lung disease (emphysema, chronic bronchitis, or pulmonary fibrosis).
- Obstructive sleep apnea.

Clinical Findings

The signs and symptoms of pulmonary hypertension in its early stages may not be noticeable for months or even years. As the disease progresses, symptoms become worse.

- Shortness of breath (dyspnea), initially while exercising and eventually while at rest.
- Fatigue.
- Dizziness or fainting spells (syncope).
- Chest pressure or pain.
- Swelling (edema) in ankles, legs and eventually in your abdomen (ascites).
- Bluish color to your lips and skin (cyanosis).
- Racing pulse or heart palpitations.
- Weakness.

Diagnosis

Echocardiogram: An ultrasound picture of the beating heart. An echocardiogram can estimate pulmonary artery pressures and check the function of the heart's right and left ventricles.

Computed tomography (CT scan): Detailed X-ray films of the chest provided by a CT scan may show enlarged pulmonary arteries. A CT scan may also identify other problems in the lungs that could cause shortness of breath.

Ventilation-perfusion scan (V/Q scan): A nuclear medicine test that can help identify blood clots in the lungs (pulmonary emboli), one cause of pulmonary hypertension.

Electrocardiogram (ECG or EKG): An electrical tracing of the heart's activity. ECG may show evidence of strain on the right side of the heart, a clue to the presence of pulmonary hypertension.

Chest X-ray: An X-ray cannot diagnose pulmonary hypertension, but may provide helpful clues. Chest X-ray films can help identify any other contributing lung or heart conditions.

Treatment
Medications

- Endothelin receptor antagonists (ERAs) to stop the harmful effects of endothelin, a hormone that helps control blood flow and cell growth in blood vessels. Patients with PAH often have high levels of endothelin.
- Phosphodiesterase-5 inhibitors (PDEI) to relax the muscles and reduce abnormal cell growth in blood vessels.
- Prostacyclins to relax blood vessels, reduce abnormal cell growth, and help prevent blood clots.
- Anticoagulants to prevent blood clots in the lungs.
- Calcium channel blockers to reduce constriction in the pulmonary arteries.
- Diuretics to improve how effectively the heart works by reducing the volume of blood it must pump.
- Digoxin to help the heart pump more forcefully.
- Inhaled oxygen to reduce shortness of breath.

Surgery

- Lung or heart-lung transplantation: Patients who fail standard therapies may be candidates for heart-lung transplantation. Transplantation can be life-saving, but the supply of donor organs is very limited.
- Atrial septostomy: In this treatment, a surgeon creates a hole between the top chambers of the heart. This allows blood to be pumped to the rest of the body without going through the lungs first. This can reduce strain on the heart, but it also greatly reduce the amount of oxygen that can be delivered to the body.

▦ BIBLIOGRAPHY

1. Badesch DB, Champion HC, Sanchez MA, Hoeper MM, Loyd JE, Manes A, et al. "Diagnosis and assessment of pulmonary arterial hypertension." Journal of the American College of Cardiology, 2009.

2. James R. Gossage and Ghassan Kanj "Pulmonary Arteriovenous Malformations", American Journal of Respiratory and Critical Care Medicine. 1998;158(2)643-61.
3. Mason RJ, Broaddus VC, Martin T, King T Jr., Murray JF, DSc(Hon), FRCP and Jay A. Nadel, MD, DSc(HON).
4. Midelton GT, Frishman WH, Passo SS. Congestive heart failure and continuous positive airway pressure therapy: support of a new modality for improving the prognosis and survival of patients with advanced congestive heart failure. Heart Disease. 2002;4(2):102-9.
5. Plant P, Owen J, Elliott M. Early use of non-invasive ventilation for acute exacerbations of chronic obstructive pulmonary disease on general respiratory wards: a multicentre randomised controlled trial. The Lancet. 2000;355(Issue 9219):1931-5.
6. Ryland BP. emedicine- Ventilation, Mechanical. Retrieved Nov, 24, 2006 from http://www.emedicine.com/med/topic3370.htm
7. Sharma S. emedicine- Respiratory Failure. Retrieved Nov., 24, 2006 from http://www.emedicine.com/med/topic2011.htm
8. The Acute Respiratory Distress Syndrome Network. Ventilation with lower tidal volumes as compared with traditional tidal volumes for acute lung injury and the acute respiratory distress syndrome. New England Journal of Medicine. 2000;342(18):1301-8.
9. Tobin MJ. Principles and Practice of Mechanical Ventilation.

ARTERIAL BLOOD GAS ANALYSIS

■ INTRODUCTION

It is a common investigation in emergency departments and intensive care units for monitoring patients with acute respiratory failure. It also has some application in general practice, such as assessing the need for domiciliary oxygen therapy in patients with chronic obstructive pulmonary disease. An arterial blood gas result can help in the assessment of a patient's gas exchange, ventilatory control and acid–base balance. However, the investigation does not give a diagnosis and should not be used as a screening test. It is imperative that the results are considered in the context of the patient's symptoms.

While noninvasive monitoring of pulmonary function, such as pulse oximetry, is simple, effective and increasingly widely used, pulse oximetry is no substitute for arterial blood gas analysis. Pulse oximetry is solely a measure of oxygen saturation and gives no indication about blood pH, carbon dioxide or bicarbonate concentrations.

■ ARTERIAL PUNCTURE

Blood is usually withdrawn from the radial artery as it is easy to palpate and has a good collateral supply. The patient's arm is placed palm-up on a flat surface, with the wrist dorsiflexed at 45°. A towel may be placed under the wrist for support. The puncture site should be cleaned with alcohol or iodine, and a local anesthetic (such as 2% lignocaine) should be infiltrated. Local anesthetic makes arterial puncture less painful for the patient and does not increase the difficulty of the procedure. The radial artery should be palpated for a pulse, and a preheparinized syringe with a 23 or 25 gauge needle should be inserted at an angle just distal to the palpated pulse. A small quantity of blood is sufficient. After the puncture, sterile gauze should be placed firmly over the site and direct pressure applied for several minutes to obtain hemostasis. If repeated arterial blood gas analysis is required, it is advisable to use a different site (such as the other radial artery) or insert an arterial line.

To ensure accuracy, it is important to deliver the sample for analysis promptly. If there is any delay in processing the sample, the blood can be stored on ice for approximately 30 minutes with little effect on the accuracy of the results.

Complications of arterial puncture are infrequent. They include prolonged bleeding, infection, thrombosis or arteriospasm.

The analysis of arterial blood gas values (ABG's) can detect the presence and identify the causes of acid-base and oxygenation disturbances. The body operates efficiently within a fairly narrow range of blood pH (acid-base balance). Even relatively small changes can be detrimental to cellular function. The normal range of pH is maintained by removing acids from the blood via two organ systems.

Respiratory: Ventilation at the lungs removes carbon dioxide in exhaled air.

Metabolic: Excretion of acids in urine by the kidney.

Acid-base abnormalities, therefore, are due to imbalances in one or both of these systems.

Respiratory mediated changes in acid-base status occur as a result of increases or decreases in the exhalation of carbon dioxide. These changes occur within minutes. When the rate and depth of ventilation increases, the CO_2 level falls, more acid is removed and the blood pH will rise becoming more alkalemic (less acidic). When ventilation decreases, CO_2 levels rise, less acid is removed and blood pH falls (more acidic).

Metabolic regulation of acid-base occurs in the kidney where bicarbonate is conserved while acids (H^+) are secreted into the urine. Metabolic-mediated changes in acid-base tend to occur more slowly than respiratory, taking several hours to days rather than minutes. So it is the balance between the respiratory and metabolic regulators that maintains the acid-base status within normal limits. We analyze arterial blood to determine if an acid-base disturbance is present and which system, either respiratory, metabolic or both is responsible for the problem. Arterial blood gases should never be interpreted by themselves. You must always interpret them in light of the patient's history and clinical presentation.

Terms used in connection with ABG's
- Acid-base balance: A homeostatic mechanism in the human body that strives to maintain the optimal pH, so that body process may function optimally (normal pH of arterial blood = 7.35–7.45).
- Buffer system: Combination of body systems that work to keep optimal acid-base balance.
- Partial pressure: The amount of pressure exerted by each gas in a mixture of gases.
- PO_2—partial pressure of oxygen.
- PCO_2—partial pressure of carbon dioxide.
- PAO_2—partial pressure of alveolar oxygen.
- PaO_2—partial pressure of arterial oxygen.

- $PACO_2$—partial pressure of alveolar carbon dioxide
- $PaCO_2$—partial pressure of arterial carbon dioxide
- PvO_2—partial pressure of venous oxygen
- $PvCO_2$—partial pressure of venous carbon dioxide
- P50—oxygen tension at 50% hemoglobin saturation.

Reference Ranges and Interpretation (Table 4.1)

These are typical reference ranges, although various analyzers and laboratories may employ different ranges.

Table 4.1: Reference ranges and interpretation

Analyte	Range	Interpretation
pH	7.35–7.45	The pH or H^+ indicates if a patient is acidemic (pH < 7.35; H^+ > 45) or alkalemic (pH >7.45; H^+ < 35)
H^+	35–45 nmol/L	See above
PO_2	9.3–13.3 kPa or 80–100 mmHg	A low O_2 indicates that the patient is not respiring properly, and is hypoxemic. At a PO_2 of less than 60 mmHg, supplemental oxygen should be administered. At a PO_2 of less than 26 mmHg, the patient is at risk of death and must be oxygenated immediately
PCO_2	4.7–6.0 kPa or 35–45 mmHg	The carbon dioxide and partial pressure (PCO_2) indicate a respiratory problem: for a constant metabolic rate, the PCO_2 is determined entirely by ventilation. A high PCO_2 (respiratory acidosis) indicates underventilation, a low PCO_2 (respiratory alkalosis) hyper- or overventilation. PCO_2 levels can also become abnormal when the respiratory system is working to compensate for a metabolic issue so as to normalize the blood pH
HCO_3^-	22–26 mmol/L	The HCO_3^- ion indicates whether a metabolic problem is present (such as ketoacidosis). A low HCO_3^- indicates metabolic acidosis, a high HCO_3^- indicates metabolic alkalosis. HCO_3^- levels can also become abnormal when the kidneys are working to compensate for a respiratory issue so as to normalize the blood pH
SBC_e	21 to 27 mmol/L	The bicarbonate concentration in the blood at a CO_2 of 5.33 kPa, full oxygen saturation and 37 degrees Celsius
Base excess	– 2 to + 2 mmol/L	The base excess indicates whether the patient is acidotic or alkalotic. A negative base excess indicates that the patient is acidotic. A high positive base excess indicates that the patient is alkalotic
Total CO_2 (tCO_2 (P)c)	25 to 30 mmol/L	$tCO_2 = [HCO_3^-] + \alpha \times pCO_2$, where $\alpha = 0.226$ mM/kPa, HCO_3^- is expressed in molar concentration (M) (mol/L) and PCO_2 is expressed in kPa
Total O_2 (tO_{2e})		This is the sum of oxygen dissolved in plasma and chemically bound to hemoglobin

The main variables of arterial blood gases are:

- pH: A measure of how acidic or alkaline the blood is.
  The normal range is 7.35–7.45.
  - If the pH is <7.35—acidemia
  - When the pH falls below 7.20, the acidemia is severe
  - If the pH is >7.35—alkalemia
  - When the pH is >7.50, the alkalemia is severe.
  So, the pH idea of acid-base abnormality is present and whether it is an acidemia or an alkalemia.
- $PaCO_2$ is the partial pressure of carbon dioxide in the blood. The normal range is 35–45 mmHg. The $PaCO_2$ indicates the adequacy of ventilation at the lungs. An increase in CO_2 due to hypoventilation causes a fall in pH (acidemia), while a fall in CO_2 due to hyperventilation causes a rise in pH (alkalemia).
- PaO_2: The partial pressure of oxygen dissolved in the blood. This value reflects how effectively the lungs are moving oxygen into the blood. The normal range of PaO_2 is 80–100 mmHg depending on the age of the patient.
- HCO_3^- is the actual bicarbonate level in the blood. It only reflects changes in the bicarbonate buffer system, the most important of the blood buffers. The normal is 24 mmol.
  - If the bicarbonate is <24—acidemia
  - If the bicarbonate is >24—alkalemia.
- The base excess or base deficit: Reflects the change in all blood buffering systems. It is the most reliable indicator of the metabolic component of an acid-base disturbance. The normal value range – 5 to + 1.
  - If the BE is > + 1—alkalemia
  - If the BE is < – 5—acidemia
- Percent HbO_2 (SaO_2): Reflects how much oxygen is being transported on hemoglobin. Normal range is 92–95%. Clinically we need to be concerned if a patient cannot maintain a saturation of >90%.

  For example, if you hypoventilate and retain CO_2, the pH will fall producing a respiratory acidemia. If this condition persists for several hours, the kidneys will begin to compensate by retaining HCO_3^- thus raising the pH back towards normal. If the pH is just within normal limits but the $PaCO_2$ or BE is outside normal limits, there is full compensation. Sometimes the pH cannot be returned to normal limits and there is only partial compensation.

Example: If a patient is demonstrating signs and symptoms of respiratory acidosis and the ABG results are something like: pH 7.27 and a $PaCO_2$ of 58 mmHg and the body is compensating for this 'primary' abnormality, the other buffer system (primarily HCO_3) will be changed (e.g. elevated HCO_3^-: 30mEq/L).

The convenience is that the 'other buffer system' change will be in the 'same direction' as the 'primary problem.' In this example, the $PaCO_2$ is elevated and the compensatory system (HCO_3) is above the normal range. Consequently, they are both elevated. This tells that the human body is compensating for the 'primary problem!'

Therefore, you were able to determine that there was an elevated $PaCO_2$ (increase in acid or a respiratory acidosis) and an increased HCO_3^- (increased base or metabolic alkalosis). But you were able to determine respiratory acidosis as the 'primary problem' due to the pH being less than 7.35! This example illustrates a respiratory acidosis with a compensatory metabolic alkalosis.

Determine if the patient is demonstrating an acidotic (remember: pH less than 7.35) or alkalotic (pH greater than 7.45).

- What is the 'primary problem'
- If it is acidotic with a $PaCO_2$ greater than 45 mmHg, it is RESPIRATORY
- If it is acidotic with a HCO_3 less than 22 mEq/L, it is METABOLIC!
- If it is alkalotic with a $PaCO_2$ less than 35 mmHg, it is RESPIRATORY!
- If it is alkalotic with a HCO_3 greater than 26 mEq/L, it is METABOLIC!
- Is the patient compensating?

Are both components (HCO_3 and $PaCO_2$) shifting in the same direction? Up or down, above or below the normal ranges? If this is noted, then the patient's buffering systems are functioning and are trying to bring the acid-base balance back to normal.

ETIOLOGY AND CLINICAL MANIFESTATIONS

Respiratory Acidosis

Findings:
- Excess CO_2 retention
- pH <7.35
- HCO_3^- >28 mEq/L (if compensating)
- $PaCO_2$ >45 mm Hg.

Possible causes:
- CNS depression from drugs, injury, or disease
- Airway obstruction
  - Upper/lower COPD
  - Asthma
  - Other obstructive lung disease
- OSA
- Asphyxia
- Hypoventilation due to pulmonary, cardiac, musculoskeletal, or neuro-muscular disease.

Signs and symptoms:
- Diaphoresis
- Headache
- Tachycardia
- Confusion
- Restlessness
- Apprehension.

Respiratory Alkalosis

Findings:
- Excess CO_2 excretion
- pH >7.45
- HCO_3^- <24 mEq/L (if compensating)
- $PaCO_2$ <35 mmHg.

Possible causes:
- Hyperventilation due to anxiety, pain, or improper ventilator settings
- Respiratory stimulation caused by drugs, disease, hypoxia, fever, or high room temperature
- Gram-negative bacteremia
  - Pregnancy, liver disease, sepsis, hyperthyroidism.

Signs and symptoms:
- Rapid, deep breathing
- Paresthesia
- Light-headedness
- Twitching
- Anxiety
- Fear.

Metabolic Acidosis

Findings:
- HCO_3^- loss (acid retention)
- pH <7.35
- HCO_3^- <24 mEq/L
- $PaCO_2$ >35 mmHg (if compensating).

Possible causes:
- HCO_3^- depletion due to renal disease, diarrhea, or small-bowel fistulas
- Elevated anion gap:
  - Methanol intoxication
  - Uremia
  - Diabetic ketoacidosis, alcoholic ketoacidosis, starvation ketoacidosis
  - Paraldehyde toxicity
  - Isoniazid
  - Lactic acidosis
    - Type A: Tissue ischemia
    - Type B: Altered cellular metabolism
  - Ethanol or ethylene glycol intoxication
  - Salicylate intoxication
- Normal anion gap: will have increase in [Cl⁻]
  - GI loss of HCO_3^-
  - Diarrhea, ileostomy, proximal colostomy, ureteral diversion

  - Renal loss of HCO_3^-
  - Carbonic anhydrase inhibitor (acetazolamide)
  - Renal tubular disease
  - Chronic renal disease
  - Aldosterone inhibitors or absence
  - NaCl infusion, TPN, NH_4^+ administration
- Excessive production of organic acids due to hepatic disease
- Endocrine disorders including diabetes mellitus, hypoxia, shock, and drug intoxication.

Signs and symptoms
- Rapid, deep breathing
- Fatigue
- Fruity breath
- Headache
- Drowsiness
- Lethargy
- Nausea
- Vomiting
- Coma (if severe).

Metabolic Alkalosis

Findings:
- HCO_3^- retention (acid loss)
- pH >7.45
- HCO_3^- >28 mEq/L
- $PaCO_2$ >45 mmHg.

Possible causes:
- Inadequate excretion of acids due to renal disease
- Loss of hydrochloric acid from prolonged vomiting or gastric suctioning
- Loss of potassium due to increased renal excretion (as in diuretic therapy) or steroid overdose
- Excessive alkali ingestion.

Signs and symptoms:
- Slow, shallow breathing
- Confusion
- Hypertonic muscles
- Twitching
- Restlessness
- Apathy
- Irritability

- Tetany
- Coma (if severe)
- Seizures.

Selected Mixed and Complex Acid-base Disturbances (Table 4.2)

Is there appropriate compensation for the primary disturbance? Usually, compensation does not return the pH to normal (7.35–7.45).

If the observed compensation is not the expected compensation, it is likely that more than one acid-base disorder is present.

■ RULES FOR RESPIRATORY ACID-BASE DISORDERS (TABLE 4.3)

Rule 1: The 1 for 10 Rule for Acute Respiratory Acidosis

The (HCO_3) will increase by 1 mmol/L for every 10 mm Hg elevation in pCO_2 above 40 mm Hg.

Expected (HCO_3) = $24 + [(\text{Actual } pCO_2 - 40)/10]$

Comment: The increase in CO_2 shifts the equilibrium between CO_2 and HCO_3 to result in an acute increase in HCO_3. This is a simple physicochemical event and occurs almost immediately.

Example: A patient with an acute respiratory acidosis (pCO_2 60 mm Hg) has an actual (HCO_3) of 31 mmol/L. The expected (HCO_3) for this acute elevation

Table 4.2: Mixed and complex acid-base disturbances

Disorder	Characteristics	Selected situations
Respiratory acidosis with metabolic acidosis	$\downarrow$ in pH $\downarrow$ in HCO_3 $\uparrow$ in $PaCO_2$	• Cardiac arrest • Intoxications • Multi-organ failure
Respiratory alkalosis with metabolic alkalosis	$\uparrow$ in pH $\uparrow$ in HCO_3^- $\downarrow$ in $PaCO_2$	• Cirrhosis with diuretics • Pregnancy with vomiting • Over ventilation of COPD
Respiratory acidosis with metabolic alkalosis	pH in normal range $\uparrow$ in $PaCO_2$, $\uparrow$ in HCO_3^-	• COPD with diuretics, vomiting, NG suction • Severe hypokalemia
Respiratory alkalosis with metabolic acidosis	pH in normal range $\downarrow$ in $PaCO_2$ $\downarrow$ in HCO_3	• Sepsis • Salicylate toxicity • Renal failure with CHF or pneumonia • Advanced liver disease
Metabolic acidosis with metabolic alkalosis	pH in normal range HCO_3^- normal	• Uremia or ketoacidosis with vomiting, NG suction, diuretics, etc.

Table 4.3: Expected compensation

Disorder	Expected compensation	Correction factor
Metabolic acidosis	Expected $pCO_2 = 1.5 \times (HCO_3) + 8$	±2
Acute respiratory acidosis	Expected $(HCO_3) = 24 + [(\text{Actual } pCO_2 - 40)/10]$	±3
Chronic respiratory acidosis (3–5 days)	Expected $(HCO_3) = 24 + 4 [(\text{Actual } pCO_2 - 40)/10]$	
Metabolic alkalosis	Expected $pCO_2 = 0.7 [HCO_3] + 20$	±3
Acute respiratory alkalosis	Expected $(HCO_3) = 24 - 2 [(40 - \text{Actual } pCO_2)/10]$	
Chronic respiratory alkalosis	Expected $(HCO_3) = 24 - 5 [(40 - \text{Actual } pCO_2)/10]$	±2

of pCO_2 is 24 + 2 = 26 mmoi/L. The actual measured value is higher than this indicating that a metabolic alkalosis must also be present.

Rule 2: The 4 for 10 Rule for Chronic Respiratory Acidosis

The (HCO_3) will increase by 4 mmol/L for every 10 mm Hg elevation in pCO_2 above 40 mm Hg.

Expected $(HCO_3) = 24 + 4 [(\text{Actual } pCO_2 - 40)/10]$

Comment: With chronic acidosis, the kidneys respond by retaining HCO_3, that is, renal compensation occurs. This takes a few days to reach its maximal value.

Example: A patient with a chronic respiratory acidosis (pCO_2 60 mm Hg) has an actual (HCO_3) of 31 mmol/L. The expected (HCO_3) for this chronic elevation of pCO_2 is 24 + 8 = 32 mmol/L. The actual measured value is extremely close to this so renal compensation is maximal and there is no evidence indicating a second acid-base disorder.

Rule 3: The 2 for 10 Rule for Acute Respiratory Alkalosis

The (HCO_3) will decrease by 2 mmol/L for every 10 mm Hg decrease in pCO_2 below 40 mm Hg.

Expected $(HCO_3) = 24 - 2 [(40 - \text{Actual } pCO_2)/10]$

Comment: In practice, this acute physicochemical change rarely results in a (HCO_3) of less than about 18 mmol/s. (After all there is a limit to how low pCO_2 can fall as negative values are not possible!) So a (HCO_3) of less than 18 mmol/l indicates a coexisting metabolic acidosis.

Rule 4: The 5 for 10 Rule for a Chronic Respiratory Alkalosis

The (HCO_3) will decrease by 5 mmol/L for every 10 mm Hg decrease in pCO_2 below 40 mm Hg.

Expected $(HCO_3) = 24 - 5 [(40 - \text{Actual } pCO_2)/10]$ (range: ± 2)

Comments:
- It takes 2 to 3 days to reach maximal renal compensation
- The limit of compensation is a (HCO_3) of about 12 to 15 mmol/L.

■ RULES FOR METABOLIC ACID-BASE DISORDERS

Rule 5: The One and a Half plus Eight Rule—for a Metabolic Acidosis

The expected pCO_2 (in mm Hg) is calculated from the following formula:

Expected $pCO_2 = 1.5 \times (HCO_3) + 8$ (range: ± 2)

Comments:
- Maximal compensation may take 12–24 hours to reach
- The limit of compensation is a pCO_2 of about 10 mm Hg
- Hypoxia can increase the amount of peripheral chemoreceptor stimulation.

Example: A patient with a metabolic acidosis [(HCO_3) 14 mmol/L] has an actual pCO_2 of 30 mm Hg. The expected pCO_2 is $(1.5 \times 14 + 8)$ which is 29 mm Hg. This basically matches the actual value of 30 so compensation is maximal and there is no evidence of a respiratory acid-base disorder (provided that sufficient time has passed for the compensation to have reached this maximal value). If the actual pCO_2 was 45 mm Hg and the expected was 29 mm Hg, then this difference (45–29) would indicate the presence of a respiratory acidosis and indicate its magnitude.

Rule 6: The Point Seven plus Twenty Rule—for a Metabolic Alkalosis

The expected pCO_2 (in mm Hg) is calculated from the following formula:

Expected $pCO_2 = 0.7 (HCO_3) + 20$ (range: ± 5)

Comment:
The combination of a low (HCO_3) and a low pCO_2 occurs in metabolic acidosis and in respiratory alkalosis. If only one disorder is present it is usually a simple matter to sort out which is present. The factors to consider are:
- The history usually strongly suggests the disorder which is present
- The net pH change indicates the disorder if only a single primary disorder is present (e.g. acidemia $\geq$ acidosis)
- An elevated anion gap or elevated chloride define the 2 major groups of causes of metabolic acidosis.

■ FURTHER ANALYSIS IN CASES OF METABOLIC ACIDOSIS

Metabolic acidosis:
- Calculate the anion gap:

  Anion gap = $Na^+ - [Cl^- + HCO_3^-]$

  Difference between calculated serum anions and cations.

Based on the principle of electrical neutrality, the serum concentration of cations (positive ions) should equal the serum concentration of anions (negative ions).

However, serum Na^+ ion concentration is higher than the sum of serum Cl^- and HCO_3^- concentration.

$Na^+ = Cl^- + HCO_3^- +$ unmeasured anions (gap).

Normal anion gap: 12 mmol/L (10–14 mmol/L).

- Based on the anion gap and patient history—review potential causes.

Normal Anion Gap (Hyperchloremic) Metabolic Acidosis

The most common causes of normal anion gap acidosis are GI or renal bicarbonate loss and impaired renal acid excretion. Normal anion gap metabolic acidosis is also called hyperchloremic acidosis, because instead of reabsorbing HCO_3^- with Na, the kidney reabsorbs Cl^-. Many GI secretions are rich in bicarbonate (e.g. biliary, pancreatic, and intestinal fluids); loss from diarrhea, tube drainage, or fistulas can cause acidosis. In ureterosigmoidostomy (insertion of ureters into the sigmoid colon after obstruction or cystectomy), the colon secretes and loses bicarbonate in exchange for urinary Cl^- and absorbs urinary ammonium, which dissociates into NH_3^+ and H^+.

Loss of HCO_3^- ions is accompanied by an increase in the serum Cl^- concentration. The anion gap remains normal. Disease processes that can lead to normal anion gap (hyperchloremic) acidosis. Useful mnemonic (DURHAM):

- Diarrhea (HCO_3^- and water is lost).
- Ureteral diversion: Urine from the ureter may be diverted to the sigmoid colon due to disease (uretero-colonic fistula) or after bladder surgery. In such an event, urinary Cl^- is absorbed by the colonic mucosa in exchange for HCO_3^-, thus increases the gastrointestinal loss of HCO_3^-.
- Renal tubular acidosis: Dysfunctional renal tubular cells cause an inappropriate wastage of HCO_3^- and retention of Cl^-.
- Hyperalimentation
- Acetazolamide
- Miscellaneous conditions: They include pancreatic fistula, cholestyramine, and calcium chloride (CaCl) ingestion, all of which can increase the gastrointestinal wastage of HCO_3^-.

Increased Anion Gap Metabolic Acidosis

High anion gap acidosis: The most common causes of a high anion gap metabolic acidosis are ketoacidosis, lactic acidosis, renal failure, and toxic ingestions. Renal failure causes anion gap acidosis by decreased acid excretion and decreased bicarbonate reabsorption. Accumulation of sulfates, phosphates, urate, and hippurate accounts for the high anion gap. Toxins may have acidic metabolites or trigger lactic acidosis.

In increased anion gap metabolic acidosis, the nonvolatile acids are organic or other inorganic acids (e.g. lactic acid, acetoacetic acid, formic acid, sulfuric acid). The anions of these acids are not Cl⁻ ions. The presence of these acid anions, which are not measured, will cause an increase in the anion gap.

Methanol poisoning: Methanol is metabolized by alcohol dehydrogenase in the liver to formic acid.

Uremia: In end-stage renal failure in which glomerular filtration rate falls below 10–20 mL/min, acids from protein metabolism are not excreted and accumulate in blood.

Diabetic ketoacidosis: Incomplete oxidation of fatty acids causes a build up of beta-hydroxybutyric and acetoacetic acids (ketoacids).

Paraldehyde poisoning.

Ischemia: It causes lactic acidosis.

Lactic acidosis: Lactic acid is the end-product of glucose breakdown if pyruvic acid, the end product of anaerobic glycolysis, is not oxidized to CO_2 and H_2O via the tricarboxylic acid cycle. (Causes: hypoxia, ischemia, hypotension and sepsis).

Ethylene glycol poisoning: Ethylene is metabolized by alcohol dehydrogenase to oxalic acid in the liver. Usually there is also a coexisting lactic acidosis.

Buffer Systems

The lungs, kidneys, and the buffer system are the primary considerations in the homeostatic process. The lungs can control certain small amounts of carbon dioxide in the blood.

Carbon dioxide in the blood chemically produces carbonic acid. Thus, in cases where the lungs do not function properly, CO_2 builds up, causing increased carbonic acid. This increase in acid can affect the blood pH, leading to acidosis. The main function of kidneys is retaining or excreting of the bicarbonate ion (HCO_3^-). This is the ion which neutralizes the excess acid in the blood. If both organs are working properly, the natural build-up of acids can be neutralized effectively by the buffer system.

The buffer system in the body is able to work very quickly to maintain proper pH of the blood and body tissues. The prime buffer system is the system of carbonic acid and bicarbonate. Bicarbonate will neutralize the correct numbers of carbonic acid molecules to maintain the correct ratio of 20:1 acid molecules. This 20:1 ratio will preserve the blood pH at the normal range of 7.35 to 7.45. Bicarbonate ions and carbonic acid are constantly being produced and combined in order to keep the optimal pH.

The respiratory system also works to maintain the proper blood pH. When the bicarbonate/carbonic acid buffer system cannot work fast enough to compensate for pH disturbances, the respiratory system has a mechanism for buffering the blood. Hyperventilation and hypoventilation can be used by the body to control the amount of carbonic acid in the blood.

The respiratory center in the brain responds to changing levels of carbonic acid in the blood. When the acid level of blood increases, and is not controlled by the first buffer system, the respiratory system responds.

Hyperventilation causes the body to exhale and "get rid of" CO_2 from the blood, through the lungs. This reduction of CO_2 causes the blood pH to become less acid. Reduce the CO_2 and the acid level of the blood is reduced. This is how the body responds to excess acid in the blood.

The opposite mechanism occurs with hypoventilation. Hypoventilation will cause the retention of CO_2 in the blood. As we discussed earlier, this CO_2 becomes carbonic acid when it remains in the blood and mixes with water. If you retain CO_2, the acid level of the blood will go up. This increased acid could "buffer" any excess base that is present in the blood. If the blood becomes alkaline, then hypoventilation may be another way to neutralize it and get the blood pH back to normal. These respiratory conditions will be discussed in more detail later in this text.

In the lab, pH is measured directly using an electrode placed in the blood sample. The 'p' of pH is actually defined as 'percent Hydrion' or called the negative logarithm of the hydrogen concentration. The concentrations can be expressed as 10^{-7}, for example; this means: 0.0000001. This negative logarithm can also be expressed as the inverse ratio (Cooper, 1987). The more hydrogen ions there are, the lower the pH, or acid. On the other hand, as the hydrogen ion concentration decreases in the blood, the pH increases (alkalinity).

A third buffer system exists that will react if the first two methods fail to correct an abnormal blood pH. This third and powerful buffer system is the kidney. The kidneys will react to sustained and/or high levels of acid and/or alkalinity. The kidney buffer system responds to these dangerous levels, called 'metabolic' conditions. These conditions are metabolic acidosis and alkalosis, and will be discussed later:

$$CO_2 + H_2O \Leftrightarrow H_2CO_3 \Leftrightarrow HCO_3^- + H^+$$

(Normal HCO_3^- is: 24 to 28 mEq/L)

Compensation

We have seen how imbalance in the levels of CO_2 and HCO_3 can disturb the blood pH. However, the body has mechanisms to counteract these imbalances. Compensation is the process of the body's response to these imbalances, and tries to bring the pH back to normal.

If there is hypo- or hyperventilation causing a rise or fall in the CO_2 levels, the pH will also change. The response of the kidneys would be to conserve or excrete bicarbonate, in order to get the pH back to normal.

As an example: a patient is hyperventilating, CO_2 is "blown off" thus causing lowered acid levels, and alkalosis. The kidneys respond by excreting HCO_3^-, to try to restore the normal pH.

The ABG's might be: pH – 7.45; CO_2 – 36: HCO_3^- 22

As you see, the pH is high normal, indicating that the patient is borderline alkalotic. The low normal is trying to compensate. Another ABG will be needed soon to see if the patient has stabilized or if they are now in full blown alkalosis. If it was recognized that the patient was in compensation, the patient would be watched very carefully and probably have frequent ABG determinations to see if they were able to handle the mild hyperventilation which lead to the alkalosis.

As another example, if we are dealing with a serious metabolic problem, the condition can be much more unstable. For example, with renal failure, the kidneys will not be able to excrete even normal amounts of HCO_3^-. This renal failure will cause alkalosis as bicarbonate builds up in the blood. The body's initial response will be hypoventilation, in an effort to build up CO_2 and thus neutralize the bicarbonate with acid.

The ABG's might be: pH–7.45; CO_2– 45; HCO_3^- 25

You can see that the patient is in compensation now, but if the kidneys continue to fail, the situation will become worse, rapidly. Compensation is a delicate situation. The patient can easily go into acidosis or alkalosis with little or no reserve power to fight the situation. Also, compensatory situations can last for only a short time.

When the lungs or the kidneys respond to a pH change, they have limits to what they can do to correct the situation. If the person is already sick, and then they also develop a pH disturbance, they are probably in serious trouble. The lungs and the kidneys will only be able to compensate for a short time, due to low body reserves.

In completing our discussion on compensation, we also have to remember the patient. He/she will need to be treated as soon as possible. Since the body's own defense mechanism will last just a short time, the nurse must look for and accurately report symptoms. The susceptible patient must be identified and observed for life-threatening complications in the acid-base balance. However, do not forget the patient's oxygenation status. Up to this point, we have primarily been concerned with pH of the blood. We should also remember that changes in the acid-base balance may also affect the oxygen content.

In cases of compensation, the patient's respiratory status may be severely compromised. For example, if the patient begins to hypoventilate, it may be due to the primary cause of reduced CO_2 in the blood. However, hypoventilation may still occur in a person who is going into metabolic alkalosis. In that case, the patient may be severely hypoxic and needs to hyperventilate, but the overpowering effect of alkalosis still causes the patient to slow respirations instead of increasing them. Therefore, the patient may show signs of hypoxia (cyanosis, lethargy, etc.), but they may still be unable to breathe on their own due to the pH problem which affects the respiratory center in the brain.

Clinically, the patient looks terrible, and cannot breathe well. In fact, the breathing may become erratic. First, there may be hyperventilation which changes rapidly to hypoventilation, the patient may experience long periods of eupnea, even though they may actually be hypoxic and in alkalosis. This is why nurses must also be aware of the delicate situation the compensation creates.

■ SUMMARY

Arterial blood gas analysis is used to measure the pH and the partial pressures of oxygen and carbon dioxide in arterial blood. The investigation is relatively easy to perform and yields information that can guide the management of acute and chronic illnesses. This information indicates a patient's acid-base balance, the effectiveness of their gas exchange and the state of their ventilatory control. Interpretation of an arterial blood gas result should not be done without considering the clinical findings. The results change as the body compensates for the underlying problem. Factors relating to sampling technique, specimen processing and environment may also influence the results.

■ BIBLIOGRAPHY

1. Aaron SD, Vandemheen KL, Naftel SA, Lewis MJ, Rodger MA. "Topical tetracaine prior to arterial puncture: A randomized, placebo-controlled clinical trial". Respir Med. 2003;97(11):1195-9. doi:10.1016/S0954-6111(03)00226-9. PMID 14635973.
2. Adrogué HJ and Madias NE. Management of life-threatening acid-base disorders—first of two parts. N Engl J Med. 1998;338:26-34.
3. Baillie JK. "Simple, easily memorized "rules of thumb" for the rapid assessment of physiological compensation for acid-base disorders". Thorax. 2008;63(3): 289–90. doi:10.1136/thx.2007.091223. PMID 18308967.
4. Baillie K. "Arterial Blood Gas Interpreter". Apex (Altitude Physiology Expeditions). Retrieved on 2007-07-05. Online arterial blood gas analysis
5. Baillie K, Simpson A. "Altitude oxygen calculator". Apex (Altitude Physiology Expeditions). Retrieved on 2006-08-10. Online interactive oxygen delivery calculator.
6. Fidkowski C And Helstrom J. Diagnosing metabolic acidosis in the critically ill: bridging the anion gap, Stewart and base excess methods. Can J Anesth. 2009;56:247-56.
7. Mahoney JJ, Harvey JA, Wong RL, Van Kessel AL. "Changes in oxygen measurements when whole blood is stored in iced plastic or glass syringes". Clin Chem. 1991;37(7):1244-8. PMID 1823532.
8. Rose BD, Post TW. Clinical physiology of acid-base and electrolyte disorders, 5th ed. New York: McGraw Hill Medical Publishing Division, c2001.

INDICATION FOR VENTILATION

Following are the conditions, which indicate the need for ventilation:
- Hypoxemia
- Hypoxia
- Hypoventilation
- High work of breathing
- Ventilation-perfusion mismatch
- Ventilatory failure
- Other conditions
- Criteria for intubation and ventilation.

Apart from supportive role in patient's undergoing operative procedure, mechanical ventilatory support is indicated in critically ill patients whose spontaneous ventilation is inadequate for the sustenance of life.

Mechanical ventilation is not a cure for the disease for which it is instituted: It is a best form of support, offering time and rest to the patient until the underlying disease processes are resolved.

The indications for the mechanical ventilation may be viewed as falling under several broad categories.

■ HYPOXEMIA

Hypoxemia is reduced oxygen in the blood. The PaO_2 is most often used to evaluate a patient's oxygenation status. Since PaO_2 reflects on the oxygen that is dissolved in the plasma, it does not represent all oxygen carried by the blood (Hb and plasma). For assessment, oxygen content should be used as it includes the oxygen combined with hemoglobin as well as oxygen dissolved in the plasma.

Hypoxemia is different from hypoxia, which is an abnormally low oxygen availability to the body or an individual tissue or organ.

The type of hypoxia that is caused by hypoxemia is referred to as hypoxemic hypoxia. Because of the frequent incorrect use of hypoxemia, this is sometimes erroneously stated as hypoxic hypoxia.

Low inspired oxygen partial pressure (low PiO₂): If the partial pressure of oxygen in the inspired gas is low, then a reduced amount of oxygen is delivered to the gas exchanging parts (alveoli) of the lung each minute. The reduced oxygen partial pressure can be a result of reduced fractional oxygen content (low FiO_2) or simply a result of low barometric pressure, as can occur at high altitudes. This reduced PiO_2 can result in hypoxemia even if the lungs are normal. Additionally, it is the inspired oxygen content that is important in this case rather than the atmospheric concentration as the person may not be breathing atmospheric gas (e.g. during an anesthetic). NOTE: People will often simplify this concept and state low FiO_2 as one of the 6 principal causes of hypoxemia, but this fails to account for important circumstances such as high altitude induced hypoxemia, where indeed FiO_2 is normal.

Alveolar Hypoventilation

If the alveolar ventilation is low, there may be insufficient oxygen delivered to the alveoli each minute. This can cause hypoxemia even if the lungs are normal, as the cause may be outside the lungs (e.g. airway obstruction, depression of the brain's respiratory center, or muscular weakness).

Definition of the partial pressure (P) of a gas: P = Fraction of the molecules in the air of that gas multiplied by atmospheric pressure.

Example: 21% of the air we breathe is oxygen. The atmospheric pressure here in Boston is about 760 mm Hg. Therefore $PO_2 = 0.21 \times 760 = 160$ mm Hg.

Some other definitions:
- Hypercarbia refers to an elevated $PaCO_2$
- Hypoxemia refers to a decrease in PaO_2.

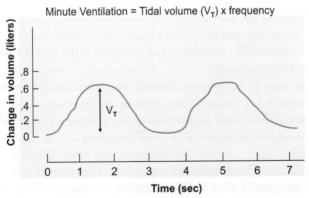

Minute Ventilation = Tidal volume (V_T) x frequency

Breathing frequency: 1 breath/ 4 sec= 15 breaths/min
V_T = 0.6 liters

Fig. 5.1: Volume vs time

Causes of Hypercarbia

The primary determinant of $PaCO_2$ is $PaCO_2$ (alveolar partial pressure for CO_2). The primary determinant of $PaCO_2$ is **alveolar ventilation**. To understand **alveolar ventilation**, we first have to understand **minute ventilation.**

Definition of ventilation: Movement of air between the atmosphere and the lungs. How much air we breathe each minute is called the Minute Ventilation (V_E). It's the product of the size of a breath (tidal volume, V_T) and the number of breaths we breathe per minute (frequency, f) (Fig. 5.1).

Minute ventilation (V_E): $= V_T \times f$.

V_T: Tidal volume (size of a breath).

f: frequency (number of breaths/min).

Important concept: Not all the air that we breathe is useful.

Dead space (V_D): Amount of air that goes into the lungs with each breath but does not reach the gas exchange region of the lung. There are several kinds of dead space:

- **Anatomic dead space:** The volume of all the airways that are not involved in gas exchange
- **Physiologic dead space:** The volume of any air spaces that do not receive a blood supply (e.g. pulmonary embolism) plus the anatomic dead space.
- **Equipment dead space:** The volume of any equipment between the subject and the atmosphere (snorkel, tubes from a ventilator, mask used in certain occupational settings). Air has to fill up this space before reaching the lungs.

Alveolar ventilation (V_A): Amount of fresh air that reaches the gas exchange region of the lung per minute. The alveolar ventilation and not the minute ventilation is what matters in terms of how much CO_2 you can get rid of and how much O_2 you can take up.

$V_A = (V_T - V_D) \times f_1$. In the Figure 5.2A, the gray area represents air that contains CO_2. The CO_2 is made in the tissues, is transported through the blood, and diffuses across the alveolar wall. As you breathe out, this CO_2-containing gas fills all the airways, so at the end of a breath, the airways and all the airspaces of the lung are full of CO_2-containing gas. Note that at the end of a breath, there is still lots of air in the lungs.

- Now you start to breathe-in. The air you breathe-in comes from the atmosphere and contains no CO_2 (represented by white area in the Figures 5.2B and C). This 'fresh' air, first has to fill up in the airways before it gets to the gas exchange region of the lung, the alveoli.
- At the end of taking a breath-in (end inspiration below), the airways are full of fresh air and the gas exchange region of the lung has received a volume of 'fresh' air equal to the size of the breath (tidal volume) minus the amount of air in the airways (the dead space).
- Now, when you breathe-out, the first air that comes out is the fresh air that was still in the airways. So this air never got to the gas exchange region of

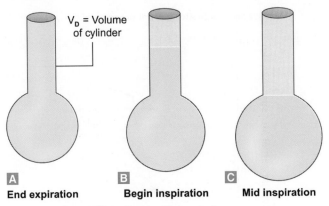

V_D = Volume of cylinder

A	B	C
End expiration	**Begin inspiration**	**Mid inspiration**

Figs 5.2A to C: Alveoli: Inspiration process

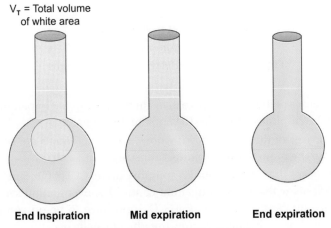

V_T = Total volume of white area

End Inspiration	**Mid expiration**	**End expiration**

Fig. 5.3: Alveoli: Expiration process

the lung and is effectively useless as far as getting O_2 into your blood is concerned (Fig. 5.3).

Relationship between Alveolar Ventilation and Alveolar Partial Pressure for CO_2 (Fig. 5.4)

$$PaCO_2 = VCO_2/V_A \times K$$

- $PaCO_2$ is the partial pressure for CO_2 in the alveolar space
- VCO_2 is the rate of CO_2 production by the body
- K is a constant.

NOTE: $PaCO_2$ is equal to $PaCO_2$. That's why we care about $PaCO_2$.
Because $PaCO_2$ is equal to $PaCO_2$, the primary determinant of hypercarbia is hypoventilation.
- Examples of things that can cause hypoventilation
  - Drugs (i.e. morphine) that suppress respiratory drive

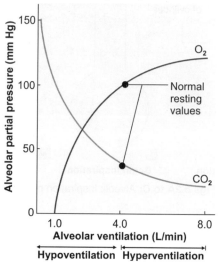

Fig. 5.4: Alveolar ventilation vs partial pressures

- Diseases of the muscles (like myasthenia gravis) that impair the ability of the respiratory muscles to ventilate the lungs
- Diseases of the nerves down whose action potentials are conducted from the brain to the respiratory muscles
- Diseases that affect central respiratory drive: CCHS (Ondine's curse). Patients with CCHS (congenital central hypoventilation syndrome), have no central sensitivity to CO_2, and have to be on ventilator at night, but during the day time, breathe normally because they control ventilation consciously.

You need to review the control of breathing to understand how the brain normally adjusts ventilation to keep $PaCO_2$ constant. See general respiratory physiology notes.

Note: you can have a minute ventilation that is very high and still be hypoventilating if the dead space is very high. Remember that for a given minute ventilation, the higher the dead space, the lower the alveolar ventilation. It is minute ventilation, not alveolar ventilation that determines $PaCO_2$ and therefore, $PaCO_2$.

Examples of Factors that Affect Dead Space

- **Breathing through a tube** (a snorkel, a mask, a tube that connects your lungs to a ventilator).
- **Pulmonary embolus:** Something that is lodged in one of the arterioles feeding the lung (examples: a clot that has been dislodged from somewhere else in the circulation; an air bubble).

Example: Deep vein thrombosis (DVT). Sitting upright and still for long periods of time (an airplane ride) causes blood to pool in the lower extremities. When blood pools and does not move much, it has a tendency to clot. The clot can become dislodged and get released into the circulation. Since these form in veins, the diameter of the vessels that the clot encounters will be increasing progressively through the smaller veins to larger veins, the vena cave and finally the right heart. But once it reaches the right heart, the clot moves into the pulmonary artery and then to pulmonary arterioles and the size of these vessels will start getting smaller and smaller. The clot will get stuck when it reaches a vessel whose diameter is the same size as the clot. Clots can also form and get released into the circulation sometimes after surgeries.

Risk factors for DVT:

– Hip or leg fractures
– Standing or sitting still for long periods of time, such as on a long plane trip or car ride. Contraction of the muscles in your legs typically helps return blood from your legs back to your heart. Otherwise blood tends to pool in the lower extremities by gravity. Blood pooling (remaining stagnant/not moving) makes it more likely to clot. Get up and walk or flex your legs frequently on long plane rides or car trips. Drink plenty of fluids: dehydration increases the risk of clotting.
– Obesity
– Smoking
– Pregnancy, taking birth control pills, or taking estrogen replacement therapy.

• **Other lung diseases:** Any disease that alters the distribution of blood flow and ventilation to different parts of the lungs can result in an effective increase in dead space (i.e. the disease affects the lung in such a way that a certain part of the lung now gets more of the tidal volume, even though it does not get more of the blood flow).

Causes of Hypoxemia

There are four primary causes of hypoxemia (low PaO_2):

• **Hypoventilation:** The definition of hypoventilation is a ventilation which results in increased $PaCO_2$ >40 mm Hg. Decreased ventilation also decreases alveolar PO_2 as follows (see brownish line in graph immediately below for a graphical representation of this relationship).

$$PaO_2 = PiO_2 - (K.VO_2/V_A)$$

– PaO_2 is the partial pressure for O_2 in the alveolar space
– PiO_2 is the partial pressure for O_2 in the inhaled air
– VO_2 is the oxygen consumption
– K is a constant
– Blood circulating through the pulmonary capillaries comes into equilibrium with air in alveoli. When alveolar PO_2 (PaO_2) is reduced,

the PO_2 of the blood leaving these capillaries and draining into the left heart is also reduced.

- Examples of things that can cause hypoventilation (same as above)
    - Drugs (i.e. morphine) that suppress respiratory drive
    - Diseases of the muscles (like myasthenia gravis) that impair the ability of the respiratory muscles to ventilate the lungs
    - Diseases of the nerves down whose action potentials are conducted from the brain to the respiratory muscles
    - Diseases that affect central respiratory drive: CCHS (Ondine's curse). Patients with CCHS (congenital central hypoventilation syndrome), have no central sensitivity to CO_2, and have to be on ventilators at night, but during the day time, breathe normally because they control ventilation consciously.

Special case: Ventilation is normal, but the PO_2 of the inspired gas is lower than normal.

Example: Breathing at altitude (See general respiratory notes)

- **Diffusion impairment:** The rate of diffusion of O_2 across the respiratory epithelium is dependent on:
    - The surface area of the lung
    - The thickness of the pulmonary epithelial/capillary endothelial barrier
    - The difference in PO_2 between the alveolar gas and the capillary blood.

Examples of diseases in which there is an increase in the time It takes for O_2 to diffuse from the alveoli into red blood cells:

- Pulmonary fibrosis: Scarring of the lung and thickening of the alveolar walls.
- Emphysema: Destruction of alveolar walls results in a decrease in the total surface area of the lung.

NOTE: There is a very large gas exchange reserve in the lung. Consequently, diffusion impairment is practically never the primary cause of hypoxemia, even in disease.

Exception: Exercise in patients with severe fibrosis. During exercise, the amount of time that red blood cells spend in the pulmonary capillaries decreases, so not only does diffusion take more time in severe fibrosis, but there is less time available.

- **Shunt:** This is a situation in which blood passes from the right heart to the left heart without being oxygenated. This can occur:
    - Because the blood goes directly from the right to the left heart without passing through the lungs.
        - The bronchial arteries are one form of a small shunt found in normal subjects.
        - In fetuses, the ductus arteriosus is another form of a normal shunt.
    - The blood does go through the lungs, but it never comes into contact with alveolar gas.

- A foreign object is lodged in an airway. All of the lung tissue subtended by that airway receives no air if the air cannot get past the obstruction. The pO_2 in the airspaces beyond the obstruction becomes the same as venous pO_2.
- Pneumonia: Alveolar airspaces become filled with pus and fluid instead of air.

■ OXYHEMOGLOBIN DISSOCIATION CURVE
Understanding the Dissociation Curve

In its basic form, the oxyhemoglobin dissociation curve describes the relation between the partial pressure of oxygen (x-axis) and the oxygen saturation (y-axis) (Fig. 5.5). Hemoglobin's affinity for oxygen increases as successive molecules of oxygen bind. More molecules bind as the oxygen partial pressure increases until the maximum amount that can be bound is reached. As this limit is approached, very little additional binding occurs and the curve levels out as the hemoglobin becomes saturated with oxygen. Hence the curve has a sigmoidal or S-shape. At pressures above about 60 mm Hg, the standard dissociation curve is relatively flat, which means that the oxygen content of the blood does not change significantly even with large increases in the oxygen partial pressure. To get more oxygen to the tissue would require blood transfusions to increase the hemoglobin count (and hence the oxygen carrying capacity), or supplemental oxygen that would increase the oxygen dissolved in plasma.

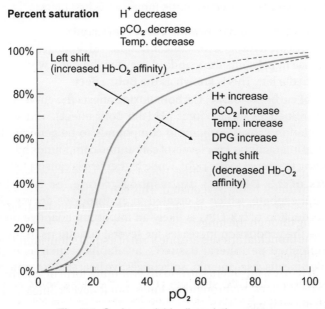

Fig. 5.5: Oxyhemoglobin dissociation curve

Although binding of oxygen to hemoglobin continues to some extent for pressures below about 60 mm Hg, as oxygen partial pressures decrease in this steep area of the curve, the oxygen is unloaded to peripheral tissue readily as the hemoglobin's affinity diminishes.

The partial pressure of oxygen in the blood at which the hemoglobin is 50% saturated, typically about 26.6 mm Hg for a healthy person, is known as the P_{50}. The P_{50} is a conventional measure of hemoglobin affinity for oxygen. In the presence of disease or other conditions that change the hemoglobin's oxygen affinity and, consequently, shift the curve to the right or left, the P_{50} changes accordingly. An increased P_{50} indicates a rightward shift of the standard curve, which means that a larger partial pressure is necessary to maintain a 50% oxygen saturation. This indicates a decreased affinity. Conversely, a lower P_{50} indicates a leftward shift and a higher affinity.

- A left shift will increase oxygen's affinity for hemoglobin.
  - In a left shift condition (alkalosis, hypothermia, etc.), oxygen will have a higher affinity for hemoglobin.
  - SaO_2 will increase at a given PaO_2, but more of it will stay on the hemoglobin and ride back through the lungs without being used. This can result in tissue hypoxia even when there is sufficient oxygen in the blood.
- A right shift decreases oxygen's affinity for hemoglobin.
  - In a right shift (acidosis, fever, etc.), oxygen has a lower affinity for hemoglobin. Blood will release oxygen more readily.
  - This means more O_2 will be released to the cells, but it also means less oxygen will be carried from the lungs in the first place.

List of factors that indicate how the curve is affected:
- Variation of the hydrogen ion concentration. This changes the blood's pH. A decrease in pH shifts the standard curve to the right, while an increase shifts it to the left. This is known as the **Bohr effect**.
- **Effects of carbon dioxide.** Carbon dioxide affects the curve in two ways: first, it influences intracellular pH (the Bohr effect), and second, CO_2 accumulation causes carbamino compounds to be generated through chemical interactions. Low levels of carbamino compounds have the effect of shifting the curve to the right, while higher levels cause a leftward shift.
- **Effects of 2,3-DPG:** 2,3-diphosphoglycerate, or 2,3-DPG, is an organophosphate, which is created in erythrocytes during glycolysis. The production of 2,3-DPG is likely an important adaptive mechanism, because the production increases for several conditions in the presence of diminished peripheral tissue O_2 availability, such as hypoxemia, chronic lung disease, anemia, and congestive heart failure, among others. High levels of 2,3-DPG shift the curve to the right, while low levels of 2,3-DPG cause a leftward shift, seen in states such as septic shock and hypophosphatemia.

- **Temperature:** Temperature does not have so dramatic effect as the previous factors, but hyperthermia causes a rightward shift, while hypothermia causes a leftward shift.
- **Carbon monoxide:** Hemoglobin binds with carbon monoxide 240 times more readily than with oxygen, and therefore the presence of carbon monoxide can interfere with the hemoglobin's acquisition of oxygen. In addition to lowering the potential for hemoglobin to bind to oxygen, carbon monoxide also has the effect of shifting the curve to the left. With an increased level of carbon monoxide, a person can suffer from severe hypoxemia while maintaining a normal PO_2.
- **Effects of methemoglobinemia** (a form of abnormal hemoglobin). Methemoglobinemia causes a leftward shift in the curve.
- **Fetal hemoglobin:** Fetal hemoglobin (HbF) is structurally different from normal hemoglobin (Hb). The fetal dissociation curve is shifted to the left relative to the curve for the normal adult. Typically, fetal arterial oxygen pressures are low, and hence the leftward shift enhances the placental uptake of oxygen.

Shunt can have a big effect on PaO_2!

Effect of increasing ventilation on PaO_2 in someone with a shunt: An increase in ventilation will increase PaO_2 in the 'good' parts of the lung but will do nothing to the 'bad' parts of the lung, since none of the ventilation goes there. Since the good parts of the lung have hemoglobin that is already fully saturated, increasing PaO_2 in those regions will not increase the O_2 content of the blood coming from the areas and therefore will have no effect of the PaO_2 of the arterial blood, which is a mixture of the blood from the good and bad parts of the lung.

Effect of increasing the O_2 concentration of the gas that a patient with a shunt is breathing: The blood going through the 'bad' lung still returns to the systemic arterial blood as it was, i.e. with 150 mL O_2/L because it never sees the gas with higher concentration of O_2 because it is not being ventilated. The well ventilated parts of the lung will have a higher PaO_2. Thus blood returning from those regions will have a higher PaO_2, but that blood was already fully saturated, so the O_2 content will still be about 200 mL O_2/L. Thus, the mixed arterial blood will have the same O_2 content and the same PaO_2.

Note: This is not precisely true since there will be slightly more O_2 dissolved in the blood from the good parts of the lung when the PaO_2 in those regions is higher, but dissolved O_2 represents such a small fraction of overall blood O_2 (See general respiratory physiology notes) that this will have very little effect on PaO_2.

- V/Q abnormalities: Most common cause of hypoxemia in patients with lung disease.
- Upper parts of the lung receive less blood supply than the lower parts (gravity).

- Upper parts of the lung also receive less of the tidal volume (because they are already more inflated and so are on a steeper part of their PV curve, so less compliant).
- The difference is greater for blood flow than for ventilation.
- The result is that the upper parts of the lung receive relatively more ventilation than they do blood flow, while the lower parts of the lung receive relatively less ventilation than they do blood flow.
- Upper parts of the lung have greater PaO_2 and lower $PaCO_2$ than average.
- Lower parts of the lung have lower PaO_2 and greater $PaCO_2$ than average.
- The net effect is a PaO_2 that is lower than it would be if there were uniform ventilation and perfusion to all parts of the lung.

Normal subjects: PaO_2 is slightly less than average PaO_2 as a result of this, but the difference is not very big (may be 3 mm Hg).

Lung disease: Because of inhomogeneities in the distribution of disease, not all units of the lung are similarly affected by the disease. Blood flow and ventilation can be distributed very unevenly resulting in big decreases in PaO_2.

Hypoxia: Hypoxia is reduced oxygen in the body organs and tissues. It is important to understand that hypoxia can occur with a normal PaO_2 (Table 5.1). For example, cyanide poisoning causes aerobic metabolism. The important signs of hypoxia include hypoxemia, dyspnea, tachypnea, tachycardia and cyanosis.

Symptoms of generalized hypoxia depend on its severity and acceleration of onset. In the case of altitude sickness, where hypoxia develops gradually, the symptoms include headaches, fatigue, shortness of breath, a feeling of euphoria and nausea. In severe hypoxia, or hypoxia of very rapid onset, changes in levels of consciousness, seizures, coma, and death occur. Severe hypoxia induces a blue discoloration of the skin, called cyanosis. Because hemoglobin is a darker red when it is not bound to oxygen (deoxyhemoglobin), as opposed to the rich red color that it has when bound to oxygen (oxyhemoglobin), when seen through the skin it has an increased tendency to reflect blue light back to the eye. In cases where the oxygen is displaced by another molecule, such as carbon monoxide, the skin may appear 'cherry red' instead of cyanotic.

Hypoxic hypoxia results from a deficiency of O_2 (or reduced partial pressure) in the air being inspired. Histotoxic hypoxia is caused by poisons that disrupt the cytochrome oxidase system which impedes the utilization of

Table 5.1: Interpretation of oxygenation status using PaO_2

Hypoxemia status	PaO_2
Normal	80–100 mm Hg
Mild	60–79 mm Hg
Moderate	40–59 mm Hg
Severe	Less than 40 mm Hg

O_2 at the cellular level. The classic example is cyanide poisoning. Exposure to cyanide could occur inflight if there were a fire; it could also occur in the aerospace maintenance work place.

Hypemic hypoxia occurs when the capacity of the blood to transport O_2 is reduced. For example, CO has an affinity for Hb over 200 times that of O_2. Consequently, if an individual is exposed to CO, it will displace O_2 on the Hb molecule thereby reducing the amount of O_2 delivered to the tissues even if the Hb and RBC levels are normal.

Stagnant hypoxia occurs if blood circulation is inadequate. This can be caused by illness such as congestive heart failure, but it can also be caused by accelerative forces inflight (+Gz) and by positive pressure breathing (PPB). In the former, positive G loads will force blood to the legs and decrease venous return. Likewise, PPB will inhibit venous return by increasing intrathoracic pressure. In both cases, cardiac output will be reduced, thereby decreasing the transportation of oxyhemoglobin.

Because the physiological effects of hypoxia were described in a previous section, we will now turn to its signs and symptoms. As shown in Table 5.2, the signs and symptoms of hypoxic hypoxia are extremely varied. Furthermore, there is significant interindividual variability. In any event, with increasing altitude and an increasingly deficient amount of ambient O_2, the more severe are the effects of hypoxia. However, even hypoxia with mild signs and symptoms is unwelcome in any cockpit because it can cause performance decrement.

Hypoventilation: A major indication for mechanical ventilation is where the alveolar ventilation falls short of the patient's requirements and condition that depress the respiratory center which produce a decline in alveolar ventilation with a rise in arterial CO_2 tension. A rising $PaCO_2$ can also result from the hypoventilation that results when fatiguing respiratory muscles are unable to sustain ventilation, such as in a patient who is expending considerable effort in moving air into stiff or obstructed lungs. Under such problems, mechanical ventilation may be used to support gas exchange until the patient's respiratory drive has been restored and the inciting pathology significantly resolved.

Table 5.2: Signs and symptoms of hypoxic hypoxia

Signs	Symptoms
Hyperventilation	Headache
Cyanosis	Dizziness
Intellectual impairment	Fatigue
Poor judgment	Reduced visual field
Behavioral changes	Decreased night vision
Delayed reaction time	Drowsiness
Unconsciousness	Paresthesias
	Tingling

High work of breathing: The assisted ventilation is used in those situations in which excessive work of breathing results in hemodynamic compromise. Even though gas exchange may not be impaired, the increased work of breathing by reason of either high airway resistance or poor lung compliance may impose a substantial burden, for example, a compromised myocardium.

When oxygen delivery to the tissue is compromised on account of impaired myocardium function, mechanical ventilation by resting the respiratory muscle, can reduce the work of breathing. This reduces the oxygen consumption of the respiratory muscle, and results in better perfusion of the myocardium itself.

Ventilation-perfusion mismatch (V/Q): It is when certain groups of alveoli experience a decrease in ventilation which causes a higher concentration of carbon dioxide (CO_2) and a lower concentration of oxygen (O_2). The inequality refers to the fact that perfusion has remained constant, the amount of blood flowing to and from the healthy alveoli and unhealthy alveoli is still the same. The body's natural reaction to this is to constrict the pulmonary arterioles that lead to the unhealthy alveoli; by doing this, the body increases the amount of blood travelling to healthy alveoli. This is generally caused by hypoxic conditions or asthma.

The ventilation-perfusion ratio is the ratio between the amount of air getting to the alveoli (the alveolar ventilation, V, in mL/min) and the amount of blood being sent to the lungs (the cardiac output or Q—also in mL/min).

V/Q = Alveolar ventilation/Cardiac output.

- 'Normal' V/Q = 0.8
    - V = Alveolar ventilation
    - Q = Pulmonary blood flow (perfusion).
- 'Normal' V/Q depends on 'normal' respiratory rate, tidal volume, and cardiac output
    - PaO_2 = 100 mm Hg
    - $PaCO_2$ = 40 mm Hg.
- Ventilation/perfusion matching is essential for ideal gas exchange of O_2 and CO_2

$$V/Q = (4\ L/min)/(5\ L/min)$$
$$V/Q = 0.8$$

As we know the V/Q ratio is the balance between the ventilation (bringing oxygen into/removing CO_2 from the alveoli) and the perfusion (removing O_2 from the alveoli and adding CO_2). The V/Q ratio is important because the ratio between the ventilation and the perfusion is one of the major factors affecting the alveolar (and therefore arterial) levels of oxygen and carbon dioxide.

There are two ways to change the V/Q ratio:

The first way is to **decrease the V/Q ratio:** A decrease in the V/Q ratio is produced by either decreasing ventilation or increasing blood flow (without altering the other variable). These will both have the same effect—the alveolar (and therefore arterial) levels of oxygen will decrease and the CO_2 will increase. The reason for each of these changes is simple:

- A decrease in ventilation (without a compensatory change in perfusion) means not bringing in enough oxygen to meet our metabolic need for oxygen (the oxygen consumption) as well as not blowing enough CO_2 to get rid of the CO_2 produced. It is easy to figure out why the alveolar and arterial blood gases change the way they do with a decrease in ventilation.
- An increase in perfusion will have the same effect on the blood gases because an increase in perfusion (without a compensatory change in ventilation) means more blood cells are coming to remove oxygen from the alveolus as they deliver more CO_2 than will be exhaled.

Decrease in the V/Q ratio means:
- Ventilation is not keeping pace with perfusion.
- The alveolar oxygen levels will decrease, which will lead to a decrease in arterial oxygen levels (PaO_2).
- The alveolar CO_2 levels will increase (we are not getting rid of it as fast), also leading to an increase in arterial CO_2.

We can also increase the ventilation-perfusion ratio. Increasing the V/Q ratio does exactly the opposite of a decrease.

To produce an increase in the ventilation-perfusion ratio:
- Increase ventilation (bring in more oxygen to the alveoli, blow off more CO_2 from the lungs).
- Decrease the perfusion (so the blood takes away less oxygen, delivers less CO_2).
- This will lead to an increase in the PaO_2 (and therefore PaO_2) and a decrease in $PaCO_2$ and $PaCO_2$.

An increase in the V/Q ratio means that ventilation is in excess of the metabolic needs being met by perfusion, so we blow off CO_2 (lower $PaCO_2$) and increase our PaO_2 (and PaO_2).

V/Q Defects

- Dead space
  - For example, pulmonary embolism (blood flow obstruction)
  - Ventilation of lung regions that are not perfused
    - Wasted ventilation
    - Physiologic dead space
    - No gas exchange occurs
    - PaO_2 has same composition as humidified, inspired air (= 150 mm Hg)
    - $PaCO_2 = 0$ mm Hg
  - 100% O_2 improves PaO_2
- Shunt (V/Q = 0)
  - For example, airway obstruction

- – Dependent portion of lung in ARDS can act as 'shunt'
- – Perfusion of lung regions that are not ventilated
  - - Wasted perfusion
  - - No gas exchange
  - - Pulmonary capillary blood has same composition as venous blood
- • 100% O_2 does not improve PaO_2.

Ventilatory failure: It is a rise in $PaCO_2$ (hypercapnia) that occurs when the respiratory load can no longer be supported by the strength or activity of the system. The most common causes are acute exacerbations of asthma and COPD, overdoses of drugs that suppress ventilatory drive, and conditions that cause respiratory muscle weakness (e.g. Guillain-Barré syndrome, myasthenia gravis, botulism). Findings include dyspnea, tachypnea, and confusion. Diagnosis is by ABGs and patient observation; chest X-ray and clinical evaluation may help delineate cause. Treatment varies by condition but often includes mechanical ventilation.

Pathophysiology

Hypercapnia occurs when alveolar ventilation either falls or fails to rise adequately in response to increased CO_2 production. A fall in alveolar ventilation is the result of a decrease in minute ventilation or an increase in dead space ventilation.

Other conditions: In addition to these indications, mechanical ventilation may be valve in certain specific conditions. The vasoconstriction produced by deliberate hyperventilation can reduce the volume of the cerebral vascular compartment, helping to reduce raised intracranial pressures. In flail chest, mechanical ventilation can be used to provide internal stabilization of the thorax when multiple rib fractures compromise the integrity of the chest wall. In such cases, mechanical ventilation using PEEP normalizes thoracic and lung mechanics so that adequate gas exchange becomes possible. Where neuromuscular disease or postoperative pain limits lung expansion, mechanical ventilation can be used to preserve a functional residual capacity within the lungs and prevent atelectasis.

Criteria for intubation and ventilation: The need of intubation and ventilation of a patient in respiratory failure have met general acceptance, these are based upon the assessment of a patient's condition.

The respiratory rate in excess of 32 breaths per minute would mean an unacceptably high work of breathing and a substantial degree of respiratory distress and is recognized as one of the criteria for intubation and ventilation. A $PaCO_2$ in excess of 55 mm Hg (especially if rising and in the presence of acidemia) can cause respiratory muscle fatigue. Except in habitual CO_2 retainers, a $PaCO_2$ of 55 mm Hg and over would normally reflect severe respiratory muscle dysfunction.

Indications for intubation:
- Need of secure airway
- Imperfect airway reflexes
- Depressed sensorium
- Decreased airway patency
- Upper airway instability after trauma
- Need for sedation in a situation of poor airway control (imaging CT, MRI, transportation of the patient).

Indications for ventilation:
- Hypoxemia
- Hypoxia
- Hypoventilation
- Unacceptably high work of breathing
- Hemodynamic compromise
- Cardiorespiratory failure
- Refractory shock
- Raised intracranial pressure
- Flail chest.

■ RESPIRATORY FAILURE

Respiratory failure exists whenever the exchange of O_2 for CO_2 in the lungs cannot keep up with the rate of O_2 consumption and CO_2 production in the cells of the body. This results in a fall in arterial O_2 tension (hypoxemia) and a rise in arterial CO_2 tension (hypercapnia).

Respiratory failure is considered acute if the lungs are unable to maintain adequate oxygenation in a previously healthy person, with or without an impairment of carbon dioxide elimination and the lung usually returns to its normal original states; but in chronic respiratory failure, the structure damage is irreversible.

- The cause of respiratory failure often is evident after a careful history and physical examination.
  - Cardiogenic pulmonary edema usually develops in the context of a history of left ventricular dysfunction or valvular heart disease.
  - A history of previous cardiac disease, recent symptoms of chest pain, paroxysmal nocturnal dyspnea, and orthopnea suggest cardiogenic pulmonary edema.
  - Noncardiogenic edema [e.g. acute respiratory distress syndrome (ARDS)] occurs in typical clinical contexts such as sepsis, trauma, aspiration, pneumonia, pancreatitis, drug toxicity and multiple transfusions.

Physical: The signs and symptoms of acute respiratory failure reflect the underlying disease process and the associated hypoxemia or hypercapnia.

Localized pulmonary findings reflecting the acute cause of hypoxemia, such as pneumonia, pulmonary edema, asthma, or COPD, may be readily apparent. In patients with ARDS, the manifestations may be remote from the thorax, such as abdominal pain or long-bone fracture. Neurological manifestations include restlessness, anxiety, confusion, seizures, or coma.

- Asterixis may be observed with severe hypercapnia. Tachycardia and a variety of arrhythmias may result from hypoxemia and acidosis.
- Once respiratory failure is suspected on clinical grounds, arterial blood gas analysis should be performed to confirm the diagnosis and to assist in the distinction between acute and chronic forms. This helps assess the severity of respiratory failure and also helps guide management.
- Cyanosis, a bluish color of skin and mucous membranes, indicates hypoxemia. Visible cyanosis typically is present when the concentration of deoxygenated hemoglobin in the capillaries or tissues is at least 5 g/dL.
- Dyspnea, an uncomfortable sensation of breathing, often accompanies respiratory failure. Excessive respiratory effort, vagal receptors, and chemical stimuli (hypoxemia and/or hypercapnia) all may contribute to the sensation of dyspnea.
- Both confusion and somnolence may occur in respiratory failure. Myoclonus and seizures may occur with severe hypoxemia. Polycythemia is a complication of long-standing hypoxemia.
- Pulmonary hypertension frequently is present in chronic respiratory failure. Alveolar hypoxemia potentiated by hypercapnia causes pulmonary arteriolar constriction. If chronic, this is accompanied by hypertrophy and hyperplasia of the affected smooth muscles and narrowing of the pulmonary arterial bed. The increased pulmonary vascular resistance increases afterload of the right ventricle, which may induce right ventricular failure. This, in turn, causes enlargement of the liver and peripheral edema. The entire sequence is known as cor pulmonale.
- Criteria for the diagnosis of acute respiratory distress syndrome
    - Clinical presentation: Tachypnea and dyspnea; crackles upon auscultation.
    - Clinical setting: Direct insult (aspiration) or systemic process causing lung injury (sepsis).
    - Radiologic appearance: Three-quadrant or 4-quadrant alveolar flooding.
    - Lung mechanics: Diminished compliance (<40 mL/cm water).
    - Gas exchange: Severe hypoxia refractory to oxygen therapy (PaO_2/FiO_2 <200).
    - Normal pulmonary vascular properties: Pulmonary capillary wedge pressure <18 mm Hg.

Causes: These diseases can be grouped according to the primary abnormality and the individual components of the respiratory system, as follows:
- Central nervous system disorders

- – A variety of pharmacological, structural, and metabolic disorders of the CNS are characterized by depression of the neural drive to breathe.
  - – This may lead to acute or chronic hypoventilation and hypercapnia.
  - – Examples include tumors or vascular abnormalities involving the brain stem, an overdose of a narcotic or sedative, and metabolic disorders such as myxedema or chronic metabolic alkalosis.
- Disorders of the peripheral nervous system, respiratory muscles, and chest wall
  - – These disorders lead to an inability to maintain a level of minute ventilation appropriate for the rate of carbon dioxide production.
  - – Concomitant hypoxemia and hypercapnia occur.
  - – Examples include Guillain-Barré syndrome, muscular dystrophy, myasthenia gravis, severe kyphoscoliosis, and morbid obesity.
- Abnormalities of the airways
  - – Severe airway obstruction is a common cause of acute and chronic hypercapnia.
  - – Examples of upper airway disorders are acute epiglottitis and tumors involving the trachea; lower airway disorders include COPD, asthma, and cystic fibrosis.
- Abnormalities of the alveoli
  - – The diseases are characterized by diffuse alveolar filling, frequently resulting in hypoxemic respiratory failure, although hypercapnia may complicate the clinical picture.
  - – Common examples are cardiogenic and noncardiogenic pulmonary edema, aspiration pneumonia, or extensive pulmonary hemorrhage. These disorders are associated with intrapulmonary shunt and an increased work of breathing.
- Common causes of type I (hypoxemic) respiratory failure
  - – Chronic bronchitis and emphysema (COPD)
  - – Pneumonia
  - – Pulmonary edema
  - – Pulmonary fibrosis
  - – Asthma
  - – Pneumothorax
  - – Pulmonary embolism
  - – Pulmonary arterial hypertension
  - – Pneumoconiosis
  - – Granulomatous lung diseases
  - – Cyanotic congenital heart disease
  - – Bronchiectasis
  - – Adult respiratory distress syndrome
  - – Fat embolism syndrome
  - – Kyphoscoliosis
  - – Obesity

- Common causes of type II (hypercapnic) respiratory failure
  - Chronic bronchitis and emphysema (COPD)
  - Severe asthma
  - Drug overdose
  - Poisonings
  - Myasthenia gravis
  - Polyneuropathy
  - Poliomyelitis
  - Primary muscle disorders
  - Porphyria
  - Cervical cordotomy
  - Head and cervical cord injury
  - Primary alveolar hypoventilation
  - Obesity hypoventilation syndrome
  - Pulmonary edema
  - Adult respiratory distress syndrome
  - Myxedema
  - Tetanus.

■ CLASSIFICATION OF RESPIRATORY FAILURE

Based on the pattern of blood gas abnormality:

Type I Hypoxemic Respiratory Failure

- Commonly defined as a PaO_2 <60 mm Hg when the patient is receiving an inspired O_2 concentration >60%.
- Disorders that interfere with O_2 transfer into the blood include pneumonia, pulmonary edema, pulmonary emboli, heart failure, shock, and alveolar injury related to inhalation of toxic gases and lung damage related to alveolar stress/ventilator-induced lung injury.
- Four physiologic mechanisms may cause hypoxemia and subsequent hypoxemic respiratory failure: (1) mismatch between ventilation and perfusion, commonly referred to as V/Q mismatch; (2) shunt; (3) diffusion limitation; and (4) hypoventilation.
- Hypoxemic respiratory failure frequently is caused by a combination of two or more of these mechanisms.

Type II Hypercapnic/Hypoxemic Respiratory Failure

- Also referred to as ventilatory failure since the primary problem is insufficient CO_2 removal.
- Commonly defined as a $PaCO_2$ >45 mm Hg in combination with acidemia (arterial pH <7.35).
- Disorders that compromise CO_2 removal include drug overdoses with central nervous system (CNS) depressants, neuromuscular diseases, acute

asthma, and trauma or diseases involving the spinal cord and its role in lung ventilation.

- Hypercapnic respiratory failure results from an imbalance between ventilatory supply and ventilatory demand. Ventilatory supply is the maximum ventilation that the patient can sustain without developing respiratory muscle fatigue, and ventilatory demand is the amount of ventilation needed to keep the $PaCO_2$ within normal limits.
- Though PaO_2 and $PaCO_2$ determine the definition of respiratory failure, the major threat of respiratory failure is the inability of the lungs to meet the oxygen demands of the tissues. This may occur as a result of inadequate tissue O_2 delivery or because the tissues are unable to use the O_2 delivered to them.

Distinctions Between Acute and Chronic Respiratory Failure

Acute hypercapnic respiratory failure develops over minutes to hours; therefore, pH is less than 7.3. Chronic respiratory failure develops over several days or longer, allowing time for renal compensation and an increase in bicarbonate concentration. Therefore, the pH usually is only slightly decreased.

The distinction between acute and chronic hypoxemic respiratory failure cannot readily be made on the basis of arterial blood gases. The clinical markers of chronic hypoxemia, such as polycythemia or cor pulmonale, suggest a long-standing disorder.

- Manifestations of respiratory failure:
  - These are related to the extent of change in PaO_2 or $PaCO_2$, the rapidity of change (acute versus chronic), and the ability to compensate to overcome this change.
  - Clinical manifestations are variable and it is important to monitor trends in ABGs and/or pulse oximetry to evaluate the extent of change.
  - A change in mental status is frequently the initial indication of respiratory failure.
  - Tachycardia and mild hypertension can also be early signs of respiratory failure.
  - A severe morning headache may suggest that hypercapnia may have occurred during the night, increasing cerebral blood flow by vasodilation and causing a morning headache.
  - Cyanosis is an unreliable indicator of hypoxemia and is a late sign of respiratory failure because it does not occur until hypoxemia is severe ($PaO_2 \leq 45$ mm Hg).
  - Hypoxemia occurs when the amount of O_2 in arterial blood is less than the normal value, and hypoxia occurs when the PaO_2 falls sufficiently to cause signs and symptoms of inadequate oxygenation.
  - Hypoxemia can lead to hypoxia if not corrected, and if hypoxia or hypoxemia is severe, the cells shift from aerobic to anaerobic metabolism.

Clinical Manifestations

- Clinical findings include a rapid, shallow breathing pattern or a respiratory rate that is slower than normal. A change from a rapid rate to a slower rate in a patient in acute respiratory distress such as that seen with acute asthma suggests extreme progression of respiratory muscle fatigue and increased probability of respiratory arrest.

- The position that the patient assumes is an indication of the effort associated with breathing.
  - The patient may be able to lie down (mild distress), but prefer to sit (moderate distress), or be unable to breathe unless sitting upright (severe distress). The patient may require pillows to breathe when attempting to lie flat and this is termed orthopnea.
  - A common position is to sit with the arms propped on the overbed table.

- Pursed-lip breathing may be used.

- The patient may speak in sentences (mild or no distress), phrases (moderate distress), or words (severe distress).

- There may be a change in the inspiratory (I) to expiratory (E) ratio. Normally, the I:E ratio is 1:2, but in patients in respiratory distress, the ratio may increase to 1:3 or 1:4.

- There may be retractions of the intercostal spaces or the supraclavicular area and use of the accessory muscles during inspiration or expiration. Use of the accessory muscles signifies moderate distress.

- Paradoxic breathing indicates severe distress and results from maximal use of the accessory muscles of respiration.

- Breath sounds:
  - Crackles and rhonchi may indicate pulmonary edema and COPD.
  - Absent or diminished breath sounds may indicate atelectasis or pleural effusion.
  - The presence of bronchial breath sounds over the lung periphery often results from lung consolidation that is seen with pneumonia.
  - A pleural friction rub may also be heard in the presence of pneumonia that has involved the pleura.

Diagnostic Studies

- ABGs are done to obtain oxygenation (PaO_2) and ventilation ($PaCO_2$) status, as well as information related to acid-base balance.

- A chest X-ray is done to help identify possible causes of respiratory failure.

- Other diagnostic studies include a complete blood cell count, serum electrolytes, urinalysis, and electrocardiogram.
  - Cultures of the sputum and blood are obtained as necessary to determine sources of possible infection.

- For the patient in severe respiratory failure requiring endotracheal intubation, end-tidal CO_2 ($EtCO_2$) may be used to assess tube placement within the trachea immediately following intubation.
- In severe respiratory failure, a pulmonary artery catheter may be inserted to measure heart pressures and cardiac output, as well as mixed venous oxygen saturation (SvO_2).

■ PATHOPHYSIOLOGY

Hypoxemia is the result of impaired gas exchange and is the hallmark of acute respiratory failure. Hypercapnia may be present, depending on the underlying cause of the problem. The main causes of hypoxemia are alveolar hypoventilation, ventilation/perfusion (V/Q) mismatching, and intrapulmonary shunting. Type I respiratory failure usually results from V/Q mismatching and intrapulmonary shunting, whereas type II respiratory failure usually results from alveolar hypoventilation, which may or may not be accompanied by V/Q mismatching and intrapulmonary shunting.

Alveolar hypoventilation: Alveolar hypoventilation occurs when the amount of oxygen being brought into the alveoli is insufficient to meet the metabolic needs of the body. This can be the result of increasing metabolic oxygen needs or decreasing ventilation. Hypoxemia caused by alveolar hypoventilation is associated with hypercapnia and commonly results from extrapulmonary disorders.

Ventilation/Perfusion (V/Q) mismatching: V/Q mismatching occurs when ventilation and blood flow are mismatched in various regions of the lung in excess of what is normal. Blood passes through alveoli that are underventilated for the given amount of perfusion, leaving these areas with a lower-than-normal amount of oxygen. V/Q mismatching is the most common cause of hypoxemia and is usually the result of alveoli that are partially collapsed or partially filled with fluid.

Intrapulmonary shunting: The extreme form of V/Q mismatching, intrapulmonary shunting, occurs when blood reaches the arterial system without participating in gas exchange. The mixing of unoxygenated (shunted) blood and oxygenated blood lowers the average level of oxygen present in the blood. Intrapulmonary shunting occurs when blood passes through a portion of a lung that is not ventilated. This may be the result of alveolar collapse secondary to atelectasis or alveolar flooding with pus, blood, or fluid. If allowed to progress, hypoxemia can result in a deficit of oxygen at the cellular level. As the tissue demands for oxygen continue and the supply diminishes, an oxygen supply/demand imbalance occurs and tissue hypoxia develops. Decreased oxygen to the cells contributes to impaired tissue perfusion and the development of lactic acidosis and multiple organ dysfunction syndrome.

■ TREATMENT

Hypoxemia is the major immediate threat to organ function. Therefore, the first objective in the management of respiratory failure is to reverse and/or prevent tissue hypoxia. Hypercapnia unaccompanied by hypoxemia generally is well tolerated and probably is not a threat to organ function unless accompanied by severe acidosis. Many experts believe that hypercapnia should be tolerated until the arterial blood pH falls below 7.2. Appropriate management of the underlying disease obviously is an important component in the management of respiratory failure.

A patient with acute respiratory failure generally should be admitted to a respiratory care or intensive care unit. Most patients with chronic respiratory failure can be treated at home with oxygen supplementation and/or ventilatory assist devices along with therapy for their underlying disease.

- Airway management
  - Assurance of an adequate airway is vital in a patient with acute respiratory distress.
  - The most common indication for endotracheal intubation (ETT) is respiratory failure.
  - ETT serves as an interface between the patient and the ventilator.
  - Another indication for ETT is airway protection in patients with altered mental status.
- Correction of hypoxemia
  - After securing an airway, attention must turn to correcting the underlying hypoxemia, the most life-threatening facet of acute respiratory failure.
  - The goal is to assure adequate oxygen delivery to tissues, generally achieved with a PaO_2 of 60 mm Hg or an arterial oxygen saturation (SaO_2) of greater than 90%.
  - Supplemental oxygen is administered via nasal prongs or face mask; however, in patients with severe hypoxemia, intubation and mechanical ventilation often are required.
- Coexistent hypercapnia and respiratory acidosis may need to be addressed. This is done by correcting the underlying cause or providing ventilatory assistance.
  - Mechanical ventilation is used for two essential reasons: (1) To increase PaO_2 and (2) to lower $PaCO_2$. Mechanical ventilation also rests the respiratory muscles and is an appropriate therapy for respiratory muscle fatigue.

Treatment of underlying cause
- After the patient's hypoxemia is corrected and the ventilatory and hemodynamic status have stabilized, every attempt should be made to identify and correct the underlying pathophysiologic process that led to respiratory failure in the first place.
- The specific treatment depends on the etiology of respiratory failure.

■ BIBLIOGRAPHY

1. Bhangwanjee S. Theory and practical issues in ventilatory support of the trauma victim. Trauma and Emergency Medicine. 1999;16:35-9.
2. Gali B, Deepi GG. Positive pressure mechanical ventilation. Emerg Med Clin N Am. 2003;21:453-73.
3. Goldstein RS. Management of the critically ill patient in the emergency department: Focus on safety issues. Critical Care Clin. 2005;21:81-9.
4. Kumar P, Clark M. Clinical Medicine. Fourth Ed. WB Saunders, 1998.pp.849-56.
5. Orebaugh Sl. Initiation of mechanical ventilation in the emergency department. Am J Emerg Med. 1996;14:59-69.
6. Phipps P, Garrard CS. The pulmonary physician in critical care: Acute severe asthma in the intensive care unit. Thorax. 2003;58:81-8.
7. Spritzer CJ. Unravelling the mysteries of mechanical ventilation: A helpful step-by-step guide. J Emerg Nurs. 2003;29:29-36.
8. Ware LB, Matthay MA. Medical progress: the acute respiratory distress syndrome. NEJM. 2000;342:1334-49.

MODES OF VENTILATION

■ INTRODUCTION

A mechanical ventilator is a machine that generates a controlled flow of gas into a patient's airways. Oxygen and air are received from cylinders or wall outlets, the gas is pressure reduced and blended according to the prescribed inspired oxygen tension (FiO_2), accumulated in a receptacle within the machine, and delivered to the patient using one of many available modes of ventilation.

1. **Control:** How the ventilator knows how much flow to deliver

    Either

    Volume controlled (volume limited, volume targeted) and pressure variable.

    or

    Pressure controlled (pressure limited, pressure targeted) and volume variable.

    or

    Dual controlled [volume targeted (guaranteed) pressure limited].

2. **Cycling:** How the ventilator switches from inspiration to expiration: The flow has been delivered to the volume or pressure target—how long does it stay there?

    Time cycled: Such as in pressure controlled ventilation.

    Flow cycled: Such as in pressure support.

    Volume cycled: The ventilator cycles to expiration once a set tidal volume has been delivered: this occurs in volume controlled ventilation. If an inspiratory pause is added, then the breath is both volume and time cycled.

3. **Triggering:** What causes the ventilator to cycle to inspiration. Ventilators may be time triggered, pressure triggered or flow triggered.

    Time: The ventilator cycles at a set frequency as determined by the controlled rate.

    Pressure: The ventilator senses the patient's inspiratory effort by way of a decrease in the baseline pressure.

    Flow: Modern ventilators deliver a constant flow around the circuit throughout the respiratory cycle (flow-by). A deflection in this flow by patient inspiration is monitored by the ventilator and it delivers a breath. This mechanism requires less work by the patient than pressure triggering.

4. **Breaths are either mandatory or spontaneous:** What causes the ventilator to cycle from inspiration.
   Mandatory (controlled): Which is determined by the respiratory rate.
   Assisted (as in assist control, synchronized intermittent mandatory ventilation, pressure support).
   Spontaneous (no additional assistance in inspiration, as in CPAP).
5. **Flow pattern:** Constant, accelerating, decelerating or sinusoidal.
   Sinusoidal: This is the flow pattern seen in spontaneous breathing and CPAP.
   Decelerating: The flow pattern seen in pressure targeted ventilation: Inspiration slows down as alveolar pressure increases (there is a high initial flow). Most intensivists and respiratory therapists use this pattern in volume targeted ventilation also, as it results in a lower peak airway pressure than constant and accelerating flow, and better distribution characteristics.
   Constant: Flow continues at a constant rate until the set tidal volume is delivered.
   Accelerating: Flow increases progressively as the breath is delivered. This should not be used in clinical practice.

▉ NEGATIVE PRESSURE VENTILATION

The iron lung (Fig. 6.1), also known as the Drinker and Shaw tank, was developed in 1929 and was one of the first negative-pressure machines used for long-term ventilation. It was refined and used in the 20th century largely as a result of the polio epidemic that struck the world in the 1940s. The machine is effectively a large elongated tank, which encases the patient up to the neck. The neck is sealed with a rubber gasket so that the patient's face (and airway) is exposed to the room air.

While the exchange of oxygen and carbon dioxide between the bloodstream and the pulmonary airspace works by diffusion and requires no external work, air must be moved into and out of the lungs to make it available to the gas exchange process. In spontaneous breathing, a negative pressure is created in the pleural cavity by the muscles of respiration, and the resulting gradient between the atmospheric pressure and the pressure inside the thorax generates a flow of air.

In the iron lung by means of a pump, the air is withdrawn mechanically to produce a vacuum inside the tank, thus creating negative pressure. This negative pressure leads to expansion of the chest, which causes a decrease in intrapulmonary pressure, and increases flow of ambient air into the lungs. As the vacuum is released, the pressure inside the tank equalizes to that of the ambient pressure, and the elastic coil of the chest and lungs leads to passive exhalation. However, when the vacuum is created, the abdomen also expands along with the lung, cutting off venous flow back to the heart, leading to pooling of venous blood in the lower extremities. There are large portholes for nurse or home assistant access. The patients can talk and eat normally, and can see the world through a well-placed series of mirrors. Some could remain in these iron lungs for years at a time quite successfully.

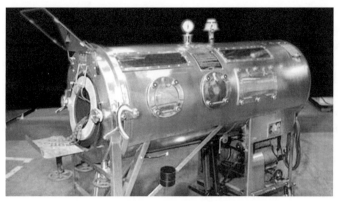

Fig. 6.1: Iron lung

The prominent device used is a smaller device known as the cuirass. The cuirass is a shell-like unit, creating negative pressure only to the chest using a combination of a fitting shell and a soft bladder. Its main use is in patients with neuromuscular disorders who have some residual muscular function. However, it was prone to falling off and caused severe chafing and skin damage and was not used as a long-term device. In recent years, this device has resurfaced as a modern polycarbonate shell with multiple seals and a high pressure oscillation pump in order to carry out biphasic cuirass ventilation.

■ POSITIVE PRESSURE VENTILATION

The design of the modern positive-pressure ventilators were mainly based on technical developments by the military during World War II to supply oxygen to fighter pilots in high altitude. Such ventilators replaced the iron lungs as safe endotracheal tubes with high volume/low pressure cuffs were developed. The popularity of positive-pressure ventilators rose during the polio epidemic in the 1950s in Scandinavia and the United States. Positive pressure through manual supply of 50% oxygen through a tracheostomy tube led to a reduced mortality rate among patients with polio and respiratory paralysis. However, because of the sheer amount of manpower required for such manual intervention, mechanical positive-pressure ventilators became increasingly popular.

Positive-pressure ventilators work by increasing the patient's airway pressure through an endotracheal or tracheostomy tube. The positive pressure allows air to flow into the airway until the ventilator breath is terminated. Subsequently, the airway pressure drops to zero, and the elastic recoil of the chest wall and lungs push the tidal volume, the breath, out through passive exhalation.

■ INDICATION FOR USE

Mechanical ventilation is indicated when the patient's spontaneous ventilation is inadequate to maintain life. It is also indicated as prophylaxis for imminent collapse of other physiologic functions, or ineffective gas exchange in the lungs. Because mechanical ventilation only serves to provide assistance for breathing and does not cure a disease, the patient's underlying condition should be correctable and should resolve over time. In addition, other factors must be taken into consideration because mechanical ventilation is not without its complications (See below).

Common medical indications for use include:
- Acute lung injury (including ARDS, trauma).
- Apnea with respiratory arrest, including cases from intoxication.
- Chronic obstructive pulmonary disease (COPD).
- Acute respiratory acidosis with partial pressure of carbon dioxide (pCO_2) > 50 mm Hg and pH <7.25, which may be due to paralysis of the diaphragm due to Guillain-Barré syndrome, myasthenia gravis, spinal cord injury, or the effect of anesthetic and muscle relaxant drugs.
- Increased work of breathing as evidenced by significant tachypnea, retractions, and other physical signs of respiratory distress.
- Hypoxemia with arterial partial pressure of oxygen (PaO_2) with supplemental fraction of inspired oxygen (FiO_2) <55 mm Hg.
- Hypotension including sepsis, shock and congestive heart failure.

■ SPONTANEOUS MODE

It is not an actual mode on the ventilators since the rate and tidal volume during spontaneous breathing are determined by the patient. The role of the ventilator during this mode is to provide the inspiratory flow to the patient in a timely manner, flow adequate to fulfill a patient's inspiratory demand and provide adjunctive mode such as PEEP to complement a patient's breathing effort.

Spontaneous mode of ventilation also named pressure support ventilation (PSV). The patient initiates every breath and the ventilator delivers support with the preset pressure value. With support from the ventilator, the patient also regulates their own respiratory rate and their tidal volume.

In pressure support, the set inspiratory pressure support level is kept constant and there is a decelerating flow. The patient triggers all breaths. If there is a change in the mechanical properties of the lung/thorax and patient effort, the delivered tidal volume will be affected. The user must then regulate the pressure support level to obtain desired ventilation. Pressure support improves oxygenation, ventilation and decreases work of breathing.

■ POSITIVE END-EXPIRATORY PRESSURE

Positive end-expiratory pressure (PEEP) is a term used in mechanical ventilation to denote the amount of pressure above atmospheric pressure present in the airway at the end of the expiratory cycle. When PEEP is applied to spontaneous breathing patients, the airway pressure is called continuous positive airway pressure (CPAP). PEEP improves gas exchange by preventing alveolar collapse, recruiting more lung units, increasing functional residual capacity, and redistributing fluid in the alveoli.

Indications

Hypoxemia due to the following:
- ARDS.
- Pneumonia.
- Pulmonary edema.
- Atelectasis.

Contraindications

- Increased intracranial pressure.
- Pneumothorax that has not been treated.
- Bronchopleural fistula.

Complications Associated with PEEP

- Decreased venous return and cardiac output.
- Barotrauma.
- Increased intracranial pressure.
- Alterations of renal functions and water metabolism.

■ CONTINUOUS POSITIVE AIRWAY PRESSURE (CPAP)

- It is a spontaneous breathing mode in which airway pressure is kept constant throughout the respiratory cycle.
- The respiratory rate, tidal volume and inspiratory time are determined by the patient. CPAP provides PEEP for the spontaneously breathing patient.
- CPAP commonly used as a weaning technique, may be given via face mask, nasal mask or endotracheal tube. In neonates, CPAP is the method of choice.

Indications

- Pulmonary edema
- Pneumonias
- Weaning from mechanical ventilation
- Post-traumatic and postoperative gas exchange disturbances.

Advantages

- Improved oxygenation through increasing functional residual capacity
- With CPAP, breathing effort is reduced because the inspiratory gas flow makes breathing easier

- Re-opening of atelectatic areas of lung
- Reduction of the intrapulmonary R-L shunt
- Improvement of the ventilation/perfusion ratio.

■ CONTROLLED MANDATORY VENTILATION (CMV) (FIG. 6.2)

In this mode, the ventilator delivers the preset tidal volume at a time triggered respiratory rate, since the ventilator controls both the patient's tidal volume and respiratory rate. Thus the ventilator controls the patient's minute volume. In this mode, patient cannot change the ventilator respiratory rate or breathe spontaneously. For example, if tidal volume and respiratory rate is 500 mL and 12 BPM respectively, the minute ventilation will be 6 liter.

The control mode should only be used when the patient is properly medicated with a combination of sedatives, respiratory depressants and neuromuscular blockers.

Indications

- The control mode is most often indicated if the patient 'fights' the ventilator in the initial stages of mechanical ventilatory support. Fighting or bucking the ventilator often means that the patient is severely distressed and struggling to breath.
- Tetanus or other seizure activities that interrupt the delivery of mechanical ventilation.
- Complete rest for patient for a period of 24 hours.
- Patients with a crushed chest injury in which spontaneous inspiratory efforts produce significant paradoxical chest wall movement.
- In surgery for paralyzed patients.

Complication

Since the patient's spontaneous respiratory drive will have been blunted with sedation in the control mode, the patient is totally dependent on the ventilator

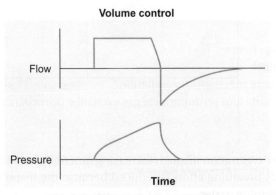

Fig. 6.2: Rectangular flow waveform

for ventilation and oxygenation. As a result, the primary hazard associated with the control mode is the potential for apnea and hypoxia.

■ PRESSURE CONTROLLED VENTILATION (FIG. 6.3)

Remember: Pressure control only refers to the flow target mechanism: pressure control can be controlled (CMV), assist-controlled or synchronized intermittent mandatory ventilation (SIMV).

Pressure control refers to the type of breath delivered, not the mode of ventilation. Many different modes are pressure controlled. Conventionally, the term 'pressure control' refers to an assist control mode (there is also an SIMV pressure control mode on some ventilators). In pressure control, a pressure limited breath is delivered at a set rate. The tidal volume is determined by the preset pressure limit and it depends on lung compliance and resistance. This is a peak pressure rather than a plateau pressure limit (easier to measure). The inspiratory time is also set by the operator. Again this is a trade-off between short times with rapid inflow and outflow of gas, and long times with gas trapping. The flow waveform is always decelerating in pressure control; this relates to the mechanics of targeting airway pressure; flow slows as it reaches the pressure limit.

Gas flows into the chest along the pressure gradient. As the airway pressure rises with increasing alveolar volume, the rate of flow drops off (as the pressure gradient narrows) until a point is reached when the delivered pressure equals the airway pressure: flow stops. The pressure is maintained for the duration of inspiration. Obviously, longer inspiratory times lead to higher mean airway

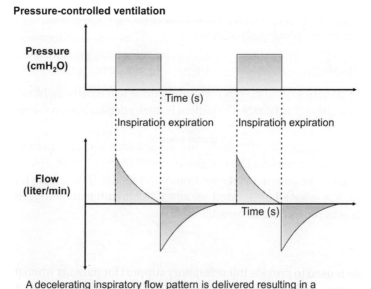

A decelerating inspiratory flow pattern is delivered resulting in a fixed pressure throughout the breath

Fig. 6.3: Process of pressure controlled mechanism

pressures (the 'i' time (Ti) is a pressure holding time after flow has stopped). The combination of decelerating flow and maintenance of airway pressure over time means that stiff, noncompliant lung units (long time constants), which are difficult to aerate are more likely to be inflated.

Pressure control does not guarantee minute ventilation, and therefore requires more monitoring by the operator. The minute ventilation is a complex mix of the peak pressure, the Ti, the lung and chest wall compliance, resistance in the airway and from other thoracic structures. If there is a rapid change in the compliance, then the patient may hypoventilate and become hypoxic.

To initiate a pressure control is slightly more difficult than volume control. Again, the PEEP and FiO_2 are determined by lung mechanics and oxygenation targets. The inspiratory pressure is determined by looking for a tidal volume of 5–6 mL/kg. The respiratory rate is determined by the minute volume requirement. The inspiratory time is usually set at 1 second, but can be increased if 1. Target tidal volume is not achieved with 2. The patient remains hypoxic in spite of a plateau pressure > 30 cm H_2O. In this way, the mean airway pressure is used to increase overall lung volumes, and improve V/Q matching. Unfortunately, there is a limit to this process, auto-PEEP. Longer inspiratory times and faster respiratory rates predispose to alveolar gas trapping. This intrinsic PEEP is present in addition to applied PEEP at the beginning of inspiration, placing the patient on a less compliant (over distended) part of the volume-pressure curve. Thus, tidal volumes fall and airway pressures rise.

■ PRESSURE ASSIST VENTILATION

Pressure assist ventilation (PAV) is pressure control without a set rate. Patients take pressure controlled breaths at the rate of their choosing, and the volumes derived are determined by the pressure preset level, the Ti and the flow demanded. This is a very comfortable mode, and is used in weaning from pressure control (the pressure limit is weaned). The Ti assures the duration of the breath, and prevents the patient from hyperventilating, which sometimes occurs in pressure support.

■ ASSIST CONTROL

With the assist control (AC) mode, the patient may increase the ventilator respiratory rate in addition to the preset mechanical respiratory rate but it does not allow the patient to take spontaneous breaths. If the breath is patient triggered, it is referred as assisted breath. If the breath is time triggered, the breath is referred as control breath.

Indication

AC mode is used to provide full ventilatory support for patients when they are first placed on mechanical ventilation. AC mode is typically used for patients who have a stable respiratory drive and can, therefore, trigger the ventilator into inspiration.

Advantages

- Patients work of breathing requirement in the AC mode is very small when the triggering sensitivity is set appropriately and the ventilator supplies an inspiratory flow that meets inspiratory flow demand.
- Allows the patient to control the respiratory rate and, therefore, MV required to normalize the patient's $PaCO_2$.

Complications

- Alveolar hyperventilation
- Hypocapnia.

▪ INTERMITTENT MANDATORY VENTILATION

Intermittent mandatory ventilation (IMV) is a mixture between spontaneous breathing and controlled ventilation. The ventilator delivers control breaths and allows the patient to breathe spontaneously at any tidal volume.

Advantages include lower airway pressure with decreased evidence of barotrauma and increased cardiac function.

Disadvantages are that the patient can breathe against the machine when the ventilator is in the process of inspiration and the patient wants to breathe out. Primary complication associated with IMV was "random chance of breath stacking". This occurs when the patient taking a spontaneous breath and ventilator delivers a time triggered mandatory breath at the same time.

▪ SYNCHRONIZED INTERMITTENT MANDATORY VENTILATION

Synchronized intermittent mandatory ventilation (SIMV) is a mixture between spontaneous breathing and mechanical ventilation. It is a mode in which the ventilator delivers either assisted breaths to the patient at the beginning of a spontaneous breath or time triggered mandatory breaths. The mandatory breaths are synchronized with the patient's spontaneous breathing efforts so as to avoid breath stacking.

SIMV Mandatory Breath Triggering Mechanism

This may be either time or patient triggered. For example, if SIMV RR is set at 12 bpm then the ventilator would time trigger a breath every 5 second. However, if patient is breathing spontaneously between the mandatory breaths and if by random chance, the patient begins to inspire just prior to the point at which ventilator would be expected to time trigger then the ventilator senses this spontaneous effort and delivers a mandatory breath as assisted patient triggered breath.

SIMV Spontaneous Breath Triggering Mechanism

In between the mandatory breath, ventilator permits the patient to breathe spontaneously to any tidal volume the patient desires. The spontaneous rate and tidal volume are totally dependent on patient's breathing effort.

SIMV-PC with PS (pressure support) (Fig. 6.4): Beyond a set background, ventilator rate and pressure spontaneous breaths are augmented (supported) with pressure.

Uses: (1) To provide mandatory backup breaths (conceptually large sighs to prevent gradual progressive atelectasis) while allowing amount of PS to be weaned slowly to 'train' respiratory muscles. (2) As a means of providing intermediate respiratory support (less than conventional modes but more than CPAP or extubation). (3) Pressure support just enough to overcome resistance of ETT and ventilator circuit and maintain minimum adequate spontaneous ventilation. Uses as above, but in 'pure pressure' support mode. (If set PIP and PS pressures are the same then essentially you have pressure AC mode). SIMV-VC with PS (pressure support): Beyond the set rate and tidal volume spontaneous breaths are augmented (supported) with pressure, usually relatively low values. The difference between this mode of ventilation (VC/PS) and the mode described above (PC/PS) is that in VC/PS the SIMV breaths are volume breaths and in PC/PS mode the SIMV breaths are pressure breaths.

■ PRESSURE REGULATED VOLUME CONTROL (PRVC)

Pressure regulated volume control (PRVC) is a ventilator mode where the breaths are delivered mandatorily to assure preset volumes, with a constant inspiratory pressure continuously adapting to the patient's condition. The flow pattern is decelerating. This mode is a form of assist control mode of ventilation, the breaths can either be ventilator initiated or patient initiated. This mode combines the advantages of volume controlled and pressure controlled ventilation.

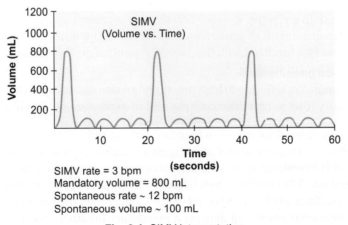

SIMV rate = 3 bpm
Mandatory volume = 800 mL
Spontaneous rate ~ 12 bpm
Spontaneous volume ~ 100 mL

Fig. 6.4: SIMV interpretation

◼ HOW THE VENTILATOR ACHIEVES PRVC MODE

The first breath delivered to the patient is a volume controlled breath. The measured plateau pressure is used as the pressure level for the next breath. The pressure is constant during the set inspiratory time and the flow is decelerating. The set tidal volume is achieved by automatic, breath-by-breath pressure regulation. The ventilator will adjust the inspiratory pressure control level, according to the mechanical properties of the airways/lung/thorax, to the lowest possible level to guarantee the preset tidal volume. If the measured tidal volume increases above the preset, the pressure level decreases in steps of maximum 3 cm H_2O between consecutive breaths until the preset tidal volume is delivered. Maximum available pressure level is 5 cm H_2O below a preset upper pressure limit.

◼ AIRWAY PRESSURE RELEASE VENTILATION

Airway pressure release ventilation (APRV-Dräger, BiVent-Maquet) has gained in popularity over the past several years as a mode of mechanical ventilation. APRV, a style of inverse-ratio ventilation, is most commonly used to support hypoxemic respiratory failure patients.

APRV mode allows the practitioner to set independent inspiratory (P High) and expiratory (PEEP) pressure settings. Time spent in each phase is controlled by adjusting inspiratory (T High) and expiratory (T PEEP) time. These set times determine the I:E ratio and the frequency of pressure releases. In the severely hypoxemic patient, the T high and T PEEP are adjusted to produce an inverse ratio that results in a higher mean airway pressure (MAP). The goal of the inverse ratio is to inflate the lungs to a set peak pressure (P High) and periodically release the pressure to a set PEEP, for a short time (T Peep), in order to allow for exhalation of CO_2 while trapping air and preventing alveolar derecruitment. Patient can breathe spontaneously at both the level that is at P high and P low.

◼ COMPLICATIONS
Respiratory

Nosocomial pneumonia.
Barotrauma: Not only due to high pressures but also due to high volumes and shear injury (due to repetitive collapse and re-expansion of alveoli) and due to tension at the interface between open and collapsed alveoli.

Causes:
- Pneumothorax
- Pneumomediastinum
- Pneumopericardium
- Surgical emphysema
- Acute lung injury.

Gas trapping: It occurs if there is insufficient time for alveoli to empty before the next breath more likely to occur:

- In patients with asthma or COPD.
- When inspiratory time is long (and therefore expiratory time short).
- When respiratory rate is high (absolute expiratory time is short).
- Results in progressive hyperinflation of alveoli and progressive rise in end-expiratory pressure (known as intrinsic PEEP).

May result in:
- Barotrauma.
- Cardiovascular compromise due to high intrathoracic pressure. In an extreme case can lead to cardiac arrest with pulseless electrical activity.

Measuring Intrinsic PEEP

Quantitative measurement of intrinsic PEEP can be obtained in an apneic patient by using the expiratory pause hold control on the ventilator. This allows equilibration of pressures between the alveoli and the ventilator allowing the total PEEP to be measured. The value for total PEEP can be read from the airway pressure dial or the PEEP display.

Intrinsic PEEP = Total PEEP-Set PEEP.

■ OTHER SUPPORTIVE MODES
Adaptive Support Ventilation

Adaptive support ventilation is the only commercially available closed-loop mode of mechanical ventilation to date that uses "optimal targeting" and was designed to minimize the work rate of breathing, mimic natural breathing, stimulate spontaneous breathing, and reduce weaning time.

■ CLOSED LOOP CONTROL

- Closed-loop control involves a positive or negative feedback of the information on the respiratory mechanics of the patient.
- It is based on measurements made almost continuously which can be modified or adapted in a more physiological and individualized ventilatory support manner.

ASV combines modes with
- PSV, if RR is higher than the target
- PCV if there is no spontaneous breathing
- SIMV when patient's RR is lower than target.

■ VENTILATOR SETTINGS

These are set by the user:
- Height of the patient (cm): Based on this it calculate the ideal body weight and dead space 2.2 mL/kg
- Gender
- Percent minimum volume: 25–350%

Normal 100%, asthma 90%, acute respiratory distress syndrome (ARDS) 120%, others 110%, Add 20% if T body >38.5°C (101.3°F) or add 5% for every 500 m (1640 feet) above sea level.

- Trigger: Flow trigger of 2 l/min
- Expiratory trigger sensitivity: Start with 25% and 40% in chronic obstructive pulmonary disease COPD
- Tube resistance compensation: Set to 100%
- High pressure alarm limit: 10 cm H_2O be the limit of ↓ and ↑ least 25 cm H_2O of PEEP/continuous positive airway pressure (CPAP)
- PEEP
- FiO_2.

Then:

- ASV selects the respiratory pattern in terms of RR, VT, inspiratory: Expiratory time (I:E ratio) for mandatory breathing and reaches the respiratory pattern selected
- Otis equation is used to determine the RR at which work of breathing is optimized
- Starts with test breaths to obtain measurements
- Ventilation is pressure and volume limited.

Advantages

- Versatile
- Can ventilate any patient group
- Safe
- Prevents tachypnea, auto-PEEP and dead space
- Less operator dependent and less need for operator involvement
- Decreases time on mechanical ventilation
- Adjusts to patient inspiratory effort.

Disadvantages

- Cannot directly program VT, RR and I:E ratio
- Limited pediatrics experience
- Algorithm tends to ventilate with low tidal volume and high RR
- Only available with Hamilton ventilators.

Automatic Tube Compensation

Automatic tube compensation (ATC) is the simplest example of a computer-controlled targeting system on a ventilator. The goal of ATC is to support the resistive work of breathing through the artificial airway.

Neurally Adjusted Ventilatory Assist

Neurally adjusted ventilatory assist (NAVA) is adjusted by a computer (servo) and is similar to ATC but with more complex requirements for implementation.

In terms of patient-ventilator synchrony, NAVA supports both resistive and elastic work of breathing in proportion to the patient's inspiratory effort as reflected by the Edi signal. This signal represents the electrical activity of the diaphragm, the body's principal breathing muscle.

The act of taking a breath is controlled by the respiratory center of the brain, which decides the characteristics of each breath, timing and size. The respiratory center sends a signal along the phrenic nerve, excites the diaphragm muscle cells, leading to muscle contraction and descent of the diaphragm dome. As a result, the pressure in the airway drops, causing an inflow of air into the lungs.

With NAVA, the electrical activity of the diaphragm (Edi) is captured, fed to the ventilator and used to assist the patient's breathing in synchrony with and in proportion to the patient's own efforts, regardless of patient category or size. As the work of the ventilator and the diaphragm is controlled by the same signal, coupling between the diaphragm and the SERVO-i ventilator is synchronized simultaneously.

NAVA: Neurally adjusted ventilatory assist (NAVA) is a new approach to mechanical ventilation based on neural respiratory output.

The act of breathing depends on rhythmic discharge from the respiratory center of the brain. This discharge travels along the phrenic nerve, excites the diaphragm muscle cells, leading to muscle contraction and descent of the diaphragm dome. As a result, the pressure in the airway drops, causing an inflow of air into the lungs. Conventional mechanical ventilators sense a patient effort by either a drop in airway pressure or a reversal in flow. The last and most slow reacting step in the chain of respiratory events is used to sense the patient effort. Hence, creating a system that is sensitive to hyperinflation, intrinsic PEEP and secondary triggering problems.

With NAVA, the electrical activity of the diaphragm (Edi) is captured, fed to the ventilator and used to assist the patient's breathing. As the ventilator and the diaphragm work with the same signal, mechanical coupling between the diaphragm and the ventilator is practically instantaneous.

Some of the potential benefits: Improved synchrony: In NAVA, the ventilator is cycled-on as soon as neural inspiration starts. Moreover, the level of assistance provided during inspiration is determined by the patient's own respiratory center demand. The same applies for the cycling-off phase—the ventilator cycles off inspiration the instant it is alerted to the onset of neural expiration. By utilizing the Edi signal, maintenance of synchrony between the patient and the ventilator is improved.

Lung protection: With NAVA, the patient's own respiratory demands determine the level of assistance. NAVA gives the opportunity to avoid over or under assistance of the patient.

Unique monitoring capability: The Edi signal is a new unique parameter in mechanical ventilation. It can be used as a diagnostic tool to monitor the electrical activity of the diaphragm (Edi). The Edi curve and its associated value can thus be used as a powerful monitoring tool in all ventilation modes, providing information on respiratory drive, volume requirements and the effect of the ventilatory settings, and to gain indications for sedation and weaning.

NAVA for infants: The Edi signal provides a tool that allows the clinicians to interpret the background of the chaotic breathing pattern so often seen in the infants. The direct access to the respiratory center output gives prompt information on the effect of any intervention relating to ventilation of the lung. PEEP adjustment and the degree of unloading can now be based on informed decisions.

Patient comfort: With NAVA, the respiratory muscles and the ventilator are driven by the same signal. The delivered assistance is matched to neural demands. This synchrony between patient and ventilator helps minimize patient discomfort and agitation, promoting spontaneous breathing.

Decision support for unloading and extubation: The Edi signal can be used as an indicator to set the support level from the ventilator, and to optimize unloading. As the patient's condition improves, Edi amplitude decreases, resulting in reduction in ventilator-delivered pressure. This pressure drop is an indicator to consider weaning and extubation.

■ HIGH FREQUENCY VENTILATION

Definition: Ventilation of lungs at a frequency >4 times of normal rate, most important difference from conventional IPPV is that it requires tidal volumes of only 1–3 mL/kg body weight to achieve normocarbia.

Three types: High frequency positive pressure (used in anesthesia), high frequency jet (anesthesia and ICU) and high frequency oscillation.

Proposed Advantages

- Reduced peak and mean airway pressures.
- Improved CVS stability due to reduced peak and mean airway pressure.
- Decreased risk of barotrauma.
- Allows adequate ventilation with a disrupted airway (e.g. bronchopleural fistula).
- Permits mechanical ventilation during bronchoscopy.
- Improves operating conditions, e.g. in thoracic surgery.
- Allows ventilation through narrow catheters and thus increases access during laryngeal and tracheal surgery.
- Reduces sedation requirements when used in intensive therapy unit (ITU).
- Avoidance of hypoxia during tracheobronchial toilet.

Disadvantages

- Specialized equipment required.
- Dangers of high pressure gas flows.
- Humidification of inspired gases difficult.
- Tidal volumes markedly affected by changes in respiratory compliance.
- Monitoring of ventilation parameters difficult.
- Difficult to predict minute ventilation from ventilator.

High Frequency Jet Ventilation

- Pulses of gas delivered at high velocity through an orifice at frequency of 10–100 Hz.
- Orifice may be in a T-piece connected to a conventional ETT, in a narrow tube incorporated in wall of a special ETT or at end of fine bore catheter placed in trachea.
- In early part of inspiratory cycle, jet entrains gas. Entrained gas develops a normal flow profile which acts as a piston in trachea.
- Expiration is passive.
- Essential to have a free expiratory pathway to prevent barotrauma.
- Entrained gas can be humidified.
- Behaves like a constant pressure generator in that tidal volume is dependent on compliance.
- Probably useful in barotrauma and in patients with a gas leak, e.g. bronchopleural fistula.
- May improve hemodynamic status of patient if it leads to a reduction of airway pressure.
- Of benefit in ARDS in combination with other methods of decreasing barotrauma.

■ HIGH FREQUENCY OSCILLATORY VENTILATION

High frequency oscillatory ventilation (HFOV) is a type of mechanical ventilation that uses a constant distending pressure (mean airway pressure [MAP] with pressure variations oscillating around the MAP at very high rates (up to 900 cycles per minute). This creates small tidal volumes, often less than the dead space. In conventional ventilation, large pressure changes (the difference between PEEP and PIP) create physiological tidal volumes and gas exchange is dependent on bulk convection (expired gas exchanged for inspired gas). HFOV relies on alternative mechanisms of gas exchange such as molecular diffusion, Taylor dispersion, turbulence, asymmetric velocity profiles, Pendelluft, cardiogenic mixing and collateral ventilation. The large pressure changes and volumes associated with conventional ventilation have been implicated in the pathogenesis of ventilator-induced lung injury (VILI) and chronic lung disease (CLD).

- 3100A high-frequency oscillatory ventilator—for adult and pediatrics
- 3100B high-frequency oscillatory ventilator—for neonates

At present, HFOV is only indicated as a rescue therapy

- Failure of conventional ventilation in the term infant persistent pulmonary hypertension of the newborn (PPHN), meconium aspiration syndrome (MAS).
- Air leak syndromes [pneumothorax, pulmonary interstitial emphysema (PIE)].
- Failure of conventional ventilation in the preterm infant (severe RDS, PIE, pulmonary hypoplasia) or to reduce barotrauma when conventional ventilator settings are high.

HFOV is not as yet proven to be of benefit in the elective or rescue treatment of preterm infants with respiratory dysfunction and may be associated with an increase in intraventricular hemorrhage. Furthermore, caution is needed when HFOV is used, as high airway pressures may result in impaired cardiac output causing hypotension requiring inotropic support or volume expansion. Some infants poorly tolerate the extra handling involved in switching ventilators or may not respond to HFOV. If there is no improvement with HFOV, consider reverting to conventional ventilation.

In this unit, HFOV will only be delivered using the SensorMedics Oscillator.

Terminology

Frequency	High frequency ventilation rate (Hz = cycles per second, i.e. 10 Hz = 10 cycles/sec = 600 cycles/min).
MAP	Mean airway pressure (cm H_2O).
Amplitude	Delta P or power is the variation around the MAP.
Oxygenation	Oxygenation is dependent on MAP and FiO_2. MAP provides a constant distending pressure equivalent to CPAP. This inflates the lung to a constant and optimal lung volume maximizing the area for gas exchange and preventing alveolar collapse in the expiratory phase.
Ventilation	In HFOV, oxygenation can be separated from ventilation as they are not dependent on each other as is the case with conventional ventilation. Ventilation or CO_2 elimination is dependent on amplitude and to a lesser degree frequency.

Initial Settings on HFOV

Optimal lung volume strategy (aim to maximize recruitment of alveoli)	Set MAP 2–3 cm H_2O above the MAP on conventional ventilation. MAP in 1–2 cm H_2O steps until oxygenation improves Set frequency to 10 Hz.
Low volume strategy (aim to minimize lung trauma)	Set MAP equal to the MAP on conventional ventilation Set frequency to 10 Hz. Adjust amplitude to get an adequate chest wall vibration.

- Obtain an early blood gas and adjust settings as appropriate.
- Obtain chest radiograph to assess inflation.

Making Adjustments Once Established on HFOV

Poor oxygenation	Over oxygenation	Under ventilation	Over ventilation
Increase FiO$_2$	Decrease FiO$_2$	Increase amplitude	Decrease amplitude
Increase MAP (1–2 cm H$_2$O)	Decrease MAP (1–2 cm H$_2$O)	Decrease frequency (1–2 Hz) if amplitude maximal	Increase frequency (1–2 Hz) if amplitude minimal

■ BASIC PRINCIPLES

Theory

HFOV utilizes much higher frequencies than CV (120–600 breaths per minute versus up to 40 breaths per minute for CV). This allows the use of tidal volumes that with conventional ventilation would lead to rising CO$_2$ levels. The principle goals for ventilating a patient with ARDS using HFOV are to prevent ventilator induced lung injury (VILI) and to achieve adequate ventilation and gas exchange with as low a fractional inspired oxygen concentration (FiO$_2$) as possible.

The key features of HFOV that are thought to be responsible for decreasing the incidence and severity of ventilator induced lung injury when compared with CV are explained below.

- Smaller tidal volumes: This helps prevent volutrauma caused by alveolar over-distension.
- Higher mean airway pressure (MAWP): The continuously high distending pressure provides improved oxygenation via improved alveolar recruitment.
- Smaller differences between inspiratory and expiratory pressures: This helps prevent atelectotrauma associated with cyclical alveolar collapse and distension that can be a feature of CV.
- Lower peak pressures: This helps reduce barotrauma.

Physiology

Gas transport on HFOV is thought to occur via 5 mechanisms.

The individual contribution of each mechanism to overall gas exchange remains debated:

1. *Bulk flow:* This is the predominant mechanism of gas transport seen in CV and it plays a part in HFOV, providing gas delivery to proximal alveoli with low regional dead space volumes.
2. *Pendelluft*: This refers to inter-regional gas mixing between alveolar units whereby there is transient movement of gas out of some alveoli and into others when flow stops at the end of inspiration and in the opposite direction at the end of expiration. This occurs where regions of the lung differ in compliance or airway resistance so that their time constants of filling in response to changes in trans-pulmonary pressure are not the same.

3. *Taylor dispersion*: This leads to mixing of fresh and residual gases along the front of a flow of gas through a tube, due to the interaction of the axial velocity profile and radial concentration gradient.

4. *Coaxial flow*: This occurs when gas in the center flows inward and the gas on the periphery flows outward. It is attributed to the asymmetry between inspiratory and expiratory velocity profiles.

5. *Augmented molecular diffusion:* This occurs at the alveolar level as a result of the added kinetic energy supplied by the oscillations.

Oxygenation on HFOV is similar to conventional ventilation (CV). It is dependent on two set variables; FiO_2 and MAWP.

CO_2 clearance on HFOV differs however. During conventional ventilation CO_2 removal is dependent on minute volume, the product of tidal volume (Vt) and respiratory rate. An increase in minute volume leads to an increase in CO_2 clearance. CO_2 clearance on HFOV is also dependent on the frequency of oscillations and tidal volume (Vt). However, as will be explained later, a decrease in frequency on HFOV leads to larger tidal volumes and subsequent increased CO_2 clearance. This is the opposite of CV.

The HFOV ventilators for both adults and pediatrics follow the same basic principles. A flow of warmed humidified gas (bias flow) is run across the proximal end of the endo-tracheal (ET) tube at 20–40 l min-1. An oscillatory piston pump vibrates this bias flow of gas so that a portion of the gas is pumped into and out of the patient. Thus, in contrast to CV, inspiration and expiration are both active processes in HFOV. The frequency of the vibration is usually between 3–10 Hz. As 1 Hz = 1 cycle per second, patients on HFOV receive respiratory rates between 180–600 breaths per minute. Occasionally a bias flow above the normal value of 20 l min-1 may be needed. Examples where a higher bias flow may be required are during suctioning, after introduction of a cuff leak in order to maintain MAWP or in the presence of specific pathology such as a broncho-pleural fistula.

Cycle volume is synonymous with tidal volume delivered. This is controlled by the distance the piston pump moves in and out, the amplitude of oscillations. On the Novalung a specific cycle volume can be set from within a range that is dependent on frequency. Altering cycle volume is another way, other than changes in frequency, in which CO_2 clearance can be altered. Vt may however vary unpredictably, particularly if a patient is making respiratory effort or there is a change in compliance such as pneumothorax or partial/total obstruction of the patient's ET tube. A clinically useful measure of tidal volume is the 'chest wiggle factor' (CWF). This refers to visible movement of the patient generated by the oscillations. Under normal circumstances such movement should be visible from chest to mid-thigh during HFOV. CWF may be used as a surrogate marker of Vt and sudden changes in observed CWF should prompt urgent patient evaluation, as discussed later in the text. Reducing frequency on HFOV leads to increased amplitude. This explains why in contrast to CV, a reduction in ventilatory rate during HFOV is associated with increased CO_2 clearance.

Adverse Effects

The adverse side effects noted during the use of high-frequency ventilation include those commonly found during the use of conventional positive pressure ventilators. These adverse effects include:

- Pneumothorax
- Pneumopericardium
- Pneumoperitoneum
- Pneumomediastinum
- Pulmonary interstitial emphysema
- Intraventricular hemorrhage
- Necrotizing tracheobronchitis
- Bronchopulmonary dysplasia.

Contraindications

High-frequency jet ventilation is contraindicated in patients requiring tracheal tubes smaller than 2.5 mm ID.

Chest Radiograph

- Initial chest radiograph at 1–2 hours to determine the baseline lung volume on HFOV (aim for 8 ribs).
- A follow-up chest radiograph in 4–6 hours is recommended to assess the expansion.
- Thereafter repeat chest radiography with acute changes in patient condition.

Weaning

- Reduce FiO_2 to <40% before weaning MAP (except when over-inflation is evident).
- Reduce MAP when chest radiograph shows evidence of over-inflation (>9 ribs).
- Reduce MAP in 1–2 cm H_2O increments to 8–10 cm H_2O.
- In air leak syndromes (low volume strategy), reducing MAP takes priority over weaning the FiO_2.
- Wean the amplitude in 2–4 cm H_2O increments.
- Do not wean the frequency.
- Discontinue weaning when MAP 8–10 cm H_2O and amplitude 20–25.
- If infant is stable, oxygenating well and blood gases are satisfactory then infant could be extubated to CPAP or switched to conventional ventilation. Discuss with consultant.

Suctioning

- Suction is indicated for diminished chest wall movement (chest wobble), elevated CO_2 and/or worsening oxygenation suggesting airway or ET tube obstruction, or if there are visible/audible secretions in the airway.

- Avoid in the first 24 hours of HFOV, unless clinically indicated.
- In-line suctioning must be used (See Suction Protocol for full procedure).
- Press the STOP button briefly while quickly inserting and withdrawing suction catheter (PEEP is maintained).

■ BIBLIOGRAPHY

1. Attar MA, Donn SM. Mechanisms of ventilator-induced lung injury in premature infants. Semin Neonatol. 2002;7:353-60.
2. Brochard LJ. "Tidal volume during acute lung injury: let the patient choose?". Intensive Care Medicine. 2009;35(11):1830–2. doi:10.1007/s00134-009-1632-z. PMID: 19760207.
3. Chamberlain D. "Never quite there: A tale of resuscitation medicine". Clinical Medicine. Journal of the Royal College of Physicians. 2003;3(6):573-7.
4. Colice, Gene L. "Historical Perspective on the Development of Mechanical Ventilation". in Martin J Tobin. Principles and Practice of Mechanical Ventilation (2 ed.). New York: McGraw-Hill, 2006. ISBN 978-0071447676.
5. MacIntyre N. "Talk to me! Toward better patient-ventilator communication". Critical Care Medicine. 2010;38(2):714–5.doi:10.1097/CCM.0b013e3181c0ddef. PMID 20083941.
6. MAQUET, NAVA, brochure, 2010 MAQUET Critical Care AB, Order No MX-0616.
7. McCulloch PR, Forkert PG, Froese AB. Lung volume maintenance prevents lung injury during high frequency oscillatory ventilation in surfactant-deficient rabbits. Am Rev Respir Dis. 1988;137(5):1185-92.
8. Navalesi P, Colombo D, Della Corte F. "NAVA ventilation". Minerva Anestesiol. 2010;76(5):346–52. PMID 20395897.
9. Otis AB, Fenn WO, Rahn H. "Mechanics of Breathing in Man." Journal of Applied Physiology. 1950;2:592-607.
10. Pillow J. High frequency oscillatory ventilation: Mechanisms of gas exchange and lung mechanics. Crit Care Med. 2005;33(3 suppl.): S135-S41.
11. Shah MR, et al. Impact of the pulmonary artery catheter in critically ill patients: Meta-analysis of randomized clinical trials. JAMA. 2005;294(13):1664-70. PMID: 16204666.
12. "Smother Small Dog to See it Revived. Successful Demonstration of an Artificial Respiration Machine Cheered in Brooklyn. Women in the Audience, But Most of Those Present were Physicians. The Dog, Gathered in from the Street, Wagged Its Tail.", New York Times (May 29, 1908, Friday). Retrieved on 25 December 2007. "An audience, composed of about thirty men and three or four women, most of the men being physicians, attended a demonstration of Prof. George Poe's machine for producing artificial respiration in the library of the Kings County Medical Society, at 1,313 Bedford Avenue, Brooklyn, last night, under the auspices of the First Legion of the Red Cross Society."
13. Tehrani FT. "Method and Apparatus for Controlling an Artificial Resirator," US Patent No. 4986268, issued on Jan. 22, 1991.
14. Vallée F, et al. Stroke output variations calculated by oesophageal Doppler is a reliable predictor of fluid response. Intensive Care Med. 2005;31(10):1388-93. Epub 2005 August 19. PMID: 16132887.

INITIATION AND MONITORING DURING MECHANICAL VENTILATION

■ INITIAL VENTILATOR SETTINGS

The following are general guidelines that may need to be modified for the individual patient.

■ TIDAL VOLUME AND INSPIRATORY PRESSURE LIMIT

- For adult patients and older children
    - Tidal volume is calculated in mL/kg. Traditionally 10 mL/kg was used but has been shown to cause barotrauma or injury to the lung by overextension. About 6–8 mL/kg is now common practice in ICU. Hence, a patient weighing 70 kg would get a TV of 450–500 mL. In adults, a rate of 12 is generally used.
    - With acute respiratory distress syndrome (ARDS)—a tidal volume of 6 mL/kg is used with a rate of 12–20/minute. This reduced tidal volume allows for minimal volutrauma but may result in an elevated pCO_2 (due to the relative decreased oxygen delivered) but this elevation does not need to be corrected (termed permissive hypercapnia).
- For infants and younger children
    - Without existing lung disease—a tidal volume of 4–8 mL/kg to be delivered at a rate of 30–35 breaths per minute.
    - With RDS—decrease tidal volume and increase respiratory rate sufficient to maintain pCO_2 between 45 and 55. Allowing higher pCO_2 (sometimes called permissive hypercapnia) may help prevent ventilator-induced lung injury.

As the amount of tidal volume increases, the pressure required to administer that volume is increased. This pressure is known as the peak airway pressure. If the peak airway pressure is persistently above 45 cm H_2O for adults, the risk of barotrauma is increased and efforts should be made to try to reduce the peak airway pressure. In infants and children, it is unclear what level of peak pressure may cause damage. In general, keeping peak pressures below 30 is desirable.

Monitoring for barotrauma can also involve measuring the plateau pressure, which is the pressure after the delivery of the tidal volume but before the patient is allowed to exhale. Normal breathing pattern involves inspiration, then expiration. The ventilator is programmed so that after delivery of the tidal volume (inspiration), the patient is not allowed to exhale for half a second. Therefore, pressure must be maintained in order to prevent exhalation, and this pressure is the plateau pressure. Barotrauma is minimized when the plateau pressure is maintained <30–35 cm H_2O.

■ RESPIRATORY RATE

The respiratory rate is set by using a dial on the machine. Normally set 12 to 20 breaths per minute. For controlled ventilation, the rate equals the total number of ventilator breaths the patient will receive. For assist control ventilation, the rate represents the minimal number of breaths; depending on the inspiratory sensitivity, the patient may initiate more than the minimal amount. For intermittent mandatory ventilation, the respiratory rate is also the total number of ventilator breaths per minute; however, between the machine breaths, the patient may breathe spontaneously.

■ INITIAL FiO$_2$

Because the mechanical ventilator is responsible for assisting in a patient's breathing, it must then also be able to deliver an adequate amount of oxygen in each breath. The FiO_2 stands for fraction of inspired oxygen, which means the percent of oxygen in each breath that is inspired. (Note that normal room air has ~21% oxygen content). In adult patients who can tolerate higher levels of oxygen for a period of time, the initial FiO_2 may be set at 100% until arterial blood gases can document adequate oxygenation. An FiO_2 of 100% for an extended period of time can be dangerous, but it can protect against hypoxemia from unexpected intubation problems. For infants, and especially in premature infants, avoiding high levels of FiO_2 (>60%) is important.

Adjusting Ventilation/Oxygenation

To increase alveolar ventilation: **Increase rate or increase tidal volume**

Minute Ventilation = Rate × Tidal Volume

To increase oxygenation: Increase FiO_2, or increase PEEP, or increase tidal volume

Oxygenation is improved by increasing MAP and/or FiO_2

Vt   PEEP

To increase ventilation: Increase rate, or increase PIP, or increase inspiratory time, or decrease PEEP (rarely done).

Minute Ventilation = Rate × Tidal Volume

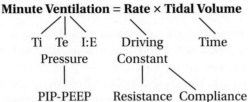

$$\text{Pulse Pressure Variation} = \frac{PP\,max - PP\,min}{\dfrac{PPmix + PP\,min}{2}}$$

To increase oxygenation: Increase FiO_2, or Increase MAP (see below)

Oxygenation is proportional to MAP × FiO_2

This equation assumes pressure vs. time is a square wave.

Ways to increase MAP (Fig. 7.1):

1. Increase PEEP
2. Increase PIP
3. Increase Ti
4. Increase RR
5. Increase flow.

■ SIGHS

An adult patient breathing spontaneously will usually sigh about 6–8 times/hour to prevent microatelectasis, and this has led some to propose that ventilators should deliver 1.5–2 times the amount of the preset tidal volume, 6–8 times/hour to account for the sighs. However, such high quantity of volume delivery requires very high peak pressure that predisposes to barotrauma. Currently, accounting for sighs is not recommended if the patient is receiving 10–12 mL/kg or is on PEEP. If the tidal volume used is lower, the sigh adjustment can be used, as long as the peak and plateau pressures are acceptable.

Sighs are not generally used with ventilation of infants and young children.

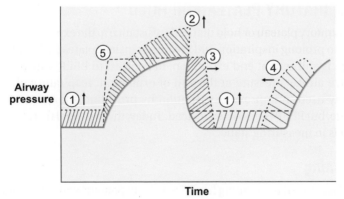

Time

Fig. 7.1: Pressure vs time

Positive End-expiratory Pressure (PEEP)

PEEP is an adjuvant to the mode of ventilation used to help maintain functional residual capacity (FRC). At the end of expiration, the PEEP exerts pressure to oppose passive emptying of the lung and to keep the airway pressure above the atmospheric pressure. The presence of PEEP opens up collapsed or unstable alveoli and increases the FRC and surface area for gas exchange, thus reducing the size of the shunt. Initially, 5 cm H_2O to be set. Excessive PEEP can, however, produce overinflation, which will again decrease compliance. Therefore, it is important to maintain an adequate, but not excessive FRC.

Peak Inspiratory Flow Rate

The peak inspiratory flow rate determines how fast each breath will be delivered to the patient and is therefore a determinant of inspiratory time. The faster the flow rate, the shorter the inspiratory time, and the more breaths that can be delivered per minute. Optimal inspiratory flow time is between 0.5 and 1.5 seconds and is usually achieved with a peak inspiratory flow rate between 40 and 70 L/min.

Sensitivity

Many volume ventilators include a dial labeled 'sensitivity' or 'inspiratory effort'; this setting determines how easily a patient can initiate a machine delivered breath. When the sensitivity dial is turned all the way to the off position, no amount of patient effort will initiate a machine breath, and the machine is in the controlled ventilatory mode. As sensitivity is 'dialed in,' the ventilator changes to the assist control mode, and it becomes much easier for the patient to initiate a machine breath. The sensitivity dial is not calibrated in units, but rather is adjusted by trial and error to the patient's own inspiratory efforts. However, the patient's inspiratory effort will show up as a negative (subatmospheric) deflection on the ventilator's pressure dial, usually 2 to 5 cm H_2O for flow trigger and – 2 to – 5 cm H_2O for pressure trigger.

■ INSPIRATORY PLATEAU OR HOLD

The inspiratory plateau or hold dial adds resistance to the expiratory circuit; the effect is to prolong inspiration and create a transient plateau pressure. Airway pressure is still zero at end expiration, in contrast to PEEP, which maintains a positive airway pressure at the end of expiration. Inspiratory plateau was originally used to improve oxygenation by providing a longer time for gas exchange, but PEEP is now used instead. Today, the principal use of inspiratory plateau is in measuring static.

Positioning

Prone (face down) positioning has been used in patients with ARDS and severe hypoxemia. It improves FRC, drainage of secretions, and ventilation-perfusion matching (efficiency of gas exchange). It may improve oxygenation in >50% of patients, but no survival benefit has been documented.

Sedation

Most intubated patients receive sedation through a continuous infusion or scheduled dosing to help with anxiety or psychological stress. Daily interruption of sedation is commonly helpful to the patient for reorientation and appropriate weaning.

Prophylaxis

- To protect against ventilator-associated pneumonia, patient's bed is often elevated to about 30°.
- Deep vein thrombosis prophylaxis with heparin or sequential compression device is important in older children and adults.
- A histamine receptor (H_2) blocker or proton-pump inhibitor may be used to prevent gastrointestinal bleeding, which has been associated with mechanical ventilation.

■ VARIABLE AND WAVEFORM CONTROL

If any one of the variables and its resultant waveform can be preset, the other two variables become dependent variables. If none can be preset, the ventilator is a time-controller.

Pressure control: Ventilator applies a set pressure with a set waveform. Flow and volume will depend on compliance, resistance and the pressure waveform chosen.

Flow control: Ventilator delivers a set flow rate and pattern independent of patient's respiratory mechanics and hence resultant volume is also constant. Pressure depends on flow rate and pattern, volume or inspiratory time, and respiratory system mechanics.

Volume control: Volume constant but specific measurement of volume distinguishes this from flow control.

Time control: Only inspiratory and expiratory times are controlled.

■ PHASE VARIABLES

Trigger Variables

Variable used to initiate inspiration, for example, fall in airway pressure or loss of basal flow (flow-by-trigger mode). During flow-by, a continuous flow of gas is presented to the patient and is vented in toto through the expiratory tubing unless the patient makes an inspiratory effort. Machine senses any difference in this basal flow and the actual flow in the expiratory limb and this triggers a mechanical breath. The difference required depends on the sensitivity setting, usually 1–3 L/min, pressure may be sensed at ventilator (underestimates effort) or at Y-piece (delays sensing by transducer sited in ventilator) with no real benefit of one over other. For given time delay flow triggering offers no advantage over pressure triggering but proper setting of flow sensitivities can reduce inspiratory work. Degree of change in variable required to trigger inspiration altered by sensitivity setting over sensitive settings will lead to autocycling.

Limit Variables

Flow, volume or pressure can be set to remain constant or reach a maximum, may be same as or unrelated to variable that terminates inspiration (i.e. cycle variable), for example, preset inspiratory pressure is achieved in PSV but usually flow terminates inspiration controversy as to whether flow should be volume or pressure limited; former has advantage of delivery of a known tidal volume but this may be at expense of high peak airway pressure. Latter has less risk of excessive peak pressures but may be fluctuations in VT and minute ventilation due to changes in impedance.

Cycle Variable

Variable used to terminate inspiration. In Europe and Australasia, this is most common. However, in the USA, it is usually volume.

Baseline Variable

Variable that is controlled during expiration pressure is most practical and common.

Conditional Variable

Some ventilators capable of delivering different patterns of pressure, volume and flow depending on what conditional variables are met. For example, in SIMV, a sensed patient effort and an open spontaneous phase ('window') will allow a spontaneous breath, otherwise a mandatory breath is delivered.

■ GOALS

- Volume ventilation modes are generally used for the majority of patients, but pressure ventilation modes should be considered if peak pressures rise over 40 cm H_2O, or if plateau pressures ($P_{plateau}$) rise >30 cm H_2O. The initial VV settings (SIMV or A/C) should be determined based upon the patient's ideal body weight (IBW), body surface area (BSA) and immediate clinical needs.
- Tidal volume (V_T) initial setting of 8 mL/kg IBW while maintaining $P_{plateau}$ <30 cm H_2O and delta P <20 cm H_2O. Necessary adjustments may range

from 4 to 12 mL/kg IBW to maintain the parameters of $P_{plateau}$ <30 cm H_2O and delta P <20 cm H_2O.

Calculate IBW:

- Males IBW (kg) = 50 + 2.3 [height (inches) – 60].
- Females IBW (kg) = 45.5 + 2.3 [height (inches) – 60].
- Minute ventilation (MV) based upon body surface area (BSA) = VE (L/min), to be achieved while maintaining $P_{plateau}$ <30 cm H_2O and delta P <20 cm H_2O.
  - Males = 4.0 × BSA = VE (L/min).
  - Female = 3.5 × BSA = VE (L/min).
  - Calculate BSA: [(Height{in} × Weight {lbs})/(3131)] × 0.5.
- Rate (f): 8 to 26 breaths/minute adjusted to achieve I: E ratio and maintain desired MV, while maintaining $P_{plateau}$ <30 cm H_2O and delta P <20 cm H_2O.
- FiO_2: Initial setting of 0.6 to 1.0 (may be less 0.4 to 1.0 for post anesthesia recovery) until ABG results are obtained.
  - Initial ABG should be obtained 15–45 minutes from start of ventilation
  - Pulse oximetry (SpO_2), and end-tidal CO_2 ($ETCO_2$ optional), should be correlated with initial ABG.
    - Once ABGs are stabilized, continue subsequent patient monitoring with continuous pulse oximetry to maintain SpO_2-desired saturation for patient's category as listed in Table 7.1.
    - Once ABGs are stabilized, continue subsequent patient monitoring with $ETCO_2$ to maintain patient's normal or within the normal $ETCO_2$ range.

  PEEP: Set initial PEEP at 5 cm H_2O, unless otherwise indicated. Higher PEEP levels may be required with acute lung injury (ALI) or acute respiratory distress syndrome (ARDS).

- Pressure support (PS): Set initial PS at 8 to 20 cm H_2O, adjusted to reduce work of breathing, patient fatigue and still support effective ventilation.
- I : E ratio: Adjust to achieve an I : E ratio greater than 1 : 1 (example 1 : 3). The I : E ratio should be optimized to provide optimum mean airway pressure, lung filling, lung emptying (minimizing air-trapping/Auto-PEEP), and patient/ventilator synchrony.

Table 7.1: Saturation levels for patients of different category

Patient Category	pH	PaCO$_2$	PaO$_2$	SpO$_2$
Normal	7.35–7.45	35–45 mm Hg	>80 mm Hg	92–97%
Chronic CO$_2$ retention	7.30–7.45	45–55 mm Hg	55–75 mm Hg	>89%
ALI/ARDS	7.25–7.45	Adjust to pH range	> 60 mm Hg	90–95%

■ PATIENT ASSESSMENT

- Initial ventilator and patient assessment will be performed within 15–45 minutes from setup.
- Assessment will include evaluation of the patient's general appearance, breath sounds, ventilating pressures and volumes, ETCO SpO_2 (optional), SpO_2, ABGs, HR, BP, and other hemodynamic data (if available).
- Adjust the ventilator settings to achieve and maintain acceptable ABG results for the following patient categories (Table 7.1).
- Select the ventilation mode that best meets the ventilatory needs and goals set for the patient, as well as the patient's general comfort.
- For a pH <7.30, evaluate to determine if the cause is respiratory.
  - If appropriate, increase rate to a maximum of 26 breaths/min until pH is >7.30.
  - If further adjustment is needed, incrementally increase VT until PIP = 40 cm H_2O or $P_{plateau}$ = 30 cm H_2O.
  - If adjustments are unable to achieve and maintain desired pH within the maximum parameters (PIP = 40 cm H_2O or $P_{plateau}$ = 30 cm H_2O), consult physician and consider allowing permissive hypercapnia.
- For a pH >7.45, evaluate to determine if the cause is respiratory.
  - If appropriate, reduce rate to a minimum of 8 breaths/minute or until pH is <7.45.
  - After rate is decreased to 8 breaths/minute, if pH is still >7.45, reduce volume to a minimum of 4 mL/kg IBW.
- PaO_2 or SpO_2 should be maintained based on patient's targeted values.
  - Hemoglobin should be checked to ensure the absence of anemia.
  - Hemodynamic data should be checked to ensure adequate perfusion.
  - Consult pulmonologist and consider the ARDS/ALI protocol if:
    - If PaO_2/FiO_2 ratio is <300
    - Settings of FiO_2 = 0.5 and PEEP = 12 cm H_2O are insufficient to maintain appropriate oxygenation.
- Insert A-line if patient requires, or is anticipated to require, more than one ABG per day.
- Change from heat moisture exchange (HME) unit to heated circuit within 48 to 72 hours on ventilator.

■ VENTILATOR SETTINGS AND ALARMS

Troubleshooting and monitoring are important parts of ventilator handling. One needs to be alert and aware of the various alarms as it guides to the proper management of the ventilated patient. For troubleshooting, various types of alarms are there in the ventilator and can be divided into the following types:

- Pressure alarms
- Volume alarms
- Respiratory rate alarms

- PEEP alarms
- Oxygenation alarms.

Low Airway Pressure

If the preset low alarm limit is set at 20 cm H_2O and circuit pressure drops below 20 cm H_2O then alarm will be triggered.

Low Expired Volume Alarm

If the limit is set at 200 mL and expired volume drops below 200 mL then the alarm will be triggered (Table 7.2).

High Airway Pressure

In addition to providing alarm, breath should be pressure limited and thus patient will only receive part of the preset tidal volume.

If pressure limit is repeatedly exceeded, patient should be disconnected and manually ventilated while problem diagnosed. Initial steps are to check for ETT blockage and ventilator malfunction. Other factors to consider are airway resistance, pneumothorax, endobronchial intubation. Normally peak pressure alarm limit is to be set at 40–50 cm H_2O.

Causes of high airway pressures include:

Asynchronous breathing

Low compliance (high peak and plateau pressures):

- Endobronchial intubation
- Pulmonary pathology
- Pneumothorax, atelectasis, ARDS

Table 7.2: Conditions that trigger low pressure or low volume alarm

Conditions	Examples
Loss of circuit pressure	Circuit disconnection ET tube cuff leak Loose circuit connection Loose humidifier connection
Loss of system pressure	Power failure Source gas failure/disconnection
Premature termination of inspiratory phase	Insufficient inspiratory time Excessive expiratory time
Inappropriate ventilator setting	Excessive rate with insufficient peak flow Low pressure alarm set too high Low volume limit set too high
Others	Asynchronous breathing Decreased compliance Increased system resistance

- Hyperinflation: Dynamic, obstructed PEEP valve or expiratory port, excessive PEEP
- Ascites.

Increased system resistance (high peak pressures only):
- Obstruction to flow in circuit, tracheal tube
- Misplaced ETT
- Bronchospasm
- Aspiration/secretions.

No specific airway pressure is guaranteed to exclude risk of barotrauma. In fact main determinant of alveolar overdistension is end-inspiratory volume rather than pressure. However, latter is easier to measure. Plateau pressure is probably a better estimate of peak alveolar pressure than peak airway pressure. Based on animal studies and the knowledge that human lungs are maximally distended at a respiratory system recoil pressure of 35 cm H_2O maintaining plateau pressure <35 recommended. NB if pleural pressure increases (e.g. due to distended abdomen) then plateau pressure will increase without an increase in alveolar pressure.

Inspiratory Flow

Tidal volume/inspiratory time: High flow rates result in high peak airway pressures. May not be of concern provided that most of the added pressure is dissipated across the ETT. Patients may find abrupt bolus of gas uncomfortable and 'fight' ventilator.

Low flows prolong inspiratory time and therefore increase mean airway pressure which may improve oxygenation but at the risk of increasing RV afterload and decreasing RV preload. Also decreases expiratory time and predisposes patient to dynamic hyperinflation. Patient may find flow insufficient and begin to 'lead' the ventilator, sustaining inspiratory effort throughout much of the inspiratory cycle.

Expiratory Flow

Cannot usually be set: Tidal volume/expiratory time. Latter is difference between cycle time and inspiratory time.

Principal ventilator-related determinant of dynamic hyperinflation.

Triggering
Flow/Pressure Triggering

Characterized by sensitivity and responsiveness (delay in providing response) even with modern sensors, there is unavoidable dyssynchrony due to the need for a certain level of insensitivity to prevent artefactual triggering and delay due to opening of demand valves.

Strategies to minimize dyssynchrony:

Ventilators with microprocessor flow controls often have significantly better valve characteristics than those on older generation ventilators.

Continuous flow systems superimposed on demand systems can improve demand system responsiveness in patients with high ventilatory drive (but can reduce sensitivity in patients with very low respiratory drive).

Flow based triggers are more sensitive and responsive to breath triggering.

Small amounts of pressure support usually ventilator's initial flow and may improve response characteristics in CPAP setting.

PEEP below PEEPi may improve triggering in patients with COPD who have an inspiratory threshold load induced by PEEPi.

◼ PATIENT-VENTILATOR DYSSYNCHRONY

Dyssynchrony is the effect of the patients respiratory demands not being appropriately met by the ventilator. The patient has their own idea about how to breathe, and the machinery supporting them, instead of making breathing easier, interferes with respiration and increases the work of breathing.

Why it is Bad?

- The work of breathing increases: Which is what you don't want with mechanical ventilation (remember, the point is to make breathing easier.)
- Thus oxygen demand increases, tachycardia develops, and bad hearts get worse.
- The patient becomes distressed (the experience of being dyssynchronous with one's ventilator resembles asphyxiation)
- The patient begins to cough and/or vomit, which is a sub-optimal level of comfort.
- If there was an intracranial pressure problem, it will get worse with all this straining. Then, your nurse will bolus the patient with a massive amount of propofol, and their blood pressure will plummet, which does nothing to improve their cerebral perfusion.

Causes of Patient-ventilator Dyssynchrony

1. Wasted Effort: Work of breathing increases because...
- The mode is mandatory but the patient is awake and fighting the ventilator
- Effort is wasted when the patient tries to initiate a breath (straining to inhale against a closed inspiratory valve)
- Effort is wasted when the patient tries to terminate a breath (straining to exhale against a closed expiratory valve)
- The trigger is too high and the ventilator fails to supply gas when the patient demands it

- Inadequate level of support: The flow rate is too low and it does not meet patient demand
- The auto-PEEP is too high and the patient expends a lot of effort trying to defeat it
- Auto-triggering: Something other than the patient's respiratory effort initiates a breath, e.g. cardiac oscillations
- Double-triggering, premature breath termination: The ventilator delivers an inappropriately short breath, and the patient wants more air.

2. Wasted effort: The mode of ventilation is mandatory; the patient wants to trigger but cannot (Fig. 7.2):
- The patient tries to breathe, but try as they may the cold indifferent ventilator refuses to help. Instead, it blows air at them when they do not want it, and closes the valve on them when they try to take a breath.
- The solution is progress the patient to a patient-triggered mode of ventilation (e.g. PSV) or to sedate them more, persisting with the same mode but abolishing their respiratory drive.

3. Wasted effort: The trigger is not sensitive enough; the patient wants to trigger but cannot (Fig. 7.3):

The patient tries to breathe, but owing to whatever patient factors they are unable to generate the effort required to deflect 2L/min of flow, or whatever your flow trigger setting is. These minor efforts may be generating some laughably small tidal volumes, but its nothing but dead space. However, it is exhausting to continue in this fashion.

The solution is to adjust the trigger to a lower setting, or sedate the patient and move to a mandatory mode. A decently low flow trigger is 0.8L/min.

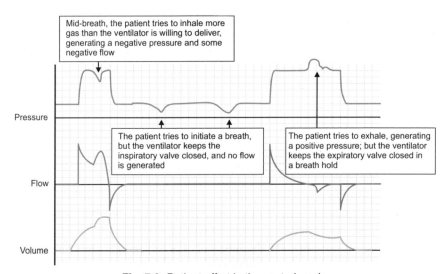

Fig. 7.2: Patient effort in the control mode

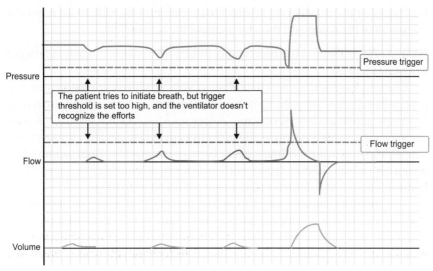

Fig. 7.3: Patient effort in high pressure trigger

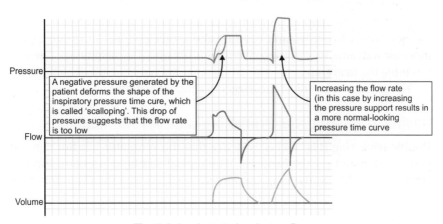

Fig. 7.4: Inadequate inspiratory flow

The Flow Rate is Inadequate to Meet the Inspiratory Flow Demand

In order to breathe comfortably, one needs a steady flow of gas, at a sufficiently high rate.

If the flow demand is not met, the patient makes an effort on top of the ventilator effort.

This appears as a 'scalloping' of the pressure-time curve, which reflects the fact that the patient is generating a negative pressure with their respiratory muscles while the ventilator turbine is generating a positive pressure (Fig. 7.4).

The solution is to increase the flow rate. Typically, a pressure controlled mode (including PSV) delivers maximal flow at the beginning of a breath. In fact, most modern machines do this. In some machines it is possible to adjust the 'ramp' of the flow curve, in which case one may be able to increase the steepness of the ramp and thereby increase the rate of flow.

Wasted effort: There is too much Auto-PEEP and it makes it harder to trigger a breath (Fig. 7.5).

If patient has a serious airflow limitation, with tightly constricted airways and hyperinflated lungs. Suppose, if intrinsic PEEP in these lungs is around 10 cm H_2O. In order to generate a breath, one must defeat one's intrinsic PEEP. Thus, this poor chest must generate a negative pressure of 11 cm H_2O to get any air movement happening (to activate the flow trigger). Perhaps the machine then supports this breath with additional flow, It does not help in terms of reducing respiratory effort, because a breath like this has taken an enormous effort to trigger.

The solution, apparently, is to adjust the PEEP to about 80–90% of the intrinsic PEEP. The additional work of breathing is the result of a pressure difference between the patient and the circuit. Increasing the circuit pressure decreases this pressure difference and therefore decreases the work of breathing.

Auto Triggering: The trigger is too sensitive: Non-respiratory factors triggers the ventilator (Fig. 7.6).

Cardiac contractions cause a small amount of air movement, and in someone with a hyperdynamic ventricle and a sufficiently sensitive flow trigger these air movements can trigger ventilator breaths. The respiratory rate will resemble the heart rate.

The solution is to adjust the trigger to a higher setting.

Double Triggering and Premature Breath Termination

Double triggering (Fig. 7.7) is evidence that the ventilator has not met the patients demand for tidal volume. The typical setting is pressure support ventilation in ARDS- the lung compliance is so low that the expiratory flow

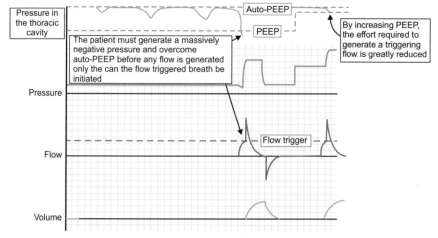

Fig. 7.5: Auto-PEEP

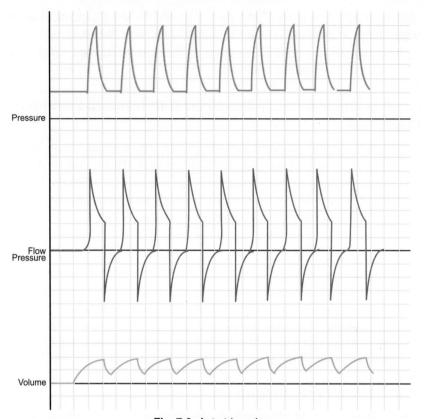

Fig. 7.6: Auto triggering

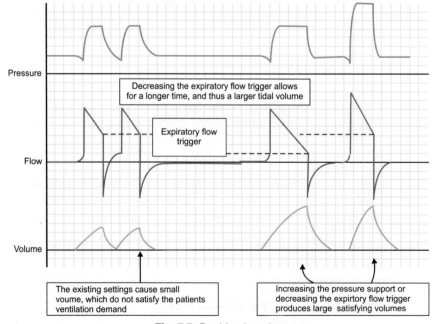

Decreasing the expiratory flow trigger allows for a longer time, and thus a larger tidal volume

Expiratory flow trigger

The existing settings cause small voume, which do not satisfy the patients ventilation demand

Increasing the pressure support or decreasing the expirtory flow trigger produces large satisfying volumes

Fig. 7.7: Double triggering

trigger is reached too soon. That trigger is usually 25–30%. Changing to a lower trigger tends to prolong insufflation time, and increase the tidal volume.

The solution is to adjust the expiratory flow trigger (Cycle off time) until the desired tidal volume is achieved.

There is too much Leak Around the Non-invasive Ventricular (NIV) Mask

- In order to generate the specified pressure, the ventilator continues to deliver flow. With a large leak, this inspiration can be very uncomfortable (as the ventilator delivers 70–80 liters per minute of gas into the patients face). The normal human response to such an experience is to cough, splutter and claw desperately at the mask/nurse/doctor.
- One can adjust the mask, to minimize the leak.
- If this does not work, one can move on to decreasing the level of pressure support (it makes sense that with less pressure there should be less leak).
- If it is not practical to decrease the pressure support level, one can increase the expiratory flow trigger. This will decrease the total inspiratory time, as the machine will cycle to expiration sooner, instead of blowing ridiculously to compensate for a leak. In some ventilators, one can actually adjust the inspiratory time directly.

High Respiratory Rate Alarm

Alarm will be triggered when exceeds the high rate limit. Usually set around 35–40 per minute. This is caused by distressed patient when need to increase rate becomes necessary. It may be cause of pain, anxiety, respiratory muscle fatigue, etc.

Apnea/Low Respiratory Rate Alarm

This alarm is triggered when the total rate drops the low rate limit. For example, disconnection of circuit, patient under respiratory depressants or muscle paralyzed agents used, respiratory center dysfunction, respiratory muscle fatigue.

High PEEP Alarm
Condition of air trapping, insufficient inspiratory flow rate (long I time or short E time).

Low PEEP Alarm
Due to leakage in the circuit or in ET tube cuff.
- Increase in airflow resistance – Patient factors
  - Bronchospasm
  - Coughing

- Patient ventilator asynchrony
- Secretions
1. Decrease in lung or chest wall compliance
   - Tension pneumothorax
   - Atelectasis
   - Pneumonia/ARDS.

■ MONITORING

Monitoring during mechanical ventilation is important from many aspects:
- Patient's clinical status in ICU changes often rapidly and unpredictably.
- Besides the underlying illness, ventilatory settings also affect the patient's status.
- Trends can be established to assess progress or deterioration of patient's condition.

Various parameters that need monitoring during mechanical ventilation include:
- Vital signs
- Heart rate, BP, respiratory rate, temperature
- Chest inspection and auscultation
- Pulse oximetery
- Arterial blood gas
  - Assessment of oxygenation status
  - Assessment of ventilatory status
- End tidal CO_2.
1. Vital signs
   A. Heart rate
      Tachycardia
      1. Pain
      2. Awake state
      3. Hypoxia
      4. Fever
      5. Low cardiac output
      6. Anxiety and stress
      7. Medications (Ionotropes)
   B. Bradycardia
      1. Hypoxia
      2. Vagal stimulation during ET suctioning
      3. Hypothermia
      4. Arrhythmias
      5. Medications (Morphine, Midazolam)
   C. Blood pressure
      Hypertension
      1. Pain
      2. Anxiety and stress
      3. Awake state

    4. Fluid overload

    5. Increased ICT

    6. Drugs (Ionotropes)

  D. Hypotension

    1. Hypoxia

    2. ET suctioning (vagal)

    3. Decreased venous return due to PPV

    4. Hypothermia

    5. Arrhythmias

    6. Drugs (Morphine, midazolam, vasodilators – SNP, NTG)

  E. Temperature

    Hyperthermia

    1. Overheated humidifier

    2. Infection (VAP)

    3. I/V fluids

    4. Sepsis

    5. Drugs

    6. After cardiopulmonary bypass

  F. Hypothermia

    1. No humidification

    2. Low cardiac output states

    3. Drugs (Adrenaline) and toxins

    4. After Cardiopulmonary bypass

    5. Induced

  G. Respiratory rate

    Tachypnea

    1. Pain

    2. Hypoxia/Hypoventilation

    3. Pneumothorax

    4. Hypovolemia

    5. Fever

    6. Low cardiac output

    7. Pulmonary embolism.

2. Chest Inspection and auscultation

  Important to rule out

  1. ET Tube position

  2. Collapse/consolidation

  3. Pneumothorax

  4. Excessive secretions

  5. Wheezing/Crepts

3. Pulse oximetery

  Advantages

  1. Measures the oxygenation status

  2. Noninvasive

3. Serial measurements can help in adjusting ventilatory settings
4. Weaning from the ventilator

Limitations

1. SpO_2 becomes less accurate when SaO_2 falls
2. Inaccurate measurement due to motion artifact
3. Inaccurate measurements due to low perfusion states, dyshemoglobinemias

4. ABG
    A. Assessment of oxygenation
        - PaO_2
        - $A\text{-}aDO_2$
        - PaO_2/FiO_2 ratio
    B. Assessment of ventilation
        - $PaCO_2$
    C. Assessment of the acid-base status
        - Acid base status
        - Anion gap
        - Electrolyte status
        - Sugars and Lactate
        - Hemoglobin/Hematocrit

5. End tidal CO_2

Advantages

- Accidental esophageal intubations
- Endotracheal tube cuff leaks
- Airway obstructions
- Weaning
- Cardiopulmonary resuscitation

Limitations:

- Dead space ventilation
- Positive pressure ventilation
- Decreased cardiac output
- Cardiac arrest.

Circuit compliance: Ventilator circuit is an important interface between the ventilator and patient. Compliance of ventilator circuit should be as low as possible. High circuit compliance leads to a higher compressible volume in the circuit during inspiration and this condition reduces the inspired tidal volume to the patient.

■ CONTRAINDICATIONS

There are no absolute contraindications to performance of a patient-ventilator system check. If disruption of PEEP or FDO_2 results in hypoxemia, bradycardia, or hypotension, portions of the check requiring disconnection of the patient from the ventilator may be contraindicated.

◼ HAZARDS/COMPLICATIONS

Disconnecting the patient from the ventilator during a patient-ventilator system check may result in hypoventilation, hypoxemia, bradycardia, and/ or hypotension.

Prior to disconnection, preoxygenation and hyperventilation may minimize these complications.

When disconnected from the patient, some ventilators generate a high flow through the patient circuit that may aerosolize contaminated condensate, putting both the patient and clinician at risk for nosocomial infection.

◼ LIMITATIONS OF PROCEDURE/VALIDATION OF RESULTS

Measurements of volumes and inspired oxygen concentration are affected by the accuracy and reproducibility of the monitoring instruments.

Volume monitoring devices should be calibrated at regular intervals. Volume monitoring accuracy should be ±10% of the measured volume.

Oxygen analyzers should be calibrated at regular intervals. Oxygen analyzer accuracy should be ±3% of actual concentration.

◼ ASSESSMENT OF NEED

Because of the complexity of mechanical ventilators and the large number of factors that can adversely affect patient-ventilator interaction, routine checks of patient-ventilator system performance are mandatory.

◼ ASSESSMENT OF OUTCOME

Routine patient-ventilator system checks should prevent untoward incidents, warn of impending events, and assure that proper ventilator settings, according to physician's order, are maintained.

◼ ARDS/ALI VENTILATOR PROTOCOL

Scope

This ventilator protocol for acute respiratory distress syndrome (ARDS) and acute lung injury (ALI) centers around tidal volumes based on the patient's IBW, derived from the patient's height.

Exclusion

This ventilator protocol is not appropriate for patients with raised intracranial pressure, spinal cord injury, tricyclic antidepressant overdose, Sickle cell disease, or other conditions where hypercapnea would not be tolerated.

ARDS/ALI Inclusion Criteria

• Choosing to Initiate ARDS/ALI protocol

- In the presence of the following criteria, the ARDS/ALI protocol is recommended.
    - PaO_2/FiO_2 ≤300.
    - Bilateral (patchy, diffuse, or homogeneous) infiltrates consistent with pulmonary edema.
    - No clinical evidence of left atrial hypertension.
- An arterial A-line is strongly recommended due to the anticipation of multiple ABGs.
- Moving from standard AVP to ARDS/ALI ventilator management
    - Select desired ventilator mode.
        - Unless current tidal volume (VT) is lower the 8 mL/kg IBW, set VT to = 8 mL/kg IBW.
        - Reduce VT by 1 mL/kg at intervals ≤2 hours until VT = 6 mL/kg IBW.
        - With a maximum respiratory rate (f) 35, set rate to achieve the required baseline MV before initiating ARDS/ALI protocol.
            - If f >35 is required to achieve the desired MV, consult physician and consider permissive hypercarbia.
            - To maintain a VT >6 mL/kg, the physician must write a medical order in the chart.
        - Adjust VT and f to achieve desired pH and plateau pressures.
        - Set the airway pressure alarm at 35 cm H_2O to limit the maximal airway pressure to 30 cm H_2O.
        - Ensure that autoflow is turned on and turn flow trigger 'on' set to 2 L/min.
        - Set flow rate (inspiratory time, if applicable) to achieve an I : E ratio of 1 : 3 without setting off the pressure limit alarm.
            - If pressure limit alarms, adjust flow rate (inspiratory time, if applicable) to allow time for delivery of the set VT without exceeding the pressure limit (e.g. 1:2, 1:1.5, 1:1).
            - If the I : E adjustment does not resolve the alarm, reduce VT in increments of one mL/kg IBW. This may be repeated every few minutes to a minimal VT of 4 mL/kg IBW. Do not reduce VT below 4 mL/kg. If a VT of 4 mL/kg is necessary, notify the physician.
            - If the patient's requisite VT is less than 6 mL/kg IBW, regular attempts should be made to increase it in increments of 1 mL/kg IBW to achieve 6 mL/kg.
            - If the patient is receiving 6 mL/kg IBW, attempts should be made to reduce the inspiratory time to give an I : E ratio of 1 : 3.
- Oxygenation goal: To keep PaO_2 55–80 mm Hg or SpO_2 88–95%.

Table 7.3: Lower PEEP/higher FiO_2

FiO₂	0.3	0.4	0.4	0.5	0.5	0.6	0.7	0.7	0.8	0.9	0.9	0.9	0.9	1.0
PEEP	5	5	8	8	10	10	10	12	14	14	14	16	18	18-24

Table 7.4: Higher PEEP/lower FIO$_2$

FiO$_2$	0.3	0.3	0.3	0.3	0.3	0.4	0.4	0.5	0.5	0.5	0.8	0.8	0.9	1.0
PEEP	5	8	10	12	14	14	16	16	18	20	22	22	22	24

- – Use a minimum PEEP of 5 cm H$_2$O.
- – Consider the following incremental FiO$_2$/PEEP combinations (not required) to achieve goal. Adjustment to oxygenation can be made on SpO$_2$ alone. It is not necessary to obtain ABGs to change FiO$_2$. However, if a PaO$_2$ is available, it shall supercede the SpO$_2$ (Tables 7.3 and 7.4).
- Plateau pressure goal: To keep P$_{plateau}$ <30 cm H$_2$O
  - – Check P$_{plateau}$ (0.5 second inspiratory pause) at least q4h and after each change in PEEP or VT
  - – Adjustments to achieve desired P$_{plateau}$.
    - - If P$_{plateau}$ >30 cm H$_2$O, decrease VT in 1 mL/kg increments to a minimum of 4 mL/kg.
    - - If P$_{plateau}$ <25 cm H$_2$O and VT <6 mL/kg, increase VT by 1 mL/kg increments until P$_{plateau}$ > 25 cm H$_2$O or VT = 6 mL/kg.
    - - If P$_{plateau}$ <30 and breath stacking or dyssynchrony occurs, consider increasing VT in 1 mL/kg increments to 7 or 8 mL/kg if P$_{plateau}$ remains <30 cm H$_2$O.
- pH goal: To keep pH 7.30–7.45
  - – Acidosis management: (pH <7.30).
    - - If pH 7.15–7.30: Increase f to achieve pH >7.30 or PaCO$_2$ <25 (Maximum set f = 35).
    - - If pH <7.15: Increase f to 35.
    - - If pH remains <7.15, VT may be increased in 1 mL/kg increments until pH >7.15 (P$_{plateau}$ target of 30 may be exceeded). Consider NaHCO$_3$.
  - – Alkalosis management: (pH >7.45).
    - - Decrease vent rate, if possible.
- I : E ratio goal: To achieve a duration of inspiration < duration of expiration.

Recruitment Maneuvers in ARDS

A maneuver designed to open up collapsed alveoli.

De-recruitment can occur with low VT ventilation, inadequate PEEP or use of high FiO$_2$.

During tidal ventilation, three distinct lung zones are produced:
- Dependent: Collapsed throughout tidal ventilation despite high levels of PEEP—chronic collapse injury.
- Intermediate: Collapse and re-expands with each breath—shear induced injury (atelectrauma).

- Least dependent: Regions that remain inflated throughout tidal ventilation and can be overinflated (volutrauma) by VT of >6 mL/kg and plateau pressures exceeding >30–35 cm H_2O.

All of these can increase cytokine release and contribute to risk of multi-organ failure and mortality.

Methods

- 40 cm H_2O of CPAP/PEEP for 40 seconds
- Consecutive sighs/min at a plateau pressure of 45 cm H_2O
- Minutes of peak pressure of 50 cm H_2O and PEEP above upper inflection point
- Obese/trauma patients may require >60–70 cm H_2O
- Stepped increase in pressure.

Advantages

- Improved gas change
- Improved compliance
- Cheap
- Quick
- Easy
- Can reduce conversion to adjuncts: iNOS, prostacycline, extracorporeal membrane oxygenation (ECMO) and oscillation.

Disadvantages

- Requires heavy sedation or paralysis
- Benefit often transient
- Hemodynamic instability (decrease in preload)
- Only some disease states respond
- Hypercapnia
- May worsen oxygenation by shunting blood to poorly aerated regions
- May contribute to overdistension and repeated opening of lung—VILI.

Prone Positioning in Recruitment

This is caused by gravity acting on heart, mediastinal, and abdominal structures to greatly increase $P_{plateau}$ in the dependent regions compared with the nondependent regions. This, in turn, creates much higher critical opening pressures in the dependent vs nondependent regions. When this effect is coupled with gravitational edema effects and the heterogeneous nature of lung disease, the supine lung is in a situation where a uniformly applied airway pressure may be unable to recruit (or prevent derecruitment) of dependent regions without overdistending nondependent regions.

In the prone position, the $P_{plateau}$ gradient between dependent and nondependent regions is greatly reduced because heart, mediastinum, and abdominal contents now 'hang' from the vertebral structures rather than lying upon them. This may be the most important effect of proning because it reduces the disparity between dependent and nondependent lung mechanics, thereby reducing the potential for regional RACE (repetitive alveolar collapse-expansion) injury in dependent regions and regional overdistention injury in nondependent regions. In addition, the prone position has several other effects. First, it stiffens the chest wall, which more evenly distributes gas as regional overdistention is limited. This often improves V/Q. Second, by repositioning abdominal contents, proning allows the diaphragm to assume a more normal curvature, which may improve muscle function.

Applying prone positioning can be done safely and relatively easily if proper planning is done. Special care must be taken to protect various lines and tubes in the turning process. In addition, suctioning may be required immediately upon turning, as secretion dislodgement can be significant. Once prone, pressure injury to facial structures is a concern but can be prevented with good nursing care. The duration of proning is controversial, but logic would suggest that it be maintained as long as patients are at significant risk for VILI.

■ BIBLIOGRAPHY

1. Bates JHT, Milic-Emili J. The flow interruption technique for measuring respiratory resistance. J Crit Care. 1991;6:227-38.
2. Bates JHT, Rossi A, Milic-Emili J. Analysis of the behavior of the respiratory system with constant inspiratory flow. J Appl Physiol. 1985;58:1840-8.
3. Bernasconi M, Ploysongsang Y, Gottfried SB, Milic-Emili J, Rossi A. Respiratory compliance and resistance in mechanically ventilated patients with acute respiratory failure. Intensive Care Medicine. 1988;14:547-53.
4. Broseghini C, Brandolese R, Poggi R, et al. Respiratory resistance and intrinsic positive end-expiratory pressure (PEEP) in patients with the adult respiratory distress syndrome (ARDS). Eur Respir J. 1988;1:726-31.
5. Irwine, Rippe's. Intensive care Medicine 7th edition, Edited by Richard S, Irwin and James M Rippe.
6. Jubran A, Tobin MJ. Passive mechanics of lung and chest wall in patients who failed or succeeded in trials of weaning. Am J Respir Crit Care Med. 1997;155:916-21.
7. Polese G, Rossi A, Appendini L, Brandi G, Bates JHT, and Brandolese R. Partitioning of respiratory mechanics in mechanically ventilated patients. J Appl Physiol. 1991;71:2425-33.
8. Slutsky A, Brochard L. Mechanical Ventilation. 2005;282-3.
9. Tobin MJ. Mechanical ventilation. N Engl J Med. 1994;330:1056-61.
10. Tobin MJ, van de Graaff WB. Monitoring of lung mechanics and work of breathing. In: Tobin MJ, ed. Principles and Practice of Mechanical Ventilation. McGraw Hill, New York, 1994:967-1003.
11. Tuxen D, et al. "Lung recruitment: Who, when and how?" Critical Care and Resuscitation. 2010;12(3):139-41.

HEMODYNAMIC WAVEFORM ANALYSIS

Hemodynamic monitoring includes arterial catheter, central venous catheter and pulmonary catheter. The central venous catheter measures central venous pressure that is right ventricular preload and pulmonary artery catheter measures pulmonary artery pressure that is right ventricular afterload and pulmonary capillary wedge pressure that is left ventricular preload.

◼ ARTERIAL CATHETER

Arterial blood pressure (BP) is most accurately measured invasively through an arterial line. Invasive arterial pressure measurement with intravascular cannulae involves direct measurement of arterial pressure by placing a cannula needle in an artery (usually radial, femoral, dorsalis pedis or brachial). The cannula must be connected to a sterile, fluid-filled system, which is connected to an electronic pressure transducer. The advantage of this system is that pressure is constantly monitored beat-by-beat, and a waveform (a graph of pressure against time) can be displayed. Cannulation for invasive vascular pressure monitoring is infrequently associated with complications such as thrombosis, infection, and bleeding. Patients with invasive arterial monitoring require very close supervision, as there is a danger of severe bleeding if the line becomes disconnected. It is generally reserved for patients where rapid variations in arterial pressure are anticipated.

Indications for Arterial Blood Pressure Measurements

- An arterial line is essential when accuracy in blood pressure measurement is needed or frequency of blood pressure is needed. Some of these are as follows:
    - Gradual or acute hypotension or hemorrhage
    - Circulatory or cardiac arrest
    - Hypertensive crisis
    - Shot regardless of the cause
    - Sepsis or respiratory failure

- Neurologic injury
- Postoperative complications
- When the patient is on vasoactive drugs such as dopamine, adrenaline, noradrenaline, dobutamine, etc.
- The arterial line may also be used when the patient requires frequent ABGs or other blood work.

Limitations of Arterial Lines

- The arterial line pressures should be 5 to 20 mm Hg higher than cuffed measurements.
- If the arterial line pressure is less than cuff pressure reading or >5–20 mm Hg over cuff pressure measurement, one of the following is occurring:
  - If the blood pressure cuff is too small for the patient's arm, then the blood pressure will read high.
  - If the blood pressure cuff is too large for the patient's arm, the blood pressure will read to low.
  - Equipment malfunction.
  - The arterial line might have poor dynamic response.
  - The patient is in severe shock, or hypothermia, which causes vasoconstriction causes lower indirect pressure measurement.
  - The patient might have occlusive peripheral vascular disease.
- The arterial pressure varies in various locations, the more peripheral the arterial line, the higher the systolic and the lower the diastolic, but the main arterial pressure will remain the same. The pedal line will have a higher systolic than the femoral line.

Physiology

The physics of the circulatory system is very complex. It says there are many physical factors that influence arterial pressure. Each of these may in turn be influenced by physiological factors, such as diet, exercise, disease, drugs or alcohol, obesity, excess weight and so-forth.

Some physical factors are:
- *Rate of pumping:* In the circulatory system, this rate is called heart rate, the rate at which blood (the fluid) is pumped by the heart. The volume of blood flow from the heart is called the cardiac output, which is the heart rate (the rate of contraction) multiplied by the stroke volume (the amount of blood pumped out from the heart with each contraction). The higher the heart rate, the higher (potentially, assuming no change in stroke volume) the arterial pressure.
- *Volume of fluid or blood volume:* The amount of blood that is present in the body. The more the blood present in the body, the higher the rate of blood return to the heart and the resulting cardiac output. There is some relationship between dietary salt intake and increased blood volume,

potentially resulting in higher arterial pressure, though this varies with the individual and is highly dependent on autonomic nervous system response.

- *Resistance:* In the circulatory system, this is the resistance of the blood vessels. The higher the resistance, the higher the arterial pressure upstream from the resistance to blood flow. Resistance is related to size (the larger the blood vessel, the lower the resistance), as well as the smoothness of the blood vessel walls. Smoothness is reduced by the buildup of fatty deposits on the arterial walls. Substances called vasoconstrictors can reduce the size of blood vessels, thereby increasing blood pressure. Vasodilators (such as nitroglycerin) increase the size of blood vessels, thereby decreasing arterial pressure.

- *Viscosity, or thickness of the fluid:* If the blood gets thicker, the result is an increase in arterial pressure. Certain medical conditions can change the viscosity of the blood. For instance, low red blood cell concentration and anemia, reduce viscosity, whereas increased red blood cell concentration increases viscosity. Viscosity also increases with blood sugar concentration— visualize pumping syrup. It had been thought that aspirin and related 'blood thinner' drugs decreased the viscosity of blood, but studies found that they act by reducing the tendency of the blood to clot instead.

Pressure in the Arterial System (Fig. 8.1)

- **Arterial pressure pulse:** Two limbs: ascending limb with a rapid rise in pressure occurring during ventricular systole and a descending limb with a rapid decrease in pressure during ventricular diastole. Characteristics include:
  - **Dicrotic notch:** Results from closing of aortic valve at the end of ejection during isovolemic relaxation phase of diastole. Two pulses = dicrotic.

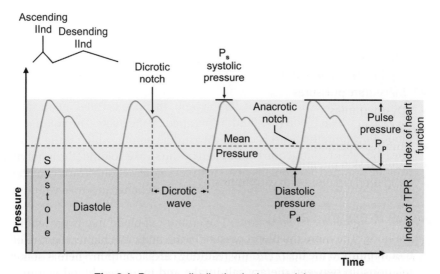

Fig. 8.1: Pressure distribution in the arterial system

– **Systolic pressure:** Peak pressure, P_s.
– **Diastolic pressure:** The pressure at the end of the diastolic wave, P_d.
- **Pulse pressure:** Difference between the systolic and diastolic pressures,
$$P_p = P_s - P_d$$
- **Mean arterial pressure (MAP):** The integrated pressure over the cycle. In practice, MAP is approximated from measures of P_s and P_d by the formula:
$$MAP = P_d + [(P_s - P_d)/3]$$

MAP depends on: (1) Arterial blood volume and; (2) Elastic properties of the arterial wall. Arterial volume, in turn, depends on the rate of blood inflow from the heart (CO) and the rate of outflow of blood from the arteries into the capillaries. If CO exceeds capillaries, arterial volume increases, the vessel walls stretch more, P rises (the ascending limb of the Fig. 8.1). As outflow from the artery exceeds inflow from the heart, the walls contract back, P drops (the descending limb of Fig. 8.1).

Pulse Pressure

The up and down fluctuations of the arterial pressure result from the pulsatile nature of the cardiac output, i.e. the heartbeat. The pulse pressure is determined by the interaction of the stroke volume of the heart, compliance (ability to expand) of the aorta, and the resistance to flow in the arterial tree. By expanding under pressure, the aorta absorbs some of the force of the blood surge from the heart during a heartbeat. In this way, the pulse pressure is reduced from what it would be if the aorta was not compliant.

The pulse pressure can be simply calculated from the difference of the measured systolic and diastolic pressures.
$$P_{pulse} = P_{sys} - P_{dias}$$

Potential Complications

- Hemorrhage
- Air emboli
- Equipment malfunction
- Inaccurate pressures
- Dysrhythmias
- Infections
- Tubing separation
- Altered skin integrity
- Impaired circulation to extremities.

Pulse Pressure Variation

The arterial pulse pressure variation (PPV) induced by mechanical ventilation has been found to be one of the most accurate and specific predictors of fluid responsiveness in patients.

Pulse pressure (PP) is defined as the difference between systolic pressure and diastolic arterial pressure. Maximal PP (PP_{max}) and Minimal PP (PP_{min}) are calculated over a single respiratory cycle. Additionally it has been observed that (PP_{max}) is always featured during the inspiratory period, while (PP_{min}) occurs during the expiratory period.

$$\text{Pulse Pressure Variation} = \frac{PP_{max} - PP_{min}}{\dfrac{PP_{max} + PP_{min}}{2}} \times 100$$

(PP_{max}): Pulse pressure where the pulse pressure is at its maximum.

(PP_{min}): Pulse pressure where the pulse pressure is at its minimum.

It is very important to point out that pulse pressure variation (PPV) is not an indicator of the volume status, nor a marker of cardiac preload, but is an indicator of the position on the Frank–Starling curve to predict fluid responsiveness.

PPV can be utilized to predict the hemodynamic effects of blood loss as well as fluid loading. In other word's a large PPV or an increase in PPV can be interpreted as operating on the steep portion of Frank-Starling curve warning the responsible clinician to counteract further fluid depletion to avoid hemodynamic instability.

Frank-Starling Curve or Cardiac Function Curve

The Frank-Sterling curve or cardiac function curve is a graph illustrating the relationship between the preload (plotted along the x-axis) and the cardiac output or stroke volume. Preload is defined physiologically as the stretch of cardiac muscle fibers before contraction. Right arterial pressure (RAP) or pulmonary capillary wedge pressure (PCWP) are often used as a surrogate measure. From the above mentioned, it should be clear that preload is better represented by mean systemic filling pressure (P_{ms}) subtracted by (RAP):

$$\text{Preload} = P_{ms} - RAP$$

■ CENTRAL VENOUS CATHETER

Central venous catheter is placed into a large vein in the neck (internal jugular vein), chest (subclavian vein) or groin (femoral vein). It is used to administer medication or fluids, obtain blood tests (specifically the "mixed venous oxygen saturation"), and directly obtain cardiovascular measurements such as the central venous pressure. Certain medications, such as inotropes and amiodarone, are preferably given through a central line.

- A catheter (tube) that is passed through a vein to end up in the thoracic (chest) portion of the vena cava (the large vein returning blood to the heart) or in the right atrium of the heart.

Normal CVP Waveforms

The central venous waveform seen on the monitor reflects the events of cardiac contraction; the central venous catheter 'sees' these slight variations in pressure that occur during the cardiac cycle and transmits them as a characteristic waveform. There are three positive waves (a, c, and v) and two negative waves (x and y), and these correlate with different phases of the cardiac cycle and EKG.

Normal CVP can be measured from two points of reference:
- Sternum: 0–14 cm H_2O
- Midaxillary line: 8–15 cm H_2O.

CVP can be measured by connecting the patient's central venous catheter to a special infusion set, which is connected to a small diameter water column. If the water column is calibrated properly, the height of the column indicates the CVP.

In most intensive care units, facilities are available to measure CVP continuously.

Normal values are 5–10 cm H_2O.

▇ PATHOLOGIC CVP WAVEFORMS (FIG. 8.2)

Variations on the normal central venous waveform can provide information about cardiac pathology. For example:
- *In atrial fibrillation,* a waves will be absent, and in *atrioventricular* disassociation, a waves will be dramatically increased ("cannon waves") as the atrium contracts against a closed tricuspid valve.
- *In tricuspid regurgitation,* the c wave and x descent will be replaced by a large positive wave of regurgitation as the blood flows back into the right atrium during ventricular contraction. This can elevate the mean central venous pressure, but it is not an accurate measurement. A better way of estimating CVP in this case would be to look at the pressure between the regurgitation waves for a more accurate mean.
- *In cardiac tamponade,* all pressure will be elevated, and the y descent will be nearly absent.

Factors which increase CVP include:
- Hypervolemia
- Forced exhalation
- Tension pneumothorax
- Heart failure
- PA stenosis
- Positive pressure breathing, straining
- Pleural effusion
- Decreased cardiac output
- Cardiac tamponade
- Pulmonary hypertension
- Pulmonary embolism.

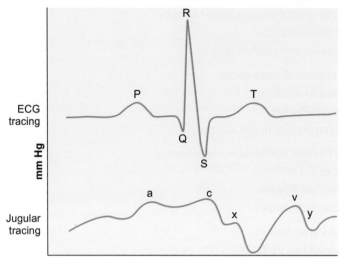

Fig. 8.2: Graph representing different pathological CVP waveforms

+ a wave: This wave is due to the increased atrial pressure during right atrial contraction. It correlates with the P wave on an EKG.

+ c wave: This wave is caused by a slight elevation of the tricuspid valve into the right atrium during early ventricular contraction. It correlates with the end of the QRS segment on an EKG.

− x descent: This wave is probably caused by the downward movement of the ventricle during systolic contraction. It occurs before the T wave on an EKG.

+ v wave: This wave arises from the pressure produced when the blood filling the right atrium comes up against a closed tricuspid valve. It occurs as the T wave is ending on an EKG.

− y descent: This wave is produced by the tricuspid valve opening in diastole with blood flowing into the right ventricle. It occurs before the P wave on an EKG.

Factors which decrease CVP include:

- Hypovolemia from hemorrhage, fluid shift and dehydration
- Deep inhalation
- Distributive shock.

Technical factors include:

- Patient positioning
- Level of transducer
- Inconsistent measurement technique with water manometer
- Inappropriate central venous catheter placement
- Against vessel wall
- In heart.

Physiologic factors include:

- Changes in intrathoracic pressure
- Respiration
- Positive end-expiratory pressure during mechanical ventilation
- Abdominal hypertension.

Changes in central venous blood volume:
• Total blood volume
• Venous return/cardiac output.

Cardiac rhythm disturbances:
• Junctional rhythm
• Atrial fibrillation
• Atrioventricular dissociation.

Changes in right ventricular compliance:
• Myocardial stiffness
• Pericardial disease
• Cardiac tamponade.

Tricuspid valve disease:
• Tricuspid regurgitation
• Tricuspid stenosis.

■ PULMONARY ARTERY CATHETER

Settings in Which to Use a Pulmonary Artery Catheter

Central venous catheters can assess cardiac function fairly accurately in a healthy patient with concordant right and left heart function, however, when there exists a dissociation between right and left heart function, a pulmonary artery catheter is necessary to 'look' at left sided cardiac function alone. Besides providing fundamental hemodynamic information for a patient, pulmonary artery catheters can be used for all of the following:

General indications are:
• Management of complicated myocardial infarction
  – Hypovolemia vs cardiogenic shock
  – Ventricular septal rupture (VSR) vs acute mitral regurgitation
  – Severe left ventricular failure
  – Right ventricular infarction
  – Unstable angina
  – Refractory ventricular tachycardia.
• Assessment of respiratory distress
  – Cardiogenic vs noncardiogenic pulmonary edema
  – Primary vs secondary pulmonary hypertension.
• Assessment of type of shock
• Assessment of therapy
  – Afterload reduction
  – Vasopressors
  – Beta-blockers
  – Intra-aortic balloon counterpulsation.
•

- Assessment of fluid requirement in critically ill patients
  - Hemorrhage
  - Sepsis
  - Acute renal failure
  - Burns.
- Management of postoperative open heart surgical patients
- Assessment of valvular heart disease
- Assessment of cardiac tamponade/constriction
  - Measure cardiac output via the thermodilution method
  - Assess the volume status of a patient
  - Measure mixed venous oxygen content
  - Derive hemodynamic indices
  - Detect venous air embolism.

  Some specialized PACs can also be utilized in the following:
- Allow drug infusions
- Perform angiography
- Obtain intracardiac EKGs
- Perform atrial and ventricular pacing
- Calculate ejection fraction.

Contraindications to pulmonary artery catheter use: Relative contraindications include Wolff-Parkinson-White syndrome and Ebstein's malformations (given that PACs can induce arrhythmias) and complete left bundle branch block (due to the risk of complete heart block).

Physiology

As we have learned, pulmonary artery catheters (PACs) can assist physicians caring for patients undergoing an array of procedures. However, in anesthesiology, one of the most important functions of a PAC is to provide accurate, precise, frequent information regarding the cardiac function and hemodynamic state of a patient undergoing a surgical procedure. Two measurements obtained with a PAC which are most helpful, and which can enable the anesthesiologist to calculate other aspects of cardiac function are:
- Pulmonary capillary wedge pressure
- Cardiac output.

Pulmonary Capillary Wedge Pressure

Pulmonary capillary occlusion pressure (PCOP, also called pulmonary artery wedge pressure) is measured when the balloon on the tip of the PAC is inflated within a pulmonary artery. This enables the catheter to obtain an indirect measurement of left ventricular end diastolic pressure (normal range: 6–12 mm Hg).

How does it do this?

Analogy: Imagine a small creek. First standing on the edge of the creek and looking at the water, it is difficult to know how that water is flowing, and what may be occurring further downstream that you cannot see. Imagine then that you could instantly place a temporary dam in the creek. Now, by looking at what the water does on the downsteam side of the dam, you can infer what may be going on further down the creek. If the water quickly drops, then you can surmise that the creek is flowing rapidly and nothing is obstructing its path. However, if the water slowly drops, you could guess that something must be holding up the flow of the creek—perhaps the water is simply flowing slowly, or perhaps a beaver has made his home downstream!

When the balloon is inflated, the pressure monitor at the tip of the catheter is shielded from all right sided pressures, and 'sees' only what is happening 'downstream', namely the pressures from the left atrium and left ventricle.

So, in cases where left and right cardiac functions are discordant, PCOP is a valuable tool with which to measure left-sided heart functions by way of filling pressures independently from right-sided cardiac function.

Limitations to pulmonary capillary occlusion pressure

The assertion that PCOP is an accurate reflection of left cardiac function is based on certain assumptions regarding the patient's cardiopulmonary function. PCWP is accurate as a predictor of left ventricular end diastolic volume only if the vascular system between the catheter tip and the left ventricle is free from any pathology, which could influence the pressures detected by the catheter. Typically, pulmonary artery wedge pressures are equivalent to left ventricular end diastolic volumes over a range of 5–25 mm Hg.

- Instances where PCWP overestimates LVED pressure include those which create an interfering pressure gradient, but do not represent the function of the left ventricle:
  - Chronic mitral stenosis
  - PEEP (Positive end expiration pressure ventilation)
  - Left atrial myxoma
  - Pulmonary hypertension.
- Instances where PCWP underestimates LVED pressure include those that increase the pressure in the left ventricle, which the catheter tip cannot detect:
  - Stiff left ventricle
  - LVED pressure >25 mm Hg
  - Aortic insufficiency.

Complications with PA catheters

- Infection and sepsis are serious problems associated with PA catheters.
  - Careful surgical asepsis for insertion and maintenance of the catheter and attached tubing is mandatory.
  - Flush bag, pressure tubing, transducer, and stopcock should be changed every 96 hours.

- Air embolus is another risk associated with PA catheters.

- Pulmonary infarction or PA rupture from: (1) balloon rupture, releasing air and fragments that could embolize; (2) prolonged balloon inflation obstructing blood flow; (3) catheter advancing into a wedge position, obstructing blood flow; and (4) thrombus formation and embolization.

  – Balloon must never be inflated beyond the balloon's capacity (usually 1 to 1.5 mL of air) and must not be left inflated for more than four breaths (except during insertion) or 8 to 15 seconds.

  – PA pressure waveforms are monitored continuously for evidence of catheter occlusion, dislocation, or spontaneous wedging.

  – PA catheter is continuously flushed with a slow infusion of heparinized (unless contraindicated) saline solution.

- Ventricular dysrhythmias can occur during PA catheter insertion or removal or if the tip migrates back from the PA to the right ventricle and irritates the ventricular wall.

- The nurse may observe that the PA catheter cannot be wedged and may need to be repositioned by the clinician.

■ PULSE OXIMETRY (FIG. 8.3)

Pulse oximetry is a simple noninvasive method of monitoring the percentage of hemoglobin (Hb), which is saturated with oxygen. The pulse oximeter consists of a probe attached to the patient's finger or ear lobe, which is linked to a computerized unit. The unit displays the percentage of Hb saturated with oxygen together with an audible signal for each pulse beat, a calculated heart rate and in some models, a graphical display of the blood flow past the probe. Audible alarms, which can be programmed by the user are provided. An oximeter detects hypoxia before the patient becomes clinically cyanosed.

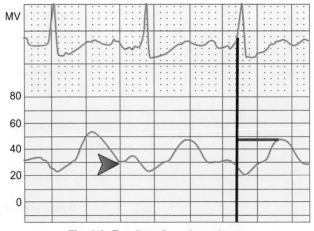

Fig. 8.3: Reading of a pulse oximeter

How does an oximeter work?

A source of light originates from the probe at two wavelengths (650 nm and 805 nm). The light is partly absorbed by hemoglobin, by amounts which differ depending on whether it is saturated or desaturated with oxygen. By calculating the absorption at the two wavelengths, the processor can compute the proportion of hemoglobin which is oxygenated. The oximeter is dependent on a pulsatile flow and produces a graph of the quality of flow. Where flow is sluggish (e.g. hypovolemia or vasoconstriction), the pulse oximeter may be unable to function. The computer within the oximeter is capable of distinguishing pulsatile flow from other more static signals (such as tissue or venous signals) to display only the arterial flow.

Calibration and performance

Oximeters are calibrated during manufacture and automatically check their internal circuits when they are turned on. They are accurate in the range of oxygen saturations of 70 to 100% ($\pm$ 2%), but less accurate under 70%. The pitch of the audible pulse signal falls with reducing values of saturation.

The size of the pulse wave (related to flow) is displayed graphically (Fig. 8.4). Some models automatically increase the gain of the display when the flow decreases and in these the display may prove misleading. The alarms usually respond to a slow or fast pulse rate or an oxygen saturation below 90%. At this level, there is a marked fall in PaO_2, representing serious hypoxia.

Pulse oximeters may be used in a variety of situations but are of particular value for monitoring oxygenation and pulse rates throughout ICU/anesthesia. They are also widely used during the recovery phase. The oxygen saturation should always be above 92%. In patients with long-standing respiratory disease, or those with cyanotic congenital heart disease readings may be lower and reflect the severity of the underlying disease.

In intensive care, oximeters are used extensively during mechanical ventilation and frequently detect problems with oxygenation before they are

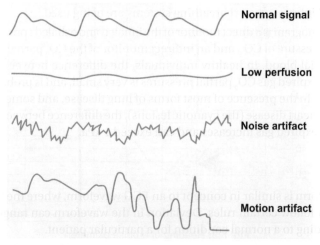

Normal signal

Low perfusion

Noise artifact

Motion artifact

Fig. 8.4: Different graphical displays of flow-related pulse wave

noticed clinically. They are used as a guide for weaning from ventilation and also to help assess whether a patient's oxygen therapy is adequate. In some hospitals, oximeters are used on the wards and in casualty departments. When patients are sedated for procedures such as endoscopy, oximetry has been shown to increase safety by alerting the staff to unexpected hypoxia.

Limitations and Advancements

Oximetry is not a complete measure of respiratory sufficiency. A patient suffering from hypoventilation (poor gas exchange in the lungs) given 100% oxygen can have excellent blood oxygen levels while still suffering from respiratory acidosis due to excessive carbon dioxide.

It is also not a complete measure of circulatory sufficiency. If there is insufficient blood flow or insufficient hemoglobin in the blood (anemia), tissues can suffer hypoxia despite high oxygen saturation in the blood that does arrive.

A higher level of methemoglobin will tend to cause a pulse oximeter to read closer to 85% regardless of the true level of oxygen saturation. It also should be noted that the inability of two-wavelength saturation level measurement devices to distinguish carboxyhemoglobin due to carbon monoxide inhalation from oxyhemoglobin must be taken into account when diagnosing a patient in emergency rescue.

■ CAPNOGRAPHY (FIGS 8.5 TO 8.9)

Capnography is the monitoring of the concentration or partial pressure of carbon dioxide (CO_2) in the respiratory gases. Its main development has been as a monitoring tool for use during anesthesia and intensive care. It is usually presented as a graph of expiratory CO_2 plotted against time, or, less commonly, but more usefully, expired volume. The plot may also show the inspired CO_2, which is of interest when rebreathing systems are being used.

The capnogram is a direct monitor of the inhaled and exhaled concentration or partial pressure of CO_2, and an indirect monitor of the CO_2 partial pressure in the arterial blood. In healthy individuals, the difference between arterial blood and expired gas CO_2 partial pressures is very small, and is probably zero in children. In the presence of most forms of lung disease, and some forms of congenital heart disease (the cyanotic lesions), the difference between arterial blood and expired gas increases and can exceed 1 kPa.

Understanding the Capnograph

This waveform is similar in concept to an ECG waveform, where the 'normal' wave must follow certain rules. Deviation in the waveform can range from a critical finding to a normal condition for a particular patient.

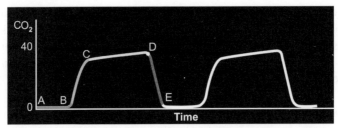

Fig. 8.5: A normal capnography waveform

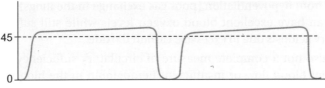

Fig. 8.6: Hypoventilation

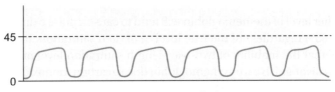

Fig. 8.7: Hyperventilation

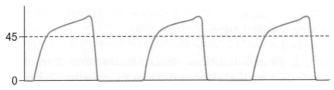

Fig. 8.8: Partial lower airway obstruction

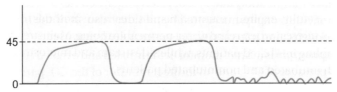

Fig. 8.9: Esophageal intubation, but also represents a dislodged ET tube, a plug in an ET tube or a mechanical failure of the capnographer

The cwapnography waveform represents various phases of inhalation and exhalation and is divided into four phases (I, II, III and inspiration). Each complex has lettering similar to the PQRST labeling associated with an ECG (Fig. 8.1). Phase I is the period between A and B and represents late phase inspiration and the beginning of exhalation. In this period, the dead air space, which typically has no substantial amount of CO_2, is emptied. Phase II is the period between B and C and represents continued exhalation of the air from the remaining dead space and proximal alveoli. This phase should rise sharply as the CO_2 content increases. Phase III is the period between C and D, which reflects airflow from the alveoli during uniform ventilation, where there is nearly a constant CO_2 level. This phase is also known as the respiratory plateau. Point D is actually considered the end-tidal point of CO_2 monitoring in which the highest concentration of carbon dioxide is typically measured. Phase IV is the last phase that identifies inspiration and is displayed from D to E. The waveform should exhibit a rapid downward slope drop as the patient inhales or is ventilated and oxygen-rich air rushes into the respiratory tract. This phase should terminate at a baseline of zero.

Indications for the Use of Capnography

One clear indication is to confirm and continuously monitor endotracheal tube placement. Moving the patient has the potential to dislodge a properly placed tube. Capnography provides excellent continuous visual waveforms and a near immediate response to dislodgment of the tube. Immediately after placement of the endotracheal tube, employ the end-tidal CO_2 monitor as a secondary confirmation method and as a monitoring device for continuous proper tube placement.

Mainstream vs Sidestream

Capnography must use exhaled gas to determine the amount of CO_2 in each breath. This is accomplished through one of three different technologies: mainstream, sidestream or microstream. Mainstream samples exhale gases directly through the endotracheal tube or a mouthpiece attachment. Sidestream and microstream are similar in that they draw a sample of gas into a small tube attached to the sampling device (endotracheal tube or nasal cannula) for analysis. One concern of sidestream is that the amount of sample withdrawn may possibly affect tidal volume in the airway circuit when using a ventilator. Additionally, microstream and sidestream methods must use filters, water condensation traps and water-permeable tubing. Mainstream works well for sampling intubated patients, while sidestream and microstream work well for both intubated and nonintubated patients.

■ CARDIAC OUTPUT

Cardiac output is the volume of blood pumped by the heart per minute and is the product of the amount of blood per heart beat (called the stroke volume) times the number of heart beats in a minute (heart rate).

Stroke volume (SV) = EDV – ESV
Ejection fraction (EF) = (SV/EDV) × 100%
Cardiac output (Q) = SV × HR
Cardiac index (CI) = Q/Body surface area (BSA) = SV × HR/BSA
HR is heart rate, expressed as BPM (beats per minute)
BSA is body surface area in square meters.

Derived hemodynamic data:

Cardiac index (CI): CO/BSA = 2.5–4.0 L/min/m^2

Stroke volume (SV): CO/HR × 1000 = 60–100 mL/beat

Increased SV is associated with bradycardia and positive inotropic agents, which increase contractility.

Stroke volume index (SVI): CI/HR × 1000 = 33–47 mL/m^2/beat

Systemic vascular resistance (SVR): 80 × (MAP – RAP)/CO = 1000–1500 dyne s/cm^5.

Systemic vascular resistance (SVR) represents the load applied to the left ventricular muscle during ejection.

Systemic vascular resistance index (SVRI): 80 × (MAP – RAP)/CI = 1970–2390 dyne s/cm^5/m^2.

Pulmonary vascular resistance (PVR): 80 × (MPAP – PAWP)/CO = <250 dyne s/cm^5.

PVR is an index of the resistance offered by the pulmonary capillaries to the systolic effort of the right ventricle.

Pulmonary vascular resistance index (PVRI): 80 × (MPAP – PAWP)/CI = 255–285 dyne s/cm^5/m^2.

There are a number of clinical methods for measurement of Q ranging from direct intracardiac catheterization to noninvasive measurement of the arterial pulse. Each method has unique strengths and weaknesses and relative comparison is limited by the absence of a widely accepted 'gold standard' measurement. Q can also be affected significantly by the phase of respiration; intrathoracic pressure changes influence diastolic filling and, therefore, Q. This is especially important during mechanical ventilation, where Q can vary by up to 50% across a single respiratory cycle. Q should, therefore, be measured at evenly spaced points over a single cycle or averaged over several cycles.

■ FICK PRINCIPLE (FIG. 8.10)

Definition

A generalization in physiology, which states that blood flow is proportional to the difference in concentration of a substance in the blood as it enters and leaves an organ and which is used to determine cardiac output from the difference in oxygen concentration in blood before it enters and after it leaves the lungs and from the rate at which oxygen is consumed—also called Fick method.

Principle

VO_2, the oxygen consumption, is simply the difference between the inspired and expired O_2. You can measure it with an exhaled gas collection bag. Conventionally, resting metabolic consumption of oxygen is 3.5 mL of O_2 per kg per minute, or 25 mL O_2 per square meter of body surface area per minute.

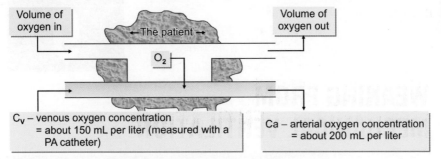

Fig. 8.10: Oxygen extraction by Fick principle

Fick teaches us that VO_2 (oxygen extraction) is determined by the following equation:

$VO_2 = (CO \times C_a) - (CO \times C_v)$; where CO = cardiac output in L/min.

We can rearrange that to form an equation, which calculates cardiac output on the basis of oxygen extraction:

$$CO = \frac{VO_2}{C_a - C_v}$$

So, in a normal person, with a body surface area of 2 m² and thus with a VO_2 of 250 mL per minute,

$$
\begin{aligned}
CO &= 250 \text{ mL}/(200{-}150 \text{ mL}) \\
&= 250/50 \\
&= 5 \text{ L/min.}
\end{aligned}
$$

■ BIBLIOGRAPHY

1. Berne RM, Levy MN. Cardiovascular physiology. 7th Ed Mosby, 1997.
2. Braunwald E (Editor). Heart Disease: A Textbook of Cardiovascular Medicine. 5th Ed. WB Saunders, 1997.
3. Fick A. Uber die messung des Blutquantums in den Hertzvent rikeln. Sitzber Physik Med Ges Wurzburg. 1870;36.
4. Johnston IG, Jane R, Fraser JF, Kruger P, Hickling K. Survey of intensive care nurses' knowledge relating to the pulmonary artery catheter. Anaesth Intensive Care. 2004;32:564-8.
5. Rowell LB. Human Cardiovascular Control. Oxford University press, 1993.
6. Shah MR, Hasselblad V, Stevenson LW, Binanay C, O'Connor CM, Sopko G, et al. Impacts of the Pulmonary Artery Catheter in Critically Ill Patients: Meta-analysis of Randomized Trials. J Am Med Ass. 2005;294:1634-70.
7. Stevenson LW and the ESCAPE investigators and ESCAPE coordinators. Evaluation Study of Congestive Heart Failure and Pulmonary Artery Catheterization Effectiveness. J Am Med Ass. 2005;294:1625-33.

WEANING FROM MECHANICAL VENTILATION

■ INTRODUCTION

Weaning is a process of withdrawing mechanical ventilatory support.

■ WEANING SUCCESS

It is defined as effective spontaneous breathing without any mechanical assistance for 24 hours or more. Supplemented oxygen, bronchodilator, PS/CPAP is often used to support and maintain adequate spontaneous ventilation and oxygenation.

■ WEANING FAILURE

Whenever a patient is placed back on the ventilator, weaning attempt has failed in one form or another. Signs of worsening clinical conditions include diaphoresis, increased respiratory effort, tachycardia, arrhythmias, and hypotension.

Conditions that may Cause Successful Weaning Failure

- Patient/Pathological: Fever, infection renal failure, sepsis.
- Cardiac/Circulatory: Arrhythmias, BP, CO, fluid balance.
- Acid-base/Electrolyte: Acid-base imbalance, electrolyte disturbances, anemia.

Mechanical ventilation refers to the use of life-support technology to perform the work of breathing for patients who are unable to do so on their own, and the majority of critically ill patients in most modern intensive care units (ICUs) require a period of this treatment. The use of prolonged mechanical ventilation is associated with nosocomial pneumonia, cardiac-associated morbidity, and death.

Discontinuing mechanical ventilation prematurely, however, may result in reintubation, which is associated with similar complications to prolonged ventilation. Thus, optimal weaning minimizing the duration of mechanical ventilation without incurring substantial risk of reintubation, and thus preventing important complications plays a crucial role in the management of critically ill patients.

The following key questions defined the parameters of the investigation:

1. When should weaning be initiated?
2. What criteria should be used to initiate the weaning process?
3. What are the most effective methods of weaning from mechanical ventilation?
4. What are the optimal roles of non-physician healthcare professionals in facilitating safe and expeditious weaning?
5. What is the value of clinical practice algorithms and computers in expediting weaning?

■ WEANING CRITERIA (TABLE 9.1)

Weaning criteria are used to assess the patient trial weaning is successful if patient meets most of the used criteria.

Ventilatory criteria: Ventilatory status of the patients to be assessed for weaning and outcome.

$PaCO_2$ (Partial pressure of CO_2) in the arterial blood is the most reliable indicator of the patient's ventilatory status. $PaCO_2$ should be less than 50 mm Hg. The normal $PaCO_2$ level should be 35–45 mm Hg and pH should be between 7.35 and 7.45. In COPD patients $PaCO_2$ is slightly higher and pH on slightly lower side.

Vital capacity (VC) and spontaneous tidal volume (Vt): The minimum VC and spontaneous Vt should be 10–15 mL/kg of body weight and 5–8 mL/kg of body weight respectively.

Spontaneous respiratory rate (RR): It should be less than 30–34 breaths while corresponding $PaCO_2$ should be less than 50 mm Hg. If RR is increased after disconnection of ventilator, it is rarely associated with weaning failure.

Table 9.1: Signs of weaning failure

Indicator	Examples
Blood gases	Increased $PaCO_2$ more than 50 mm Hg Decreased pH Decreased SpO_2 less than 85%
Respiratory parameters	Decreased Vt less than 250 mL Increased RR more than 35–40/min Decreased static compliance less than 30 mL/cm H_2O Increased RSBI more than 105 cycles/liter
Vital signs	Increasing/Decreasing BP Increasing HR Abnormal ECG (Presence of arrhythmias)

Minute volume (MV): Patient's MV should be 10–15 liter for successful weaning outcome.

Oxygenation criteria: Weaning success will be more if the patient is adequately oxygenated. PaO_2 greater than 60 mm Hg corresponds to an SaO_2 at about 92% an FiO_2 of 40% or less.

Pulmonary measurements: Airway resistance, compliance and dead space to Vt ratio are three measurements that are not dependent on a patient's effort. They are used to indicate the amount of pulmonary workload that is needed to support the spontaneous ventilation. In general, low compliance, high airway resistance and high Vd/Vt ratio all indicate to an increased workload, this may interrupt the weaning process.

How to Calculate PaO_2/FiO_2 Ratio

You take the PaO_2 value from the arterial blood gas (let's say it is 100) and you take the FiO_2 from the ventilator (let's say it is 30%) and then you divide the PaO_2 by FiO_2. Now, 30% = 0.3

So PaO_2/FiO_2 ratio would be 100/0.3 = 333 mm Hg.

If it is 300 or below, would think of ALI.

If it is 200 or below, would think of ARDS.

Protocols and Beyond

Weaning the patient from mechanical ventilation can be frustrating and potentially dangerous. There is often confusion about whether the patient is ready to wean and what is the best method to use in the weaning process. Some of the confusion may result from labeling weaning as an event rather than a process. A more useful success is to consider weaning as titration from mechanical ventilation.

To be effective, titration from mechanical ventilation must be:
- Well-planned
- Patient specific
- Implemented with a team approach
- Have specific and measurable goals.

Assess the Patient's Readiness to Wean

There are five major reasons why patients have difficulty with the titration process. These are:

1. The primary respiratory problem remains unresolved
2. The patient has excessive secretions
3. Nutrition has not been maintained
4. Electrolytes are abnormal
5. The patient has auto-PEEP.

■ METHOD OF WEANING

Before titration is begun, the method for weaning should be considered. Titration should be patient-specific, taking into consideration the patient's primary illness, length of ventilatory support, and other confounding medical conditions. Four major modes of titration are commonly used:
1. SIMV
2. T-piece
3. CPAP/BiPAP
4. Pressure support.

Synchronized intermittent mandatory ventilation (SIMV) is most useful in patients in whom a rapid change in intrathoracic pressure would cause hemodynamic instability. SIMV allows for gradual change from positive pressure ventilation to spontaneous (negative) pressure ventilation. SIMV allows patient to breathe spontaneously in between control breaths with or without pressure support.

Pressure support (PS) provides inspiratory support to help overcome airway resistance and decrease respiratory muscle fatigue. PS may be helpful in retraining respiratory muscles in a patient who has been on long-term ventilation.

Continuous positive airway pressure (CPAP) and bi-level positive airway pressure (BiPAP) are effective in providing expiratory support to maintain oxygenation and prevent alveolar collapse during titration. They also maintain a level of positive intrathoracic pressure that may be helpful in the cardiovascular patient. BiPAP adds inspiratory support to CPAP, which may be helpful in preventing respiratory muscle fatigue.

T-piece trials are usually used during weaning the patient from ventilator. During this period, we can give intermittent T-piece trials and we can observe the patients breathing pattern. T-piece trials may work best in the patient with COPD or other chronic lung conditions that cause respiratory muscle weakness.

Research does not support the use of any one of these methods for all patients. The choice should be patient specific based on the patient's primary pathology, previous cardiovascular and respiratory disease, and tolerance of the method chosen.

Before titration can begin, the patient should be 'packed up' by weaning to minimal support. Optimally, the patient would be on <40% FiO_2, <8 cm H_2O PEEP, and should be taking spontaneous breaths. At this time, the patient's hemodynamics must be evaluated carefully, and diuresis may be helpful to prevent cardiac congestion with intrathoracic pressure changes.

Usually sedation is discontinued when weaning is begun. This often results in a wide-awake, frightened patient who is 'bucking' the ventilator and pulling on the tube. Most patients say that mechanical ventilation is extremely uncomfortable, and moderately painful, therefore, it would make sense to manage the patient's pain and discomfort for the best outcome. A well-planned strategy would include sedation, pain control, and anxiety control in modest amounts to keep the patient comfortable but conscious during weaning. Use of a sedation protocol may be helpful in providing a standardized approach.

Once the previous planning has been done, the patient should be physically and psychologically prepared for weaning. Check the patient's nutritional status with the help of a dietitian. Assure adequate rest the night before weaning. Keep in mind that the average ICU patient sleeps about two hours a day. Your patient may need sedation overnight with a short-acting medication such as propofol.

Shortly before weaning, suction the patient and allow several minutes for his oxygenation to return to normal. Preoxygenate with 100% during suctioning.

Go

Start the weaning trial at the appropriate time of day. Mornings can be difficult for several reasons:

- Preload may be higher in the morning
- Respiratory function is worse in the morning (circadian effects)
- Interruptions are more frequent (rounds, shift change, etc.)

Therefore, if weaning is to begin early in the day, be aware of these variables and try to minimize their effects on the patient by:

- Assessing hemodynamics and the need for diuresis
- Recognizing that some patients may have better respiratory function in the afternoon
- Limiting interruptions, examinations, and procedures during weaning.

■ RAPID WEANING

The rapid-wean approach is generally reserved for patients without pulmonary disease who were placed on mechanical ventilation to treat an acute or postoperative condition that is expected to respond quickly to treatment.

These three considerations are key to success of rapid weaning:

1. Choosing appropriate patients to wean quickly: The rapid-weaning protocol should detail, which patients are candidates, based on hemodynamic, neurologic, and respiratory parameters. (For details, see Sample rapid-weaning protocol). A key feature to weaning is the spontaneous breathing trial. A patient who has met all the readiness criteria is placed on a T-piece. A low level of PEEP (5 cm H_2O) and low levels of pressure support (8 cm H_2O) may be used during the spontaneous breathing trial.

2. Careful use of analgesia and anesthesia: Once standard, high doses of opioids (for example, more than 20 mcg/kg of fentanyl) are now giving way to low-dose opioids (for example, 20 mcg/kg or less of fentanyl), short-acting opioids, and use of hypnotic agents for anesthesia during

cardiac surgery, without significantly increasing the rate of reintubation. Using lower doses and short-acting agents results in fewer problems with depressed respiratory drive.

3. Effective and efficient use of a well-designed protocol: Protocols for patients who have had open-heart surgery should be designed to safely reduce ventilatory support while maintaining stable hemodynamic values, adequate oxygenation and elimination of CO_2, and acceptable or appropriate neurologic status. A multidisciplinary approach involving clinicians and respiratory therapists is essential when developing, testing, implementing, and evaluating the protocol.

A protocol-based weaning process directed by respiratory therapists has been found more effective than clinician-directed weaning because the respiratory therapist are at the bedside and can make more timely changes while weaning.

APPROACH TO DIFFICULT WEANING

Aggressively seek and treat reversible causes of ventilator dependence.

- Wheeze (especially COPD and asthma)
- Heart disease and fluid overload
- Electrolytes and metabolic derangement
- Anxiety
- Neuromuscular disease and weakness
- Sepsis
- Nutrition insufficiency
- Opiates and other sedatives
- Thyroid disease.

If patient failed SBT but passed 'wean screen':

- Consider an extubation attempt to ensure that the irritant and loading effects of the artificial airway are not the cause of the SBT failure.
- Careful reevaluation of the need(s) for ongoing ventilatory support should be coupled with a daily reassessment for the appropriateness of repeat SBTs.
- Ventilatory support between SBTs should be comfortable interactive support that does not necessarily have to be 'weaned'.
- Do not perform SBTs more often than once daily to avoid fatigue.

Causes of weaning failure: When the patient's work of breathing becomes too great to sustain, this may cause weaning failure.

Increased airflow resistance: The conditions that increase airflow resistance are ET tube kinking/obstruction by secretions, abdominal distension and increased CO_2 production.

Decreased lung compliance: Low lung compliance makes lung expansion difficult and this is a major factor, which may lead to respiratory muscle fatigue and weaning failure. The conditions are ARDS, retained secretions, atelectasis, kinking ET tube, obesity, tension pneumothorax, bronchospasm, airway obstruction, etc.

Respiratory muscle fatigue: Respiratory work is a product of transpulmonary pressure and tidal volume. The transpulmonary pressure is increased in low lung compliance and high airflow resistance. So if pressure is increased, work of breathing also increases and respiratory muscle fatigue occurs.

Terminal weaning: Means withdrawal of mechanical ventilation that leads to death of patient. When terminal weaning is considered, three concerns must be evaluated and discussed:

1. Patients informed request
2. Medical fatility
3. Reduction of pain and suffering.

■ WHEN TO STOP

Determination of assessment parameters for continued weaning (Go), cautious weaning (Caution), weaning discontinuation (Stop) should be made before the trial is begun (Table 9.2). These parameters should be patient-specific and should consider: hemodynamics, underlying cardiac and respiratory disease,

Table 9.2: Weaning protocol for the medical respiratory intensive care unit

All patients receiving mechanical ventilation are assessed by using screen 1 every day, and results are documented on the weaning assessment form		
Step-1 Parameters	Results	
1. Hemodynamics stable?	Yes	No
2. Off vasopressors?	Yes	No
3. PaO_2/FiO_2 ratio ≥ 150?	Yes	No
(If ABGs not available: $SaO_2 \geq 95\%$ on FiO_2 of 0.50 or less)		
4. PEEP set at 8 cm H_2O or less?	Yes	No
5. RASS † of – 2 or higher?	Yes	No
If NO to any question, STOP! Otherwise, ALWAYS proceed to Step-2.		
Step-2: Rapid Shallow Breathing Index (RSBI). For 1 minute, through ventilator with 'flow trigger' mode rate set to 0, PSV set to 0, PEEP allowed up to 5 cm H_2O. Start measurement 1 minute after setup At the end of 1 minute, measure respiratory rate (f), and minute ventilation (VE) and calculate tidal volume (Vt) in liters. RSBI = f/Vt RSBI of 105 or less If YES, proceed to spontaneous breathing trial. If NO, rest patient until the next day and reassess starting with step-1		

Contd...

Contd...

Spontaneous breathing trial
Spontaneous breathing for 120 minutes through ventilator with 'flow trigger' mode rate set to 0, PSV set to 0, PEEP allowed up to 5 cm H_2O. A 2-hour continuous trial without termination indicates a successful spontaneous breathing trial.
Successful spontaneous breathing trial?

Termination criteria (document cause if terminated):
Respiratory rate >35/min for 5 minutes or more
SaO_2 <90%
Heart rate >140/min or sustained increase 20% greater than baseline
Systolic blood pressure >180 mm Hg or <90 mm Hg
Increased anxiety
If spontaneous breathing trial is unsuccessful, rest patient until the next day and begin with step-1 again

---

Extubation: .... **Date** .... **Time**
Reason for not extubating, if all criteria met:
ABGs, arterial blood gases; FiO_2, fraction of inspired oxygen; PEEP, positive end-expiratory pressure; PSV, pressure-support ventilation; RASS, Richmond agitation-sedation scale; SaO_2, oxygen saturation

---

Richmond Agitation-Sedation Scale

Score and term Description	
+ 4 Combative	Overtly combative or violent, immediate danger to staff
+ 3 Very agitated	Pulls on or removes tube(s) or catheter(s), or has aggressive behavior toward staff
+ 2 Agitated	Frequent nonpurposeful movement or patient-ventilator dyssynchrony
+ 1 Restless	Anxious or apprehensive but movements not aggressive or vigorous
0 Alert and calm	
– 1 Drowsy	Not fully alert, but has sustained (>10 seconds) awakening, with eye contact, to voice
– 2 Light sedation	Briefly (<10 seconds) awakens, with eye contact, to voice
– 3 Moderate sedation	Any movement (but no eye contact) to voice
– 4 Deep sedation	No response to voice, but any movement to physical stimulation
– 5 Unarousable	No response to voice or physical stimulation

respiratory muscle strength, and energy reserves. Some general guidelines are below:

- Go:
  - No respiratory distress
  - Hemodynamically stable

- Caution
  - Mild respiratory distress
  - Hemodynamic changes
- Stop
  - Respiratory distress, respiratory acidosis
  - Vital sign changes: Increased RR, HR, BP, decreased saturation.

Consider tracheostomy if likely to remain intubated for >5–10 days:
- Requiring high levels of sedation to tolerate endotracheal tubes.
- With marginal respiratory mechanics and reduced airway resistance from tracheostomy may reduce risk of muscle overload.
- That may psychologically benefit from ability to eat orally, to communicate by speaking, and enhanced mobility.
- In whom enhanced mobility may assist physiotherapy.
- Early tracheotomy's are better to reduce the length of ICU stay.

■ PROCEDURE

1. Observe the patient. Is the patient alert and calm? (Score 0). Does the patient have behavior consistent with restlessness or agitation? (Score +1 to + 4 according to criteria listed above).
2. If the patient is not alert, in a loud speaking voice, state the patient's name and direct the patient to open eyes and look at you. Repeat once, if necessary. Can prompt the patient to continue looking at you. Patient has eye opening and eye contact sustained for >10 seconds (Score 1). Patient has eye opening and eye contact, but this is not sustained for 10 seconds. (Score 2). Patient has any movement in response to voice, excluding eye contact (Score 3).
3. If the patient does not respond to voice, physically stimulate him or her by shaking his or her shoulder. If no response to shaking the shoulder, rub the sternum. Patient has any movement to physical stimulation (Score 4). Patient has no response to voice or physical stimulation (Score 5).
   Figures 9.1 to 9.4 depict the weaning process from start to finish.

■ SUMMARY

Weaning from mechanical ventilation is best achieved when it is viewed as a process of titration, and is implemented in a collaborative manner with input from the physician, respiratory therapist and nurse. When the patient is properly prepared, the plan is well-communicated, and goal-directed, then the length of ventilatory support is decreased, ICU stay is shortened, and mortality is improved.

The conceptual model described above may help to integrate many components of the complicated weaning process (Fig. 9.1). Caregiver-directed protocols shorten ventilator duration, and improve patient's outcomes. But it is important that weaning not be directed from protocols or standard methods

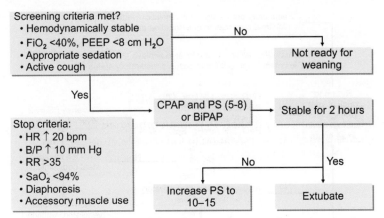

Fig. 9.1: Conceptual model describing components of weaning process

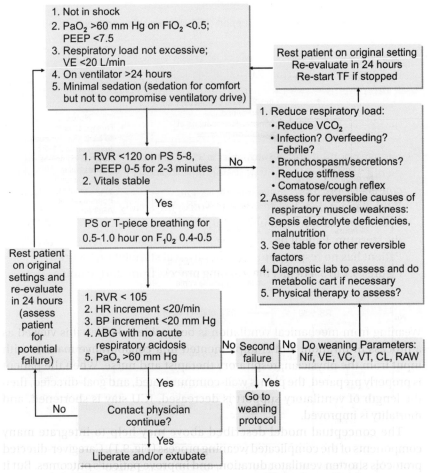

Fig. 9.2: Weaning readiness assessment/weaning protocol

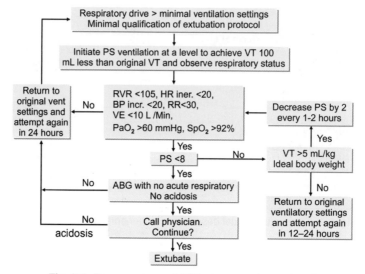

Fig. 9.3: Pressure support (PS) slow weaning protocol

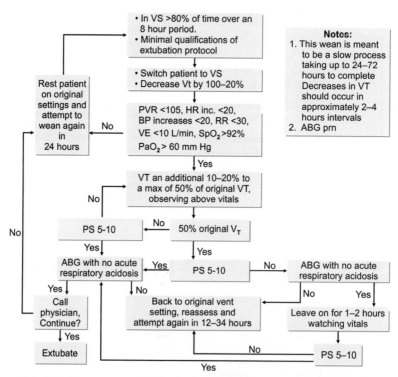

Fig. 9.4: Pressure-regulated volume control/volume support (PRVC/VS) slow weaning protocol

alone, but should instead be patient-specific, and flexible enough to allow for changes based on the patient's response to titration (Figs 9.2 to 9.4).

■ BIBLIOGRAPHY

1. Afessa B, Hogans L, Murphy R. Predicting 3-day and 7-day outcomes of weaning from mechanical ventilation. Chest. 1999;116(2):456-61.
2. Bhatt SB. Esophageal balloon manometry and weaning from mechanical ventilation. Crit Care Med. 1996;24(1):179-80.
3. Brochard L, Rauss A, Benito S, Conti G, Mancebo J, Rekik N, et al. Comparison of three methods of gradual withdrawal from ventilatory support during weaning from mechanical ventilation. Am J Respir Crit Care Med. 1994;150(4):896-903.
4. Chatila W, Ani S, Guaglianone D, Jacob B, Amoateng-Adjepong Y, Manthous CA. Cardiac ischemia during weaning from mechanical ventilation. Chest. 1996; 109(6):1577-83.
5. Cook D, Meade M, Guyatt G, Butler R, Aldawood A, Epstein S. Trials of miscellaneous interventions to wean from mechanical ventilation. Chest. 2001; 120(6 Suppl):438S-44S.
6. Cook DJ, Meade MO, Perry AG. Qualitative studies on the patient's experience of weaning from mechanical ventilation. Chest. 2001;120(6 Suppl):469S-73S.
7. Ely EW, Bennett PA, Bowton DL, et al. Large scale implementation of a respiratory therapist-driven protocol for ventilator weaning. American Journal of Respiratory and critical Care Medicine. 1999;159:439-46.

VENTILATOR GRAPHICS

■ GENERAL CONCEPTS

Ventilator graphics have become an essential tool in managing patients on mechanical ventilators. All newer mechanical ventilators are equipped with a graphic package that displays selected ventilator waveforms facilitating assessment of the patient's condition.

These graphics are displayed in two forms—scalars and loops.

Guidelines for proper interpretation and application of the most common ventilator graphics are described below.

The following waveforms will be described in this module:
A. Scalars:
  1. Flow vs time
  2. Pressure vs time
  3. Volume vs time.
B. Loops:
  1. Pressure–volume loop
  2. Flow-volume loop.

Any single variable displayed against time is known as a Scalar graphic (Fig. 10.1). The three components that make up the ventilator graphics, flow, volume and pressure are plotted against time. These three scalars are generally referred to as:
- Flow curve
- Volume curve
- Pressure curve.

When viewing scalar graphics, time is conventionally shown on the horizontal (x) axis whereas flow, volume, and pressure are plotted on the vertical axis (y) axis. The following tracings indicate the typical flow vs time, pressure vs. time and volume vs. time scalars during mechanical volume cycled ventilation with a constant (preset) flow. The next few frames discuss scalars and their clinical significance.

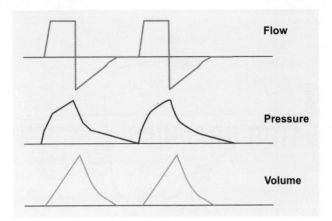

Fig. 10.1: Scalar graphic with three components placed against time

Loops are the two-dimensional graphic display of two scalar values. There are two loops available for interpretation. They are:

• Pressure-volume loop (Fig. 10.2).

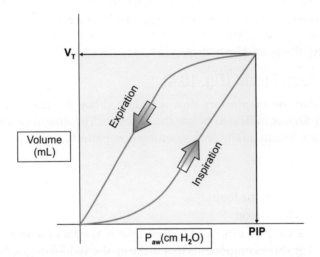

Fig. 10.2: Pressure-volume loop interpretation

• Flow-volume loop (Fig. 10.3)

When viewing the flow-volume loop, the horizontal x-axis is used to indicate volume whereas flow is displayed on the vertical y-axis. As indicated in the flow-volume loop in Figure 10.3, the inspiratory curve is plotted above the baseline and the expiratory curve is traced below the baseline. However, it is not unusual to see a completely reverse pattern where the inspiratory component is presented below the baseline.

When viewing the pressure-volume loop, pressure is usually displayed on the horizontal x-axis while volume is displayed on the vertical y-axis.

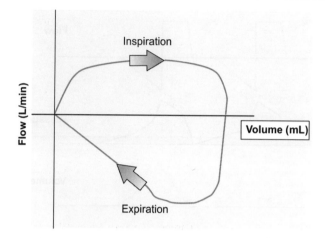

Fig. 10.3: Flow-volume loop interpretation

■ ANALYSIS OF SCALAR GRAPHICS

Each scalar will be discussed individually identifying components of the tracing and commonly observed normal and abnormal patterns.

Basics of Flow vs time Curve

Spontaneous Breath (Fig. 10.4)

Observe that the inspiratory flow is traced above the baseline whereas expiratory flow is indicated below the baseline. The flow/time curve for a spontaneous breath resembles a sinewave flow pattern.

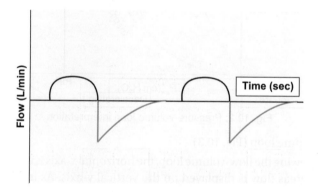

Fig. 10.4: Spontaneous breath

Mechanical Breath (Fig. 10.5)

This tracing shows components of a flow vs time curve for a mechanical volume-targeted breath.

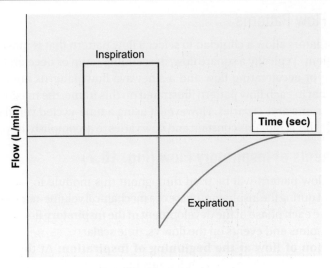

Fig. 10.5: Mechanical breath

Observe the following (Fig. 10.6):

- The inspiratory flow pattern is square, indicating a constant flow delivery. This pattern is selected by the operator.
- There is a significant tracing below the baseline representing expiratory flow, which is dependent on the patient's lung characteristics and effort.
- Only the flow vs time curve demonstrates a significant tracing below the baseline. The other scalars stay above the baseline except on a pressure vs. time curve where a very small deflection occurs below the baseline when the patient initiates inspiration.

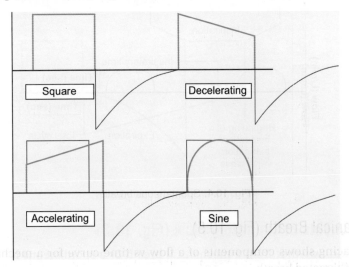

Fig. 10.6: Flow patterns

Typical Flow Patterns

Most ventilators allow a clinician to select a flow pattern that is most suitable to the patient. Typically a square flow, descending ramp or decelerating flow, ascending or accelerating flow and a sinewave flow patterns are available. Observe that in each flow pattern illustrated on this frame, the maximum flow rate is the same and Ti varies. However, if using a time-cycled ventilator (e.g. Servo 300), the TI remains constant and flow varies to accomplish the preset VT.

Components of Inspiratory Flow (Fig. 10.7)

A square flow pattern will be used throughout this module to identify each component during the inspiratory phase of a mechanical volume-targeted breath.

Observe each phase of the development of the inspiratory flow. Notice the following points and events on the flow vs. time scalar:

1. **Initiation of flow at the beginning of inspiration:** At this time, the exhalation valve closes to permit a mechanical breath to deliver volume to the patient's lungs.
2. The peak inspiratory flow (PIFR) level is reached instantaneously during a constant flow pattern. The flow remains at this level until the inspiration is terminated.
3. **End of inspiratory flow delivery and beginning of expiration:** This event occurs when the preset tidal volume is delivered. At this time, the exhalation valve opens to allow for passive exhalation.
4. Notice inspiratory time (T_I), Expiratory time (T_E) and the total cycle time (TCT) for one mechanical breath.

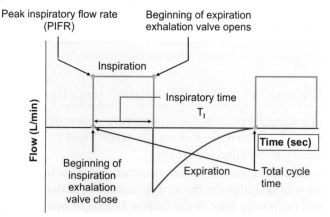

Fig. 10.7: Inspiratory flow pattern

Components of Expiratory Flow (Fig. 10.8)

Expiration, whether from a mechanical breath or a spontaneous breath, is generally a passive maneuver. Both the inspiratory and the expiratory flows reach their peak value instantaneously and both return to the baseline.

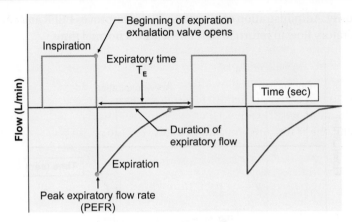

Fig. 10.8: Expiratory flow pattern

Observe the following points on the expiratory section of the flow/time tracing:

1. Initiation of expiration
2. Peak expiratory flow rate (PEFR)
3. Duration of expiratory flow
4. Expiratory time (T_E).

Notice that the expiratory flow decays to zero before the next mechanical breath is initiated. Thus, the duration of expiratory flow may be shorter than the allocated expiratory time.

Recognition of Common Abnormalities

Flow vs. time scalars help in recognizing certain disorders. Different lung disorders show different flow patterns. These abnormal flow patterns, their causes, and appropriate actions are discussed below:

Airway Obstruction vs Active Exhalation (Fig. 10.9)

Exhalation is normally passive. The expiratory flow pattern and PEFR depend upon the changes in the patient's lung compliance and airway resistance, as well as patient's active efforts to exhale.

For example, increased airway resistance due to bronchospasm or accumulation of secretions in the airway may result in decreased PEFR and a prolonged expiratory flow. If the patient begins to actively exhale using expiratory muscles, this may result in an increase in PEFR and a shorter duration of expiratory flow.

Response to Bronchodilator (Fig. 10.10)

Flow vs time tracing can verify clinically suspected bronchoconstriction. In these cases, the PEFR is reduced and the expiratory flow returns to the baseline very slowly. Administration of a bronchodilator improves PEFR and allows for an expiratory flow to return to baseline within a normal time.

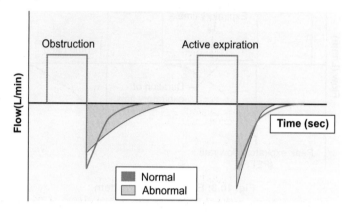

Fig. 10.9: Airway obstruction vs active exhalation

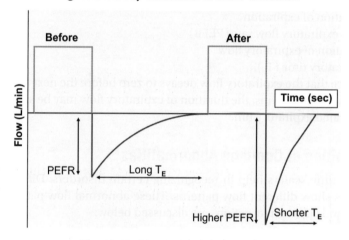

Fig. 10.10: Response to bronchodilator

Air Trapping or Auto-PEEP (Fig. 10.11)

Normally, expiratory flow returns to the baseline prior to the next breath. In the event that the expiratory flow does not return to the zero line and the subsequent inspiration begins below the baseline, auto-PEEP or air trapping is present.

The presence of auto-PEEP or air trapping may result from:

- Inadequate expiratory time
- Too high a respiratory rate
- Long inspiratory time
- Prolonged exhalation due to bronchoconstriction.

Even though auto-PEEP is best detected from the flow-time waveform, its magnitude is not directly measured from the flow-time scalar. A higher inspiratory flow rate (in volume-cycled ventilators) or short T_I (in time-cycled ventilators) allows for a longer TE and may eliminate auto-PEEP.

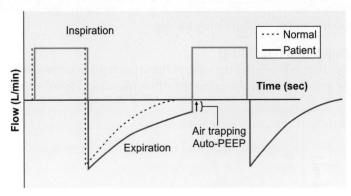

Fig. 10.11: Air trapping

Basics of Volume vs Time Curve (Fig. 10.12)

Information obtained from a volume vs time scalar graph includes a visual representation of:
- Inspiratory tidal volume
- Inspiratory phase
- Expiratory phase
- Inspiratory time.

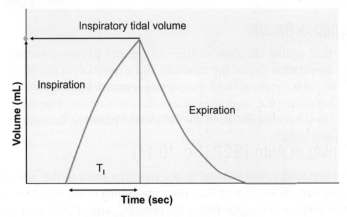

Fig. 10.12: Volume vs time scalar

Recognition of Common Abnormalities

The volume vs time scalar can be used to identify the following common abnormalities:

Presence of Air Leak
A leak in the circuit or around the tracheal tube can be detected from the volume/time curve. If the expiratory tracing smoothly descends, and then

plateaus, but does not reach baseline, it indicates the presence of a leak in the system. This pattern mandates that the leak should be located and fixed. The volume of the leak can be easily estimated by measuring the distance from the plateau to the end of the expiratory tracing.

Active Exhalation (Fig. 10.13)

Forced exhalation is seen on the volume/time tracing as a tracing that extends below the zero line. It can also occur if the flow transducer is out of calibration.

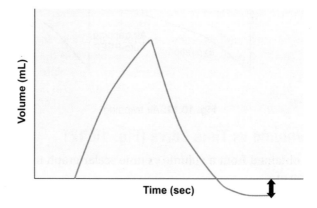

Fig. 10.13: Active exhalation

Basics of Pressure vs Time Curve (Fig. 10.14 and Table 10.1)

Spontaneous Breath

Observe that unlike the flow vs time curve, the pressure vs time scalar indicates inspiration below the baseline and expiration is traced above the baseline which is consistent with the normal spontaneous respiratory pattern. Observe that during the inspiratory phase, the pressure curve shows a negative deflection and during exhalation goes above the baseline. Compare this with a mechanical breath.

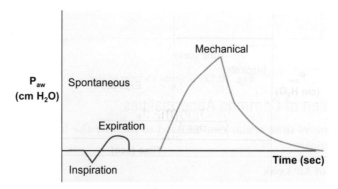

Fig. 10.14: Spontaneous vs mechanical

Table 10.1: Pressure vs time curve

Basics of Pressure vs. Time Curve	Recognition of Common Abnormalities Spontaneous Breath
Spontaneous breath	Increased airway resistance
Mechanical Breath	Effect of high inspiratory flow
Controlled vs assisted breath	Decreased lung compliance
Components of inflation pressure	Inadequate inspiratory flow

Mechanical Breath

The pressure vs time scalar is one of the most useful waveforms in the clinical setting (Fig. 10.15). It provides visual representations of the following:

Peak inspiratory pressure (PIP) is the maximum pressure achieved during a breath. PIP indicates the pressure required to deliver a set tidal volume during volume ventilation. Increased airway resistance (R_{aw}) and/or decreased lung compliance result in an increased PIP.

Positive End-expiratory Pressure

Positive end expiratory pressure (PEEP) is confirmed only on a pressure vs time scalar and a pressure-volume loop. PEEP is present when the baseline pressure is above zero.

Assisted vs Controlled Breath (Fig. 10.16)

A pressure vs time scalar verifies the triggering mechanism of the mechanical breath. If the breaths are initiated at the baseline at fixed intervals, the mode is time triggered or a control mode. In an assist mode, the patient initiates the breath by generating a negative pressure, the ventilator sensor recognizes the patient's effort and delivers a mechanical breath. This event can be observed on the pressure vs time scalar, where a small negative deflection below the baseline precedes a mechanical breath.

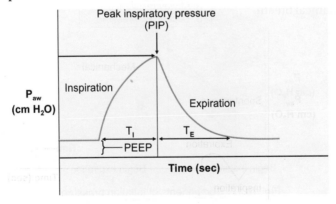

Fig. 10.15: Pressure vs time scalar

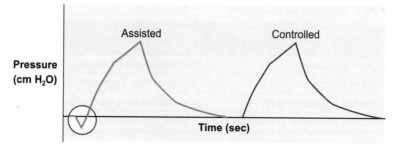

Fig. 10.16: Assisted vs controlled breath

Components of Inflation Pressure (Fig. 10.17)

Although dynamic lung mechanics can be observed from a pressure vs time curve, the addition of an inspiratory pause or inflation hold provides information to calculate static mechanics.

Plateau pressure (P_{plat}): P_{plat} or alveolar pressure is obtained upon activation of an inflation hold or inspiratory pause control. The exhalation valve is kept in a closed position and the volume is held in the lungs. For clinical purposes, the plateau pressure is the same as the alveolar pressure. This measurement provides a means of measuring static lung compliance.

Transairway pressure ($PTA = PIP - P_{plat}$): It reflects the pressure required to overcome airway resistance. Bronchospasm, airway secretions, and other types of airway obstructions are verified from an increase in the transairway pressure ($PIP - P_{plat}$). With inflation hold, the pressure required to overcome the recoiling force (lung compliance) can be determined. The static lung compliance can be obtained by dividing the volume in the lung by the plateau pressure minus PEEP, if present.

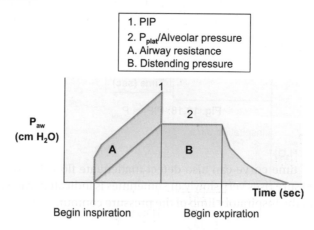

Fig. 10.17: Components of inflation pressure

Recognition of Common Abnormalities

PIP vs P$_{plat}$ (Fig. 10.18)

Changes in the pressure vs. time curve have profound clinical significance. Four common clinical situations are demonstrated in the following tracings.

Normal curve: Indicates PIP, P$_{plat}$, P$_{TA}$, and T$_I$.

High R$_{aw}$: A significant increase in the P$_{TA}$ is associated with increase in airway resistance.

High flow: Notice that the inspiratory time is shorter than normal indicating a higher inspiratory gas flow rate.

Decreased lung compliance: An increase in the plateau pressure and a corresponding increase in the PIP is consistent with decreased lung compliance.

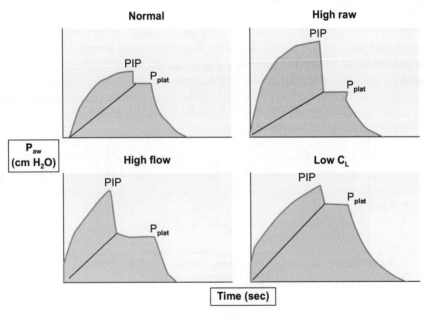

Fig. 10.18: PIP vs P$_{plat}$

Inadequate Flow (Fig. 10.19)

A pressure vs time curve can also detect inadequate flow that is indicated when the pressure rises very slowly or sometimes is indicated when there is a depression in the inspiratory limb of the pressure contour.

LOOPS

Loops are the two-dimensional graphic displays of two scalar values.

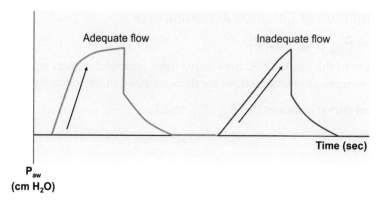

Fig. 10.19: Inadequate inspiratory flow

Pressure-volume Loop

Type of Breath (Fig. 10.20)

Observe the direction of the tracing of the loop. When the tracing is counterclockwise, the breath delivered is a mechanical breath. On the other hand, a clockwise tracing indicates a spontaneous breath. The angle, shape and size of the loop impart pertinent information to the clinician. In an assisted mechanical breath, the tracing begins clockwise indicating patient's effort and resumes in counterclockwise fashion for the mechanical delivery.

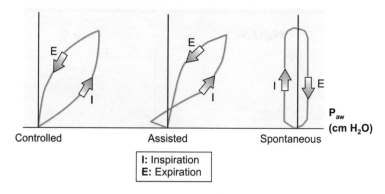

Fig. 10.20: Types of breath

FRC and P-V Loop (Fig. 10.21)

It is important to recognize that the beginning point on a pressure-volume loop is the FRC level. When PEEP is added, the FRC level increases.

Components of a P-V Loop (Fig. 10.22)

A pressure-volume loop traces changes in pressures and corresponding changes in volume. Inspiration begins from the FRC level and terminates when the preset parameter (volume or pressure) is achieved. The tracing continues during expiration and returns to FRC at end of exhalation. PIP and delivered tidal volume can readily be obtained from the pressure-volume loop.

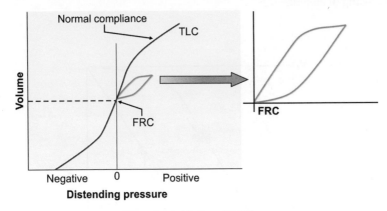

Fig. 10.21: FRC and P-V loop

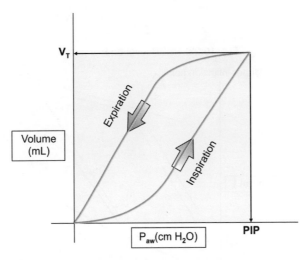

Fig. 10.22: Components of a P-V loop

PEEP (Fig. 10.23)

When PEEP is applied, the pressure-volume curve shifts to the PEEP level on the horizontal scale.

Inflection Points (Fig. 10.24)

Inflection point is the point of change in the slope of a line. The inflection points represent sudden changes in alveolar opening and closing. The lower inflection point represents the opening pressure, whereas the upper inflection point represents recoiling characteristics. The higher the opening pressure, the stiffer the lung, as indicated by the curve moving laterally to the right along the pressure axis. Setting PEEP levels at the level of the lower inflection point is recommended to optimize alveolar recruitment and prevent repeated opening and closing of alveoli.

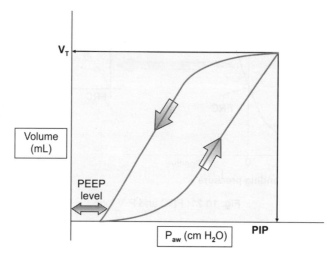

Fig. 10.23: PEEP level on P-V loop

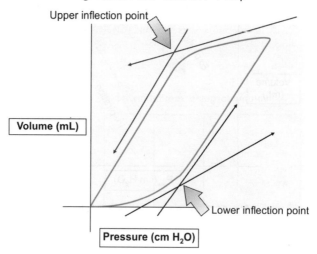

Fig. 10.24: Inflection points

Work of Breathing (Fig. 10.25)

The major advantage of a pressure-volume loop is that it provides a quick assessment of the elastic as well as resistive work of breathing.

Since work of breathing is calculated from the product of pressure and volume (WOB = Pressure × Volume). The shaded area represents elastic work of breathing.

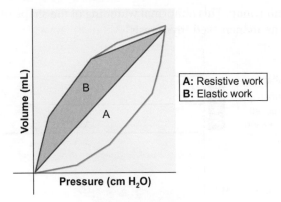

Fig. 10.25: Work of breathing

Recognition of Common Abnormalities

Decreased lung compliance

A shift of the curve to the right of a pressure-volume loop indicates decreased lung compliance and a shift to the left is associated with an increased compliance. Observe the pressure required to deliver the same tidal volume in the three graphs.

Volume targeted ventilation (Fig. 10.26)

Notice that in volume-targeted ventilation, the PIP is the changing variable. In pressure-targeted ventilation, the PIP is the constant variable, and V_T is the changing variable.

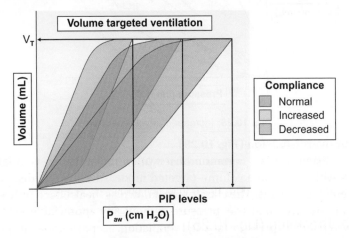

Fig. 10.26: Volume targeted ventilation

Pressure targeted ventilation (Fig. 10.27)

Increased airway resistance (A wide loop) (Fig. 10.28)

An increased airway resistance is associated with the abnormal widening of the inspiratory tracing. Patients with obstructive disorders exhibit a wide pressure-volume loop. This abnormal widening of the shape of the P-V loop is referred to as an increased "hysteresis".

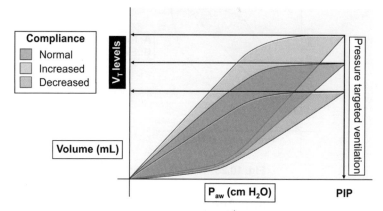

Fig. 10.27: Lung compliance changes in the P-V loop

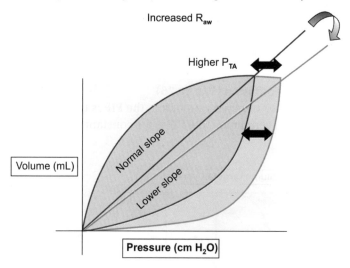

Fig. 10.28: Increased airway resistance

Alveolar overdistension (Fig. 10.29)

Alveolar distension is a common observation made during ventilation of patients with ARDS on a volume-targeted mode. Alveolar overdistension is detrimental to patients. The classic sign, known as 'beak effect' or 'Duckbill' shows an increase in airway pressure without any appreciable increase in volume. A switch to pressure targeted ventilation, at appropriate safe pressure level, or a reduction in VT are indicated.

Increased WOB

Inadequate sensitivity (Fig. 10.30)

Normally the pressure-volume loop traces in a counterclockwise direction. A clockwise tracing prior to the initiation of a mechanical breath indicates patient's effort. Adjusting the sensitivity can minimize this effort. Inadequate sensitivity setting promotes increased WOB. On the P-V loop, it is recognized by a significant clockwise deflection of the tracing with the pressure decreasing significantly (>5 cm H_2O) below the baseline pressure.

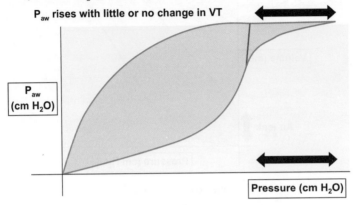

Fig. 10.29: Alveolar overdistension

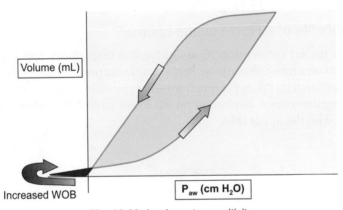

Fig. 10.30: Inadequate sensitivity

Inadequate Inspiratory Flow (Fig. 10.31)

Inappropriate inspiratory flow rates are recognized from a scooped out pattern. In some situations, the patient makes inspiratory effort in the middle of the mechanical breath exhibiting a 'notch' on the inspiratory curve.

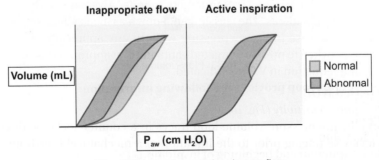

Fig. 10.31: Inadequate inspiratory flow

Air Leak (Fig. 10.32)
When the expiratory curve does not return to zero volume, an air leak is present.

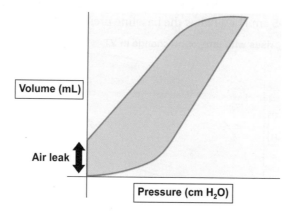

Fig. 10.32: Air leak

Flow-Volume Loop (Fig. 10.33)

Components of a Flow-volume Loop

There is no set convention in assigning the inspiratory and expiratory quadrants on a flow-volume loop. Some ventilators produce flow-volume loop with inspiration on the upper quadrant and expiration on the lower quadrant. Other ventilators plot inspiration on the lower side of the volume axis and expiration on the upper side.

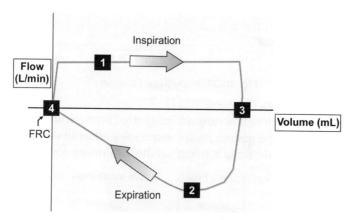

Fig. 10.33: Flow-volume loop

A flow-volume loop provides the following information:
1. PIFR
2. PEFR
3. Tidal volume
4. End expiration and beginning of inspiration.

Recognition of Common Abnormalities

Air leak (Fig. 10.34)

Ideally, expired volume should be equal to the inspired volume. With an air leak, however, expired volume is less than inspired volume. This is commonly observed in situations such as leak around the endotracheal tube, and circuit leak. A leak can be identified from a flow-volume loop when the volume does not return to the zero volume level. The deficit of volume indicates the magnitude of air leak.

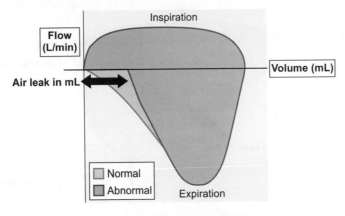

Fig. 10.34: Air leak

Auto-PEEP (Fig. 10.35)

In an air trapping or auto-PEEP situation, the flow does not return to the zero level. Since the next inspiration must begin from the zero flow level, the tracing jumps abruptly, from the trapped level to the zero level and proceeds with next breath.

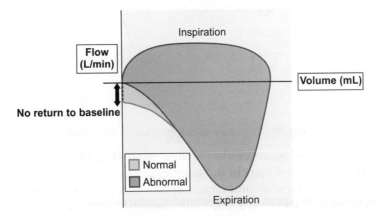

Fig. 10.35: Air trapping

Increased airway resistance (Fig. 10.36)

An increased airway resistance due to bronchospasm, such as in asthma, is shown on a flow-volume loop as a scooped out pattern on the expiratory tracing and a decreased PEFR. Effective administration of bronchodilator will show an improvement on both the configuration of the expiratory tracing and the PEFR. A continued scooped out appearance and a low PEFR indicate ineffectiveness of the bronchodilator therapy.

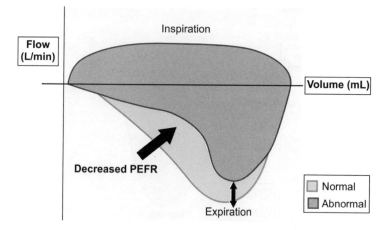

Fig. 10.36: Increased airway resistance

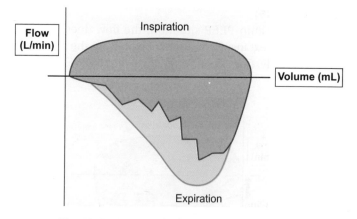

Fig. 10.37: Airway secretions/water in the circuit

Airway secretions/accumulation of condensate (Fig. 10.37)

The presence of secretions in the large airways, as well as excessive fluid condensation in the ventilator circuit, appear as a distinctive pattern in the flow-volume loop known as a 'saw-tooth' pattern, which occurs mostly on the expiratory component of the curve. However, if the situation is not corrected, this pattern will also appear on the inspiratory curve.

■ BIBLIOGRAPHY

1. Branson R, Hess D, Chatburn R. Respiratory Care Equipment. 2nd edn. St Louis: Mosby, 1999.
2. Branson R, Hess D, Chatburn R. Respiratory Care Equipment. 2nd edn. Philadelphia: Lippincott Williams & Wilkins, 1999.
3. Haas C. Volume-pressure curves during mechanical ventilation. AARC Times. 2000;24:64-8.
4. Ouellet P. Waveform and Loop Analysis in Mechanical Ventilation. Solna, Sweden: Siemens-Elema, 1997.
5. Pilbeam S. Mechanical Ventilation: Physiological and Clinical Applications. 2nd ed. St Louis: Mosby, 1998.
6. Scanlon C, Wilkins R, Stoller J. Egan's Fundamentals of Respiratory Care. 7th ed. St Louis: Mosby, 1999.

AIRWAY MANAGEMENT

■ INTRODUCTION

In cardiopulmonary resuscitation, anesthesia, emergency medicine, intensive care medicine and first aid, airway management is the process of ensuring that there is an open pathway between a patient's lungs and the outside world, and the lungs are safe from aspiration.

In nearly all circumstances, airway management is the highest priority for clinical care. This is because if there is no airway, there can be no breathing, hence no oxygenation of blood and therefore circulation (and hence all the other vital body processes) will soon cease. Getting oxygen to the lungs is the first step in almost all clinical treatments. The 'A' is for 'airway' in the 'ABC' of cardiopulmonary resuscitation.

■ MANUAL METHODS
Head Tilt/Chin Lift

The simplest way of ensuring an open airway in an unconscious patient is to use a head tilt chin lift technique, thereby lifting the tongue from the back of the throat. This is taught on most first aid courses as the standard way of clearing an airway.

Jaw Thrust

The jaw thrust is a technique used on patients with a suspected spinal injury and is used on a supine patient. The practitioner uses their thumbs to physically push the posterior (back) aspects of the mandible upwards—only possible on a patient with a GCS < 8 (although patients with a GCS higher than this should also be maintaining their own patent airway). When the mandible is displaced forward, it pulls the tongue forward and prevents it from occluding (blocking) the entrance to the trachea, helping to ensure a patent (secure) airway.

Removal of Vomit and Regurgitation

In the case of a patient who vomits or has other secretions in the airway, these techniques will not be enough. Suitably trained clinicians may elect to use suction to clean out the airway, although this may not always be possible. A unconscious patient who is regurgitating stomach contents should be turned into the recovery position when there is no suction equipment available, as this allows (to a certain extent) the drainage of fluids out of the mouth instead of down the trachea.

■ ADJUNCTS TO AIRWAY MANAGEMENT

There are a variety of artificial airways, which can be used to keep a pathway between the lungs and mouth/nose. The most commonly used in long-term or critical care situations is the endotracheal tube, a plastic tube which is inserted through the mouth and into the trachea, often with a cuff which is inflated to seal off the trachea and prevent any vomit being aspirated into the lungs. In some cases, a laryngeal mask airway (LMA) is a suitable alternative to an endotracheal tube, and has the advantage of requiring a lower level of training that an ET tube.

In the case of a choking patient, laryngoscopy or even bronchoscopy may be performed in order to visualize and remove the blockage.

An oropharyngeal airway or nasopharyngeal airway can be used to prevent the tongue from blocking the airway. When these airways are inserted properly, the rescuer does not need to manually open the airway with a head tilt/chin lift or jaw-thrust maneuver. Aspiration of blood, vomitus, and other fluids can still occur with these two adjuncts.

■ LARYNGEAL MASK AIRWAY (FIG. 11.1)

The **laryngeal mask airway** was invented in 1983 by British anesthetist, Dr Archie Brain.

Use

Laryngeal masks are used in anesthesia and in emergency medicine for airway management. They consist of a tube with an inflatable cuff that is inserted into the pharynx. They cause less pain and coughing than an endotracheal tube, and are much easier to insert. However, a standard laryngeal mask airway does not protect the lungs from aspiration, making them unsuitable for patients at risk for this complication.

The device is useful in situations where a patient is trapped in a sitting position, suspected of trauma to the cervical spine (where tilting the head to maintain an open airway is contraindicated), or when intubation is unsuccessful. It is not inserted as far as an endotracheal tube (it sits tightly over the top of the larynx, and thus does not need to be inserted into the trachea), and supports both spontaneous and artificial ventilation. It is popular in day case surgery.

However, unlike an endotracheal tube, a laryngeal mask cannot protect the airway or lungs from aspiration of regurgitated material, and deep (subglottic) suctioning cannot be performed through the mask.

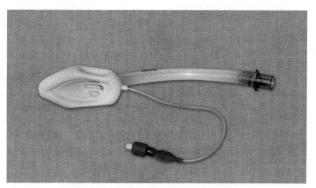

Fig. 11.1: Laryngeal mask airway

Guide to Use

Laryngeal mask airways come in a variety of sizes. The cuff of the mask is deflated before insertion and lubricated. The patient is anesthetized if conscious, and their neck is extended and their mouth opened widely. The apex of the mask, with its open end pointing downwards toward the tongue, is pushed backwards towards the uvula. It follows the natural bend of the oropharynx and comes to rest over the pyriform fossa. Once placed, the cuff around the mask is inflated with air to create a tight seal. Air entry is confirmed by listening for air entry into the lungs with a stethoscope, or by presence of end tidal carbon dioxide.

▪ ENDOTRACHEAL TUBE (FIG. 11.2)

(It also called an ET tube or ETT) is used in anesthesia, intensive care and emergency medicine for airway management and mechanical ventilation. The tube is inserted into a patient's trachea in order to ensure that the airway is not closed off and that air is able to reach the lungs. The endotracheal tube is regarded as the most reliable available method for protecting a patient's airway.

Insertion of the endotracheal tube: The ET tube is held in practitioner's right hand and the laryngoscope is held in the left. The tube is inserted into the trachea, generally via the mouth, but sometimes through the nares of the nose (e.g. in extensive mouth surgery) or even through a tracheostomy.

▪ INTUBATION (FIG. 11.3)

The process of inserting an ETT is called intubation. Intubation usually requires general anesthesia and muscle relaxation but can be achieved in the awake patient with local anesthesia or in an emergency without any anesthesia, although this is extremely uncomfortable and generally avoided in other circumstances.

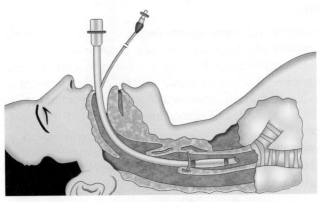

Fig. 11.2: Endotracheal tube function

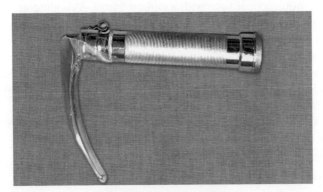

Fig. 11.3: Intubation device

Many patients who require intubation in the ICU may have poor respiratory reserves and may be hemodynamically unstable. Hence, it is important to be prepared for instability during and after the procedure; besides, intubation needs to be quick, given the possibility of worsening hypoxia and risk of regurgitation and aspiration. Intubation in the ICU is a three person procedure, with the operator at the head end coordinating the process.

Preparation

- The crash cart must be by the bedside
- Ensure working suction with a Yankauer sucker, self-inflating bag with an appropriate size mask, Guedel (oropharyngeal) airways, two working laryngoscopes, appropriate sized endotracheal tubes (size 8.0 for males and size 7.0 for females; keep smaller size, up to 6.0 in case of difficulty), bougie and Magill forceps. A laryngeal mask airway (sizes 3 and 4) must be readily available in case of difficulty.
- The capnograph must be up and running before you start—it is very important to confirm position of the endotracheal tube within the trachea.

Procedure

- The choice of induction agents depends on the clinical situation. In hemodynamically stable patients, it is appropriate to use fentanyl and propofol. In hypotensive/hypovolemic patients, it may be appropriate to use ketamine. Muscle relaxation is with succinyl choline (do not use with hyperkalemia, spinal injuries, neuromuscular disorders) or rocuronium.
- Atropine 0.5 mg/mL and adrenaline 10 mL of 1:10,000 must be readily available.
- Pre-oxygenate for about 3 minutes.
- Cricoid pressure may be required in patients at high-risk for regurgitation and aspiration.
- Confirm intubation by capnography.
- Listen to breath sounds to ensure ventilation to both lungs.
- Tie the endotracheal tube with a ribbon gauze. As a general rule, do not insert Guedel airways post intubation—it may result in trauma to the mouth, tongue, etc. and make oral hygiene difficult.
- If a gastric tube is required, insert it at this time.
- Presence of adequate ventilation in both lungs may be confirmed by pleural sliding; if in doubt, do X-rays to confirm position of the tip of the endotracheal tube.
- Always do X-rays to confirm tip of the gastric tube; do not administer feeds before confirming position of the tube within the stomach.

Macintosh Pattern Laryngoscope

It is usually performed by visualizing the larynx by means of a hand-held laryngoscope that has a variety of curved and straight blades. The intubation can also be performed 'blind' or with the use of the attendant's fingers (this is called digital intubation). A stylet can be used inside the endotracheal tube. The malleable metal stylet is a bendable piece of metal inserted into the ETT as to make the tube more stiff for easier insertion, this is then removed after the intubation and a ventilator or self-inflating bag is attached to the ETT. The goal is to position the end of the ETT 2 centimeters above the bifurcation of the lungs or the carina. If inserted too far into the trachea it often goes into the right main bronchus (the right main brochus is less angled than the left one).

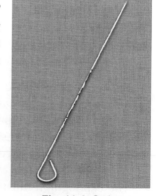

Stylet (Fig. 11.4): A stylet is a long, bendable rod that can be inserted into an endotracheal tube to facilitate intubation. It is placed into the tube prior to laryngoscopy and then the tube (with the stylet in it) is bent to resemble a hockey stick. After insertion of the tube into the trachea, the stylet is removed.

Fig. 11.4: Stylet

Document the view of the larynx obtained during laryngoscopy using the following criteria:
- Grade I: Full view of the cords
- Grade II: Partial view of the cords
- Grade III: View of the epiglottis
- Grade IV: No view of the cords or epiglottis.

Magill's Forceps (Fig. 11.5)

It can be used to:
1. Direct the endotracheal tube.
2. Remove foreign body.
3. Put some gauze to absorb fluid or blood leak.

Risk vs Benefit

Tracheal intubation is a potentially very dangerous invasive procedure that requires a lot of clinical experience to master. When performed improperly (e.g. unrecognized esophageal intubation), the associated complications may rapidly lead to the patient's death. Subsequently, tracheal intubation's role as the 'gold standard' of advanced airway maintenance was downplayed (in favor of more basic techniques like bag-valve-mask ventilation) by the American Heart Association's Guidelines for Cardiopulmonary Resuscitation in 2005, and again in 2010.

Difficult Intubations

The American Society of Anesthesiologists has developed an algorithm for handling difficult airways. Although each patient must be evaluated on an individual basis, conditions generally associated with difficult intubations include:
- Oral/pharyngeal tumors, hemangiomas or hematomas
- Infections such as submandibular or peritonsillar
- Abscesses or epiglottitis

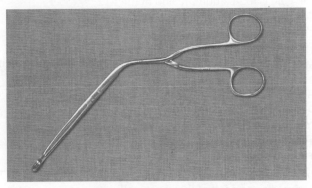

Fig. 11.5: Magill's forceps

- Congenital anomalies such as Pierre Robin syndrome, laryngeal atresia or craniofacial dysostosis
- Foreign body
- Facial trauma such as laryngeal, maxillary or mandibular fracture, cervical spine injury
- Inhalational burn
- Obesity
- Inadequate neck extension due to rheumatoid arthritis, cervical stenosis or ankylosing spondylitis.

Anatomic variations such as micrognathia, prognathism, macroglossia, arched palate, short neck, prominent incisors or buck teeth.

■ APPROACH TO THE AIRWAY IN TRAUMA PATIENTS

The A of ABC

The most immediately life-threatening complication of any trauma is loss of airway patency. Maintaining oxygenation and preventing hypercarbia are critical in managing the trauma patient, especially if the patient has sustained a head injury. Thus, the first step in evaluating and treating any trauma patient is to assess airway patency and, if compromised, restore it: the A of A (airway), B (breathing), C (circulation). Any patient who is awake, alert and able to talk has a patent airway. Whether they need supplemental oxygen can be determined by vitals and physical exam. Patients who are unconscious or have signs suggestive of respiratory compromise, however, require immediate attention. All patients should be immobilized due to increased risk of spinal injury. Assessment of the patient should be done while maintaining the cervical spine in a stable, neutral position. Begin the primary survey by rapidly assessing airway patency: rapidly assess for obstruction. Maintain an airway with jaw thrust or the chin lift maneuver. Clear the airway of foreign bodies. If the patient is likely to vomit, position them in a lateral and head down position to prevent aspiration. All trauma patients should be administered supplemental oxygen! Include and determine the patient's needs. Signs and symptoms suggestive of airway or ventilatory compromise:

- Maxillofacial trauma
- Neck trauma
- Laryngeal trauma (with hoarseness or subcutaneous emphysema).

Look for

- Obtundation
- Agitation (which may suggest hypercarbia)
- Cyanosis
- Retractions/accessory muscle use
- Symmetrical rise and fall of the chest wall.

Listen for

- Abnormal breath sounds
- Snoring
- Stridor
- Crackles
- Dysphonia
- Symmetrical breath sounds over both hemithoraces
- Tachypnea.

Feel for

- A deviated trachea
- Subcutaneous emphysema.

Risk Management

No single method for confirming tube placement has been shown to be 100% reliable. Accordingly, the use of multiple methods to confirm correct tube placement is now the standard of care. At least one of the methods utilized should be an instrument. Waveform capnography is emerging as the gold standard instrument for the confirmation of correct tube placement and maintenance of the tube once it is in place.

Predicting Ease of Intubation

- Look externally (history of craniofacial traumas/previous surgery)
- Evaluate 3,3,2—three of the patient's fingers should be able to fit into his/her mouth when open, three fingers should comfortably fit between the chin and the throat, and two fingers in the thyromental distance (distance from thyroid cartilage to chin)
- Mallampati score
- Obstructions (stridorous breath sounds, wheezing, etc.)
- Neck mobility (can patient tilt head back and then forward to touch chest).

Observational Methods to Confirm Correct Tube Placement

- Direct visualization of the tube passing through the vocal cords
- Clear and equal bilateral breath sounds on auscultation of the chest
- Absent sounds on auscultation of the epigastrium
- Equal bilateral chest rise with ventilation
- Fogging of the tube
- An absence of stomach contents in the tube.

Instruments to Confirm Correct Tube Placement

- Colorimetric end tidal CO_2 detector
- Waveform capnography
- Self-inflating esophageal bulb
- Pulse oximetry (patients with a pulse)—delay in fall of saturation, especially if preoxygenated.

Indications

Tracheal intubation is performed by practitioners in various medical conditions:

- Comatose or intoxicated patients who are unable to protect their airways. In such patients, the throat muscles may lose their tone so that the upper airways obstruct or collapse and air cannot easily enter into the lungs. Furthermore, protective airway reflexes such as coughing and swallowing, which serve to protect the airways against aspiration of secretions and foreign bodies, may be absent. With tracheal intubation, airway patency is restored and the lower airways can be protected from aspiration.
- General anesthesia: In anesthetized patients, spontaneous respiration may be decreased or absent due to the effect of anesthetics, opioids, or muscle relaxants. To enable mechanical ventilation, an endotracheal tube is often used, although there are alternative devices such as face masks or laryngeal mask airways.
- Diagnostic manipulations of the airways such as bronchoscopy.
- Endoscopic operative procedures to the airways such as laser therapy or stenting of the bronchi.
- Patients who require respiratory support, including cardiopulmonary resuscitation.

Tube Maintenance

The tube is secured in place with tape or an endotracheal tube holder. A cervical collar is sometimes used to prevent motion of the airway. Tube placement should be confirmed after each physical move of the patient and after any unexplained change in the patient's clinical status. Continuous pulse oximetry and continuous waveform capnography are often used to monitor the tube's correct placement.

Nasal Intubation

Several techniques exist. Tracheal intubation can be performed by direct laryngoscopy (conventional technique), in which a laryngoscope is used to obtain a view of the glottis. A tube is then inserted under direct vision. This technique can usually only be employed if the patient is comatose (unconscious), under general anesthesia, or has received local or topical anesthesia to the upper airway structures (e.g. using a local anesthetic drug, such as lidocaine).

Rapid sequence induction (RSI) is a variation of the standard technique for patients under anesthesia. It is performed when immediate definitive airway management through intubation is required, and especially when there is a risk of aspiration. For RSI, a short-acting sedative such as etomidate, propofol, thiopental or midazolam is normally administered, followed shortly thereafter by a paralytic such as succinylcholine or rocuronium. RSI is only correctly performed using an induction agent with a 1 arm-brain circulation time. The only agents classically used are those with 1 arm-brain circulation times and are thiopentone and etomidate. This provides the shortest induction time, and provided the appropriate dose based on body mass is used, protects against awareness during the RSI. Propofol and midazolam (in combination with other induction agents) may be used for induction where there is more time, however, propofol is increasingly being used to good effect for RSI.

Another alternative is intubation of the awake patient under local anesthesia using a flexible endoscope or by other means (e.g. using a video laryngoscope). This technique is preferred if difficulties are anticipated, as it allows the patient to breathe spontaneously throughout the procedure, thus ensuring ventilation and oxygenation even in the event of a failed intubation.

Some alternatives to intubation are:

- Tracheotomy: A surgical technique, typically for patients who require long-term respiratory support
- Cricothyrotomy: An emergency technique used when intubation is unsuccessful and tracheotomy is not an option.

Because the life of a patient can depend on the success of an intubation, it is important to assess possible obstacles beforehand. The ease of intubation is difficult to predict. One score to assess anatomical difficulties is the Mallampati score, which is determined by looking at the anatomy of the oral cavity and based on the visibility of the base of uvula, faucial pillars and the soft palate. It should, however, be noted that no single score or combination of scores can be trusted to detect all patients who are difficult to intubate. Therefore, persons performing intubation must be familiar with alternative techniques of securing the airways.

Position of Tube

The tip of tube should be at mid-trachea (between the clavicles on an AP chest X-ray). The position of the tube is checked by auscultation (equal air entry on each side and, in long-term intubation, by chest X-ray).

Types of Tubes

Uncuffed tubes (plain tubes) are commonly used in prepubescent children. In cross-section, the airway in children is circular which makes plain tracheal tube fit better than cuffed tube.

Cuffed tubes less than 6.0 mm and not inflated are accepted for use in pediatrics but generally in children less than 10 years old cuffed tubes are avoided to minimize subglottic swelling and ulceration.

■ OROPHARYNGEAL AIRWAY (FIG. 11.6)

An oropharyngeal airway (also known as an oral airway, OPA or Guedel pattern airway) is a medical device called an airway adjunct used to maintain a patent (open) airway. It does this by preventing the tongue from (either partially or completely) covering the epiglottis, which could prevent the patient from breathing. When a person becomes unconscious, the muscles in their jaw relax and may allow the tongue to obstruct the airway; in fact, the tongue is the most common cause of a blocked airway.

History and Usage

The oropharyngeal airway was designed by Arthur E. Guedel (1883-1956). Oropharyngeal airways come in a variety of sizes, from infant to adult, and are used mostly in pre-hospital emergency care. This piece of equipment is utilized by certified first responders, emergency medical technicians, and paramedics when intubation is either not available or not advisable.

Oropharyngeal airways are usually indicated for unconscious patients, because there is a high probability that the device would stimulate a conscious patient's gag reflex. This could cause the patient to vomit and potentially lead to an obstructed airway. Nasopharyngeal airways are mostly used when the patient has a gag reflex, due to the fact that it can be used on a conscious patient, whereas the oropharyngeal cannot.

Insertion

The correct size OPA is chosen by measuring against the patient's head (from the earlobe to the corner of the mouth). The airway is then inserted into the patient's mouth upside down. Once contact is made with the back of the throat,

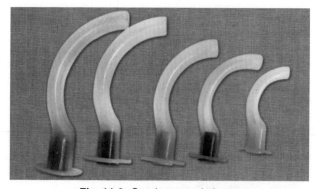

Fig. 11.6: Oropharyngeal airway

the airway is rotated 180 degrees, allowing for easy insertion, and assuring that the tongue is secured. Measuring is very important, as the flared ends of the airway must rest securely against the oral opening in order to remain secure. An alternative method for insertion, the method that is recommended for OPA use in children and infants, involves holding the tongue forward with a tongue depressor and inserting the airway right side up. The airway does not remove the need for the recovery position: it does not prevent suffocation by liquids (blood, saliva, food, cerebrospinal fluid) or the closing of the glottis, but it facilitates the insufflations (cardiopulmonary resuscitation) for patients with a thick tongue.

Key Risks of Use

The mains risks of its use are:
- If the patient has a gag-reflex, they may vomit
- When it is too large, it can close the glottis and thus close the airway
- Improper sizing can cause bleeding in the airway.

■ NASOPHARYNGEAL AIRWAY (FIG. 11.7)

In medicine, a nasopharyngeal airway, also known as an **NPA** or a **nasal trumpet** because of its flared end, a type of airway adjunct, is a tube that is designed to be inserted into the nasal passageway to secure an open airway. When a patient becomes unconscious, the muscles in the jaw commonly relax and can allow the tongue to slide back and obstruct the airway. The purpose of the flared end is to prevent the device from becoming lost inside the patient's head. A safety pin is often included in the NPA kit to be attached to the outside for just such a purpose.

Indications and Contraindications

Nasopharygeal airways are sometimes used by people who have sleep apnea. These devices are also used by emergency care professionals such as EMTs

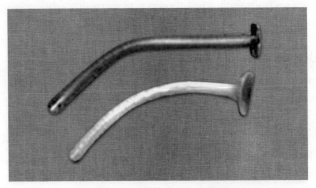

Fig. 11.7: Nasopharyngeal airway

and paramedics in situations where an artificial form of airway maintenance is necessary but it is impossible or unadvisory to use an oropharyngeal airway, the preferred type of airway adjunct. For example, in a patient having epileptic seizures whose teeth are clenched shut. In an unconscious patient, suction of the upper airways may also be applied via an NPA.

Insertion of an NPA is contraindicated in patients with severe head or facial injuries, or have evidence of a basal skull fracture (Battle's sign, Raccoon eyes, cerebrospinal fluid/blood from ears, etc.) due to the possibility of direct intrusion upon brain tissue. An oropharyngeal airway may be used instead, but these devices frequently trigger a patient's gag reflex, while nasopharyngeal airways often do not.

Insertion

The correct size airway is chosen by measuring the device on the patient: the device should reach from the patient's nostril to the earlobe or the angle of the jaw. The outside of the tube is lubricated with a water-based lubricant so that it enters the nose more easily. The device is inserted until the flared end rests against the nostril.

Indications and Contraindications

Nasopharygeal airways are sometimes used by people who have sleep apnea. These devices are also used by emergency care professionals such as EMTs and paramedics in situations where an artificial form of airway maintenance is necessary but it is impossible or unadvisory to use an oropharyngeal airway, the preferred type of airway adjunct. For example, in a patient having epileptic seizures whose teeth are clenched shut. In an unconscious patient, suction of the upper airways may also be applied via an NPA.

Insertion of an NPA is contraindicated in patients with severe head or facial injuries, or have evidence of a basal skull fracture (Battle's sign, Raccoon eyes, cerebrospinal fluid/blood from ears, etc.) due to the possibility of direct intrusion upon brain tissue. An oropharyngeal airway may be used instead, but these devices frequently trigger a patient's gag reflex, while nasopharyngeal airways often do not.

Cuffed Oropharyngeal Airway (Figs 11.8A and B)

Cuffed oropharyngeal airway (COPA) is an oropharyngeal airway with a cuff to prevent any air leak.

Laryngeal Tube (Fig. 11.9)

- Insert it in the esophagus and inflate the two cuffs.
- It has an opening above the lower cuff to ventilate the larynx.
- The lower cuff will be inflated inside the esophagus to prevent aspiration.

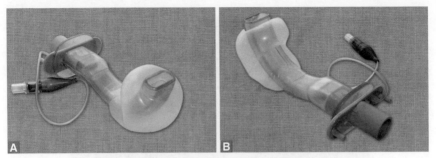

Figs 11.8A and B: Cuffed oropharyngeal airway

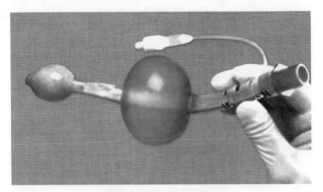

Fig. 11.9: Laryngeal tube

Disadvantages

- This opening might be inadequate to ventilate the patient to the limit he needs.
- If the patient suddenly vomits, it might cause esophageal rupture.

Bougie (Fig. 11.10)

The Bougie is a straight, semi-rigid stylette-like device with a bent tip that can be used when intubation is (or is predicted to be) difficult. During laryngoscopy, the bougie is carefully advanced into the larynx and through the cords until the tip enters a mainstem bronchus. While maintaining the laryngoscope and Bougie in position, an assistant threads an ETT over the end of the bougie, into the larynx. Once the ETT is in place, the bougie is removed.

Combitube (Fig. 11.11)

The Combitube is a twin lumen device designed for use in emergency situations and difficult airways. It can be inserted without the need for visualization into the oropharynx, and usually enters the esophagus. It has a low volume inflatable distal cuff and a much larger proximal cuff designed to occlude the oro- and nasopharynx.

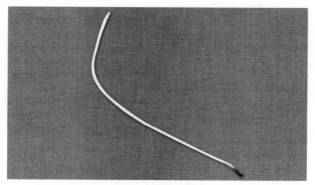

Fig. 11.10: Bougie

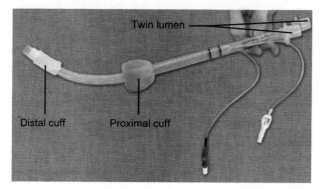

Fig. 11.11: Combitube

If the tube has entered the trachea (Fig. 11.12A), ventilation is achieved through the distal lumen as with a standard ETT. More commonly the device enters the esophagus and ventilation is achieved through multiple proximal apertures situated above the distal cuff (Fig. 11.12B). In the latter case, the proximal and distal cuffs have to be inflated to prevent air from escaping through the esophagus or back out of the oro- and nasopharynx.

The Combitube has been used effectively in cardiopulmonary resuscitation. It has been used successfully in patients with difficult airways secondary to severe facial burns, trauma, upper airway bleeding and vomiting where there was an inability to visualize the vocal cords. It can be used in patients whose cervical spine has been immobilized with a rigid cervical collar, though placement may be more difficult. Ventilation does not seem to be affected by the rigid cervical collar if the Combitube can be placed.

Complications of the Combitube include an increased incidence of sore throat, dysphagia and upper airway hematoma when compared to endotracheal intubation and LMA. Esophageal rupture is a rare complication but has been described. Known esophageal disease is a contraindication to the use of the Combitube. These complications may be partially preventable by avoiding over-inflation of the distal and proximal cuffs (See recommendations

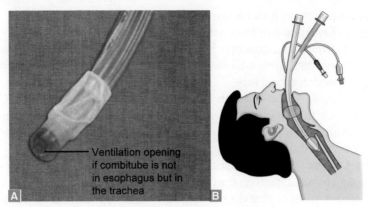

Ventilation opening
if combitube is not
in esophagus but in
the trachea

A   B

Figs 11.12A and B: (A) Ventilation opening if combitube is not in esophagus but in
the trachea; (B) Insertion of combitube

below). Compared to intubation with an endotracheal tube under direct laryngoscopy or using the LMA, the Combitube seems to exert a more pronounced hemodynamic stress response.

Although, it is possible to maintain an airway with the Combitube, endotracheal intubation is the preferred method for definitively securing the airway. Either the oral or the nasal route can be used for fiberoptic-guided airway exchange. The Combitube is left in place and the proximal cuff is partially deflated for fiberoptic intubation with an endotracheal tube.

Preparation

Little preparation is needed beyond testing both cuffs for leaks. The pilot balloon of the distal cuff is white and is marked with the number 2. Test the distal cuff by inflating with 15 mL of air. The pilot balloon of the proximal cuff is blue and is marked with the number 1. Test the proximal cuff by inflating with 85 mL of air. The available sizes are 41 Fr and 37 Fr. The original recommendation by the manufacturer is to use 41 Fr for patients taller than 5 ft (152 cm) and 37 Fr for patients below that height. However, the bulky design of the 41 Fr can make it more technically difficult to insert and some authors have reported satisfactory results using the 37 Fr Combitube on taller patients. A redesigned Combitube has been described by creating an enlarged hole in the pharyngeal lumen that allows fiberoptic access, tracheal suctioning, and tube exchange over a guide wire. However, this type of Combitube is not available in our department.

Oral Intubation: A Step-by-Step Guide

The Combitube can be inserted blindly without the aid of a laryngoscope. However, use of a laryngoscope has been reported to facilitate placement of the Combitube. It appears that the laryngoscope aids insertion by forcefully creating a greater space in the hypopharynx.

- Induce patient as if for regular intubation.
- Patient head position can be neutral.
- When direct laryngoscopy is attempted and the vocal cords can be visualized, the Combitube should be placed in the trachea and used as a regular endotracheal tube.
    - Inflate the distal cuff with just enough air until no leak is present.
    - Check for bilateral breath sounds over the lungs and confirm endotracheal placement on the capnogram.
    - Connect the breathing circuit to the white connector number 2.
- If the Combitube is placed blindly, the left hand should elevate the chin while the right hand maneuvers the Combitube. Alternatively, more space can be created in the hypopharynx by using a laryngoscope with the left hand. The Combitube should be inserted to such a depth that the upper incisors are between the two black guidelines on the external surface of the tube:
    - Inflate the distal cuff with 12 mL.
    - Ventilate through the white connector number 2 and listen for gurgling sounds over the epigastrium or breath sounds over the lungs. If breath sounds are heard over the lungs, the Combitube has been placed in the trachea and can be used as a regular ETT as described above after confirmation on the capnogram. If gurgling sounds are heard over the epigastrium, the Combitube is located in the esophagus.
    - Inflate the proximal cuff with just enough air until either no leak is present or a subjective sensation of increased resistance to cuff inflation is encountered. This is usually achieved by inflating with 50–75 mL of air. This is less than the 85 mL recommended by the manufacturer but has been found to cause less upper airway trauma (1)
    - Ventilate through the blue connector number 1, listen for breath sounds over the lungs and confirm ventilation on the capnogram.

Troubleshooting Tips

Unable to Ventilate Patient through Blue Connector Number 1

Make sure that the Combitube is not per chance in the trachea. Attempt to ventilate through connector number 2, if breath sounds are heard over the lungs then the combitube has been placed in the trachea instead of the esophagus. Deflate the large proximal pharyngeal cuff and use the Combitube as a regular ETT.

Unable to Ventilate Patient through either Connector

Confirm that the combitube has been placed in the esophagus by listening for epigastric gurgling sounds while ventilating through connector number 2. Then withdraw the combitube 2–3 cm at a time while ventilating through connector number 1 until breath sounds are heard over the lungs. The most common cause of this inability to ventilate through either connector is an excessive insertion depth of the combitube (relative to the patient). This will cause obstruction of the glottic opening by the large proximal pharyngeal cuff.

ESOPHAGEAL OBTURATOR AIRWAY

An esophageal obturator airway (EOA) is a semi-flexible large-bore tube approximately 30 cm in length, with 19 holes in the shaft and an inflatable cuff. A soft face mask is attached to one end and the other end is closed. The airway is designed for personnel who are not authorized to place endotracheal tubes. One of the distinct advantages is that it can be inserted blindly through the mouth without having to visualize the larynx. It is also helpful in the prevention of gastric regurgitation. The disadvantages are that the tracheobronchial tree cannot be adequately suctioned and there is the possibility of esophageal rupture when the cuff is inflated too fully. The following steps are to be followed when inserting the EOA:

1. Hyperventilate the patient.
2. Position the head in a neutral position or slightly flexed. Do not hyperextend the neck.
3. Lift the jaw and insert the tube until the mask is flush with the face.

Mouth-to-mask breathing: Ventilate through the tube and auscultate both lung fields. The EOA is sometimes inserted into the trachea; this is of little worry if recognized and corrected immediately. Inflate the cuff (about 35 cc of air). Overinflation can possibly rupture the esophagus or may compress the trachea causing an obstruction. Ventilate and auscultate again to ensure proper placement.

Advantages of the Esophageal Obturator Airway (EOA)

- Insertion does not require laryngeal visualization.
- Indication
- The EOA should be inserted only in apneic, comatose adult-sized patients.

Contraindications

Patients with upper airway obstruction, known esophageal disease, or caustic ingestions. They require different airway management as do patients with massive nasal or intraoral hemorrhage.

Esophageal Airway Device

It is a large-bore 34 cm tube with a rounded, occluded distal tip. A snap lock connects the tube through the center of a clear plastic oronasal mask. There are sixteen 3 mm openings in the proximal half of the tube below the mask at the hypopharyngeal level.

Technique (Figs 11.13A and B)

- The mask is attached to the proximal end of the tube.
- The patient's mandible and tongue are pulled forward with the head held in a neutral position. If a neck injury is excluded, slight neck flexion will decrease the incidence of inadvertent tracheal intubation.

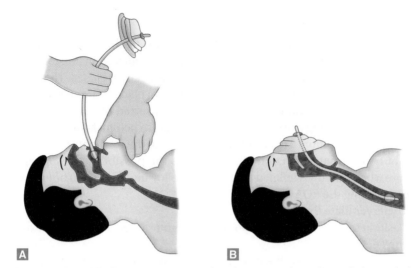

Figs 11.13A and B: Diagram demonstrating placement of esophageal airway device

- Once the mask is sealed by hand to the patient's face, ventilation is initiated. This forces air into the trachea, which is the only unobstructed orifice.
- Auscultation for bilateral breath sounds ensures esophageal placement of the tube. Then the cuff is inflated with 30 to 35 mL of air. The cuff must lie below the level of the carina or partial compression of the trachea will obstruct ventilation.

■ ESOPHAGEAL GASTRIC TUBE AIRWAY (FIG. 11.14)

The distal end of this tube is patent. There are two holes in the mask. The esophageal tube attaches to one, and a nasogastric tube can be passed down the tube through a valve into the stomach. This unit allows ventilation through the second hole.

The esophageal gastric tube airway consists of an inflatable face mask and an esophageal tube. The transparent face mask has two ports: a lower port for insertion of an esophageal tube, and an upper port for ventilation. The inside of the mask is soft and pliable; it molds to the patient's face and makes a tight seal, preventing air loss.

The proximal end of the esophageal tube has a one-way, nonrefluxing valve that blocks the esophagus. This valve prevents air from entering the stomach, thus reducing the risk of abdominal distension and aspiration. The distal end of the tube has an inflatable cuff which rests in the esophagus just below the tracheal bifurcation, preventing pressure on the noncartilaginous back of the tracheal wall.

During ventilation, air is blown into the upper port of the mask, and, with the esophagus blocked, enters the trachea and lungs.

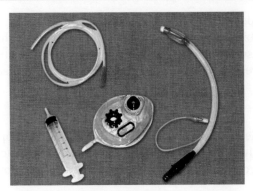

Fig. 11.14: Esophageal gastric tube airway

A gastric tube can be used to suction stomach contents before extubation. It is inserted through the masks lower port into the esophageal tube, then through a small hole in the end of the tube.

The esophageal obturator airway consists of an adjustable, inflatable face mask with a single port, attached by a snap lock to a blind esophageal tube.

When properly inflated, the transparent mask prevents air from escaping through the nose and mouth.

The esophageal tube has sixteen holes at its proximal end through which air or oxygen blown into the port of the mask, is transferred to the trachea. The tube's distal end is closed and circled by an inflatable cuff. When the cuff is inflated, it occludes the esophagus, preventing air from entering the stomach and acting as a barrier against vomitus and involuntary aspiration.

■ CRICOTHYROIDOTOMY

A cricothyroidotomy, often known as an emergency tracheotomy, consists of incising the cricothyroid membrane, which lies just beneath the skin between the thyroid cartilage and the cricoid cartilage. The cricothyroid membrane can be located easily in most cases. Hyperextend the neck so that the thyroid notch (Adam's apple) becomes prominent anteriorly. Identify the position of the thyroid notch with the index finger. This finger descends in the midline to the prominence of the cricoid cartilage. The depression of the cricothyroid membrane is identified above the superior margin of the cricoid cartilage. A small lateral incision is made at the base of the thyroid cartilage to expose the cricothyroid membrane. This membrane is then excised, taking care not to go too deeply, and a small bore airline is then inserted into the trachea. An alternate method is to use a 12 to 16 gauge intercatheter. Locate the cricothyroid membrane as above and insert the needle into the trachea. Immediately upon penetrating the cricothyroid membrane, thread the plastic catheter into the trachea and remove the needle. The catheter can then be connected to an oxygen line for translaryngeal oxygen jet insufflation. A cricothyroidotomy should not be attempted except as a last resort when other methods of opening the airway are unsuccessful.

Suctioning devices in a first-aid setting, the hospital corpsman may have access to portable or fixed suctioning devices equipped with flexible tubing, semirigid tips, suction catheters, and nonbreakable collection bottles. The suction pressure should be tested regularly and the equipment kept clean.

Technique

After testing the apparatus, attach a catheter or tip, and open the victim's mouth. Carefully insert the end into the pharynx. Apply suction, but for no more than 15 seconds. Suction may be repeated after a few breaths.

Definition

Emergency cricothyroidotomy is a surgical procedure where an incision is made through the skin and cricothyroid membrane. This allows for the placement of an endotracheal tube into the trachea when control of the airway is not possible by other methods.

Introduction

- Cricothyroid space is the key anatomic landmark between the thyroid cartilage and the circoid cartilage.
- Cricothyroid space: Trapezoidal shape; 3 cm horizontal, vertical height is variable: 5 mm–9 mm.
- Overlying tissue: Skin, subcutaneous tissue, cervical fascia, cricothyroid ligament.
- No major blood vessels in the midline at the proper location.
- Cricothyroid arteries: Transverse the superior aspect of the cricothyroid membrane but are not usually major sources of hemorrhage.
- If you hit the thyroid gland, you are too low; major bleeding from thyroid vessels can occur.

Anatomical Landmarks (Fig. 11.15)

- **Trachea:** Also known as the windpipe. It is the cartilaginous and membranous tube descending from, and continuous with, the lower part of the larynx to the bronchi.
- **Thyroid cartilage:** Also known as the "Adam's apple." The thyroid cartilage is located in the upper part of the throat. The thyroid cartilage tends to be more prominent in men than women.
- **Cricoid cartilage:** Located approximately 3/4 inch inferior to the thyroid cartilage. The cricoid and thyroid cartilage form the framework of the larynx.

- **Cricothyroid membrane:** Soft tissue depression between the thyroid and cricoid cartilage. This membrane connects the two cartilages and is only covered by skin.
- **Carotid arteries:** Two principal arteries of the neck.
- **Jugular veins:** Two principal veins of the neck.
- **Esophagus:** Musculomembranous tube extending downward from the pharynx to the stomach. The esophagus lies posterior to the trachea.
- **Thyroid gland:** Largest endocrine gland, the thyroid gland is situated in front of the lower part of the neck. Consists of a right and left lobe on either side of the trachea.

Indications

There are many reasons for which an emergency cricothyroidotomy may be required. Listed below are a few of the most common reasons:

Absolute Indication for Cricothyrotomy

- When the patient intubate, cannot ventilate, and patient is too unstable to attempt alternative airway devices.

Obstructed Airway

Obstructed airway and/or swelling of tissues will usually prevent the passage of an endotracheal tube through the airway. Therefore, a surgical airway distal to the obstruction is required. Causes of an obstructed airway include:

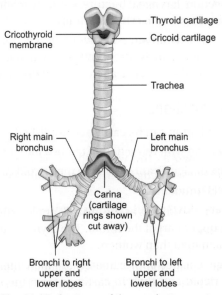

Fig. 11.15: Anatomy of the respiratory system

- Facial and oropharyngeal edema from burns
- Foreign objects (food or teeth).

Congenital Deformities

Congenital deformities of the oropharynx or nasopharynx will inhibit or prevent nasotracheal or orotracheal intubation.

Trauma to the Head and Neck

Trauma to the head and neck would preclude the use of an ambu-bag, oropharyngeal airway, nasopharyngeal airway, and endotracheal tube insertion.

Examples include:
- Facial and oropharyngeal edema from severe trauma
- Facial fractures (mandible fracture)
- Nasal bone fractures
- Cribriform fractures.

Cervical spine fractures in a patient who needs an airway but whose intubation is unsuccessful or contraindicated.

Contraindications

Absolute Contraindications

- Although textbooks list absolute contraindications to cricothyrotomy (tracheal transection, laryngeal fracture, etc.), the reality is that there is no absolute contraindication to cricothyrotomy.
- Obviously a less invasive airway is always preferred, however, if you cannot get an airway and the patient is crumping (cannot intubate, cannot ventilate), you will be forced to do a surgical airway regardless of the situation.

Relative Contraindications

- Less invasive intubation can be easily accomplished.
- Tracheal transection with retraction of trachea into mediastinum.
- Fractured larynx or significant trauma to the cricoid cartilage.
- Known laryngeal tumor.
- Children <8 years: Why? Small anatomy, very soft/compressible tissue.
- Bleeding diathesis.
- Massive neck edema.
- Severe laryngeal inflammation (laryngotracheitis, diphtheria, chemical inflammation, TB): Needs to be replaced with ETT or tracheostomy when able.

Advantages and Disadvantages

Advantages of Emergency Cricothyroidotomy

- Provides a definitive airway for ventilating the patient.
- It can be performed quickly and has few complications associated with the procedure.

Disadvantages of Emergency Cricothyroidotomy

- Need advanced training to properly perform procedure.
- Bypasses the nares function of warming and filtering the air.
- May increase respiratory resistance.
- Improper placement.
- Casualty is now totally dependent on corpsman.

Procedural Steps

Make your Decision

- Look, listen, and feel
- Attempt to secure airway by all other means
- Justify your decision.

Assemble and Check Equipment (Fig. 11.16)

- No. 11 scalpel blade
- Scalpel blade handle
- Tube
- 10 cc syringe—used to fill the cuff at the end of the endotracheal tube
- Stylet—a wire inserted into the endotracheal tube in order to stiffen the tube during passage
- Water soluble lubrication—KY Jelly or Surgilube
- Stethoscope—to check for proper placement of the endotracheal tube
- Curved Kelly hemostat—used to open the incision site
- Tissue forceps—used to retract skin tissue at the incision site
- Ambu-bag—to ventilate patient
- Sterile dressing
- Petroleum gauze
- Betadine or alcohol wipes
- Sterile or clean gloves
- Suture material
- Suction device
- Suture scissors
- Tape
- Sterile dressing.

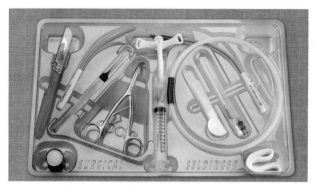

Fig. 11.16: Equipment tray for cricothyroidotomy

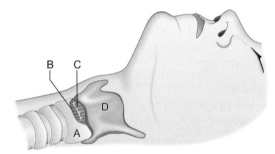

Fig. 11.17: A. Cricoid cartilage; B. Cricothyroid membrane; C. Incision site; D. Thyroid cartilage

Preparation

- Skin preparation, drape, get kit opened
- Skip the skin preparation if there is no time
- Hyperextend the neck if possible.

Palpation

- Stand on the patient's left
- Place the left elbow on the chest and use the index finger and thumb to stabilize the larynx
- Place lateral traction with fingers so that skin will spread when incision is made.

Incisions (Fig. 11.17)

- Vertical midline incision through the skin: 3–4 cm
- Horizontal incision through the inferior aspect of the cricothyroid membrane: 2 cm (Fig. 11.18)

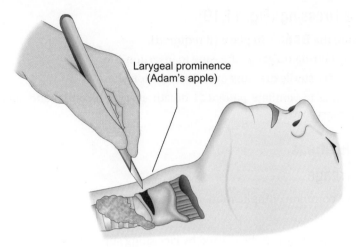

Larygeal prominence
(Adam's apple)

Fig. 11.18: Horizontal incision over the cricothyroid membrane

Traction

- While the scalpel is through the cricothyroid membrane, pass a tracheal hook through the incision with the left hand and hook the cricoid ring.
- Apply traction to the cricoid cartilage in a lifting and caudal direction.
- Remove the scalpel.

Intubation

- While applying traction with the hook (left hand), place a tube with the right hand.
- Endotracheal tube No. 6 can also be used.

Inflate balloon with 10 cc of air, this serves two purposes:
- Holds the endotracheal tube in place.
- Acts as a barrier and prevents fluids from entering the lungs.

Ventilate the patient with two breaths using bag valve mask.

Check for proper placement during these first two ventilations by:
- Observing for bilateral rise and fall of the chest with each ventilation.
- Observe the ET tube for misting, fogging, or condensation.
- Auscultate for bilateral breath sounds.

Bilateral breath sounds present: The ET tube has been properly placed causing both lungs to inflate with each ventilation.

Breath sounds in right lung field only: The tube has been placed too far down the bronchial tree and is in the right mainstem bronchus.

Pull back the endotracheal tube 1/4–1/2 inch or until bilateral breath sounds have been established.

Secure Dressing (Fig. 11.19)

- Suture the ET tube in place (if required).
- Apply petroleum gauze dressing to insertion site.
- Apply dry sterile dressing over the insertion site.
- Continue to ventilate patient (1 breath every 5 seconds) and suction as necessary.

Complications

Hemorrhage

The most common complication.

Causes
- Minor bleeding may be caused by lacerating superficial capillaries in the skin.
- Significant bleeding may be caused by the laceration of major vessels (carotid arteries and the jugular veins) within the neck.

Treatment
- Minor bleeding is treated with direct pressure and the application of a simple pressure dressing.
- Significant bleeding: Treated same as minor. However, if unable to control the bleeding, the vessel may need to be ligated.

Esophageal Perforation or Tracheoesophageal Fistula

Definition
The creation of a hole between the esophagus and trachea.

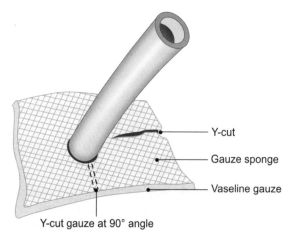

Y-cut

Gauze sponge

Vaseline gauze

Y-cut gauze at 90° angle

Fig. 11.19: Dressing for emergency cricothyroidotomy

Causes
- Creating an incision too deep through the cricothyroid membrane.
- Forcing the ET tube through the cricothyroid membrane and into the esophagus.

Treatment
Requires surgical repair at higher echelon of care.

Subcutaneous Emphysema

Definition
The presence of free air or gas within the subcutaneous tissues. Upon palpation, a crackling sensation may be felt as the air is pushed through the tissue.

Causes
- Creating too wide of an incision will allow air entrapment under the skin.
- Air leaking out of the insertion site may get trapped under the skin.

Treatment
- No treatment is necessary. The subcutaneous emphysema will resolve spontaneously within a few days.
- The placement of petroleum gauze dressing around the incision/insertion site will help reduce the incidence of subcutaneous emphysema.

■ PERCUTANEOUS TRACHEOSTOMY

- Tracheostomy: An airway that is inserted subglottically through neck tissues directly into the trachea.
- Surgical tracheostomy: Dissection and incision of trachea under direct vision.
- Percutaneous tracheostomy: Seldinger technique and dilatation of trachea between rings.
- The percutaneous tracheostomy was successfully performed bedside in ICU in all cases.

Introduction

Tracheostomy is one of the most commonly performed surgical procedures in the intensive care unit setting. Tracheostomy-related complications occur in 3–15% of patients. These are commonly divided into early and late complications. Early complications include peri-procedural hemorrhage, hypoxemia, airway loss, pneumothorax, and infection. Late complications include tracheotomy stenosis due to granulation tissue, upper airway obstruction, tracheoesophageal fistula, tracheoinnominate artery fistula (TIF), tracheomalacia, and tracheal stenosis. Fatal percutaneous tracheostomy complications are rare, but dramatic when they occur.

Percutaneous dilatational tracheostomy (PDT), first described by Ciaglia et al in 1985, is the surgical insertion of a tracheostomy tube using a modified Seldinger technique. Initially described as truly percutaneous without direct visualization of the trachea, most surgeons performing this procedure now perform a modified open technique in which a limited dissection of the central neck is performed allowing direct palpation of the anterior trachea to ensure appropriate placement. Comparative studies and meta-analyses have shown that percutaneous tracheostomy and open surgical tracheostomy are associated with similar complication rates. Percutaneous tracheostomy has largely replaced open tracheostomy in the critical care setting as it can be performed safely at the patient's bedside, does not require operating room time, and is more cost-effective.

Fiberoptic bronchoscopy and ultrasound have both been suggested to improve the safety of percutaneous tracheostomy. Fiberoptic bronchoscopy should always be performed when the classic Ciaglia percutaneous technique is employed to avoid iatrogenic injury to adjacent anatomic structures or paratracheal insertion. The modified open percutaneous tracheostomy approach negates many of the benefits of fiberoptic bronchoscopy as the trachea is directly palpated and commonly visualized. A bronchoscope should always be available at the bedside during a percutaneous tracheostomy procedure if not used routinely. Ultrasound-guided percutaneous tracheotomy facilitates identification of the tracheal midline and level of tracheal cartilages as well as identifying vulnerable adjacent anatomic structures such as the thyroid gland or blood vessels.

Percutaneous tracheotomy: It is a recent procedure which became popular especially amongst intensivists. It involves passing a needle into the tracheal lumen, through which is passed a guidewire. Dilators of increasing size are passed over the wire until a tracheostomy tube can be inserted.

The most common/popular technique which is used in intensive care unit is ciaglia (single-step dilator) technique.

Insertion Techniques

- Assess for appropriateness of PDT
- Consent
- Fast
- IV access
- Preoxygenate
- Emergency re-intubation gear
- Standard monitoring (including $EtCO_2$)
- GA + LA
- Pull ETT back to cords (LMA use)
- Sterile technique.

Technique (Figs 11.20 to 11.29)

Rhino: With this technique, there is no sharp dissection involved beyond the skin incision. The patient is positioned and prepared in the same way as for the standard operative tracheostomy.

- The patient's neck is extended.
- A horizontal incision is made halfway between the sternal notch and cricoid cartilage (a vertical midline incision may be used in emergency situation).
- Skin incision is made and the pretracheal tissue is cleared with blunt dissection in the midline.
- The thyroid isthmus then either be mobilized superiorly or inferiorly.
- Endotracheal tube is withdrawn enough to place the cuff at the level of the glottis.
- Optional but safe: Bronchoscopist places the tip of the bronchoscope such that the light from its tip shines through the surgical wound.
- Operator enters the tracheal lumen below the second tracheal ring (between 2nd and 3rd ring) with an introducer needle.
- Once needle in the trachea aspirate with syringe and saline make sure that air bubbles are passing through the saline.
- Introduce guidewire through the needle until you get the resistance.
- The tract between the skin and the tracheal lumen is then serially dilated over a guidewire and stylet.
- Initially dilate with small dilator-14F dilator, make sure air passes through the incision site.
- With stylet and bigger dilator, dilate the trachea up to black mark on the dilator.
- A tracheostomy tube is placed (under direct bronchoscopic vision, if bronchoscope is used) over a guidewire.
- Placement of the tube is confirmed again by visualizing the tracheobronchial tree through the tube with the bronchoscope if used or with end tidal carbon dioxide.
- Tube is secured with tracheostomy tape.

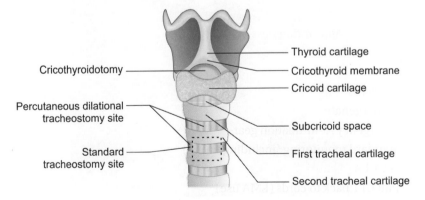

Fig. 11.20: Tracheal land mark

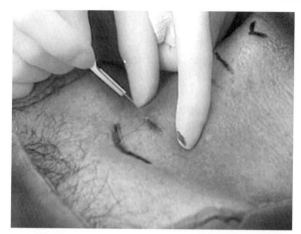

Fig. 11.21: Horizontal incision (*For color version, see Plate 2*)

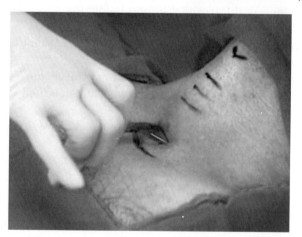

Fig. 11.22: Dilatation with forceps (*For color version, see Plate 2*)

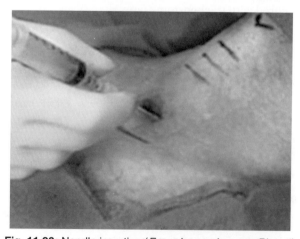

Fig. 11.23: Needle insertion (*For color version, see Plate 2*)

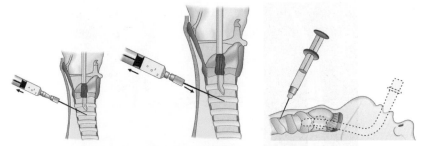

Fig. 11.24: Needle insertion

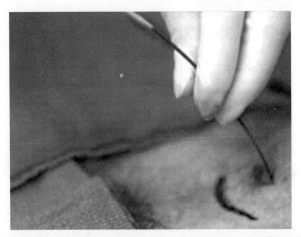

Fig. 11.25: Guidewire insertion (*For color version, see Plate 3*)

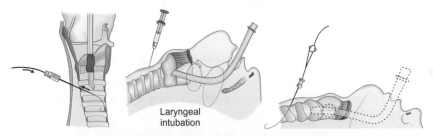

Laryngeal
intubation

Fig. 11.26: Guidewire insertion through needle

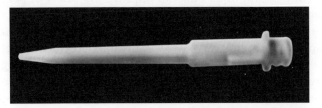

Fig. 11.27: First small dilator and dilation over guidewire

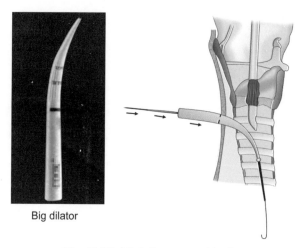

Big dilator

Fig. 11.28: Dilatation over guidewire

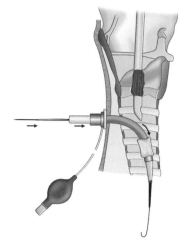

Fig. 11.29: Tube insertion over guidewire

There is one more technique, which is also been followed known as Griggs forceps (Portex) Technique—once guidewire is inserted, use of guidewire dilating forceps.

In the recent years ultrasound-guided percutaneous tracheostomy has become a routine and popular procedure in most intensive care units, 'real-time' ultrasound in an effort to improve the safety of percutaneous tracheostomy.

Patients who need prolonged ventilator support or have difficulty with maintaining and protecting airway are usual candidates for tracheostomy. Do explain the procedure in detail and possible complications including technical difficulty with possible transfer to theater to complete the procedure, bleeding during or after the procedure, and very rarely, life-threatening complications. Ensure that the consent form is signed prior to the procedure. Percutaneous tracheostomies are generally not performed in the presence of uncorrected coagulopathy and severe thrombocytopenia. If indicated, perform INR, APTT and platelet counts on the morning of the procedure.

Preparation

Take plenty of time to study the ultrasound anatomy of the neck, using the 12 MHz linear probe. The thyroid and cricoid cartilages and the first few tracheal rings must be clearly visible, on the short- as well as long-axis views. Look for abnormal vessels that may be encountered during the procedure; apply to probe gently to ensure that superficial veins do not collapse. Administer anesthesia—usually with fentanyl boluses and an infusion of propofol. Following muscle relaxant, position the patient in which neck in the extended position (if a C-spine fracture is suspected, maintain neutral position). Switch to an FiO_2 of 1.0 on an appropriate controlled mode of ventilation. Suck out the stomach tube.

The following items should be ready:
- Disposable percutaneous tracheostomy kit with a single step 'rhino' dilator
- Artery forceps, scissors and sponge holding forceps
- A Griggs dilator must be available if difficulty is encountered
- Arthroscopy sleeve to cover the ultrasound probe
- Tegaderm to stick on the probe head.

Procedure

After induction of anesthesia, cleaning and draping, view the neck with the 12 MHz linear probe. On the short-axis view, start from the thyroid cartilage and slide down gradually to view the cricoid cartilage, followed by the tracheal rings one below the other. Turn to long-axis view to see how many tracheal rings can be viewed above the suprasternal notch (3–4 rings are usually visible). Pass the introducer needle between the first and second or second and third tracheal rings, on the short-axis view. Aspirate air into the water-filled syringe to ensure needle tip within the tracheal lumen. Insert the guidewire till as far as it will go (usually it stops at the level of the carina). Inject lignocaine 2% with adrenaline 1:200,000 into the skin puncture site. Make a horizontal cut on the skin, about 2 cm wide, followed by gentle dissection of tissues. Pass the short, straight dilator over the wire till the hub; repeat about three times to ensure smooth passage. Introduce the 'rhino' dilator over the wire till the black mark is at the level of the skin. Dilate about three times to ensure smooth passage. Insert the tracheostomy tube over the wire. Confirm position of the tracheostomy tube by detection of the end tidal carbon dioxide waveform. Secure the tracheostomy tube with tapes. Check for pneumothorax with the same probe, by confirming pleural slide. Routine chest X-rays are not necessary for confirmation of tracheostomy tube position. The bronchoscope must be readily available in case of difficulty.

Indications

- Facilitate weaning from MV
- Protection from aspiration
- Airway obstruction
- Inability to protect the airway
- Access for pulmonary toilet.

Contraindications
Absolute

- Pediatric patient (<16 years)
- Midline neck mass
- Uncorrected coagulopathy or platelet dysfunction
- Infection at site
- Patient or family refusal
- Emergency.

Relative

- Suspected or known difficult intubation
- Poor respiratory function: FiO_2 >0.6, PEEP >10
- Difficult anatomy—obese/short neck/neck distortion
- Tracheomalacia
- Unstable c-spine or c-spine immobilization (cervical fusion/instability, RA).

Advantages

- Reduced sedation requirement (greater comfort than orotracheal intubation)
- Airway protection while unconscious
- Allows gradual weaning of ventilatory support (reduced work of breathing)
- Enhanced communication (written or phonation)
- Decreased ICU mortality
- Enhanced nursing care (mouth care and mobility)
- Ease of replacement of tracheal tube
- Can facilitate transfer to the ward.

Disadvantages/Complications

- Requirement for a surgical procedure.

Immediate

- Hemorrhage
- Surgical emphysema
- Pneumothorax
- Air embolism
- Cricoid cartilage damage

- Pretracheal dilation and placement
- Endobronchial placement
- Cuff herniation
- Occlusion of tip by carina or tracheal wall
- Damage to the posterior tracheal wall
- Accidental decannulation
- Death.

Delayed

- Infection (tracheostomy site, larynx, tracheobronchial tree, mediastinum)
- Obstruction with secretions
- Ulceration/perforation (mucosal, innominate artery, tracheoesophageal fistula)
- Dysphagia, complaints of mechanical compression of esophagus (requires N/G or PEG for enteral nutrition)
- Problems with decannulation—emergency airway management.

Late

- Tracheal granulomata
- Tracheal or laryngeal stenosis
- Persistent sinus at tracheostomy site
- Tracheomalacia
- Aphonia/dysphonia (recovery of voice, laryngeal or cord dysfunction)
- Tracheal dilatation.

■ BIBLIOGRAPHY

1. Benumof JL. Management of the difficult adult airway with special emphasis on awake tracheal intubation. Anesthesiology. 1991;75:1087-110.
2. Davis JM, Weeks S, Crone LA, Pavlin E. Difficult intubation in the parturient. Can J Anaesth. 1989;36:668-74.
3. Glassenberg R. General anesthesia and maternal mortality. Semin Perinatol. 1991; 15:386-96.
4. Jose C, Jahan N, Brar G, Kumar U, Moorthy R. Article: Ultrasound percutaneous tracheostomy. Intensive Care Medicine 02/2012;5.26 Impact Factor.
5. Jose C, Jahan N, Brar G, Kumar U, Moorthy R. Real-time ultrasound-guided percutaneous dilatational tracheostomy. European Journal of Intensive Care Medicine (Impact Factor: 5.17). 02/2012; 38(5):920-1. DOI:10.1007/s00134-012-2514-3.
6. Katos MG, Goldenberg D. "Emergency cricothyrotomy". Operative Techniques in Otolaryngology. June 2007;18(2):110–114. doi:10.1016/j.otot.2007.05.002. Retrieved 25 July 2010.
7. Markowitz E, Joshua, Kulkarni, Rick. "Surgical Airway Techniques" [1] Medscape Reference.
8. Merah NA, Foulkes-Crabbe DJ, Kushimo OT, Ajayi PA. Prediction of difficult laryngoscopy in a population of Nigerian obstetric patients. West Afr J Med. 2004; 23:33-41.
9. Suresh MS, Wali A. Airway management strategies. Anesthesiol Clin North Am. 1998;16:477-98.

NONINVASIVE VENTILATION AND HIGH FLOW THERAPY

■ NONINVASIVE VENTILATION

Noninvasive ventilation (NIV) refers to the technique of providing ventilatory support to a patient without an endo/orotracheal airway. It is a promising and rapidly upcoming new technique and is being used as first-line therapy in a wide variety of conditions causing respiratory failure.

Advantages

- Preservation of airway defense mechanism
- Early ventilatory support
- Intermittent ventilation
- Patient can eat, drink and communicate
- Ease of application and removal
- Patient can cooperate with physiotherapy
- Improved patient comfort
- Reduced sedation requirements
- Avoidance of complications of intubation
- Ventilation outside hospital setting possible.

Disadvantages

- Mask is uncomfortable/claustrophobic
- Time consuming for medical and nursing staff
- Airway is not protected
- No direct access to bronchial tree for suction.

Reduced Incidence of Complications

Nosocomial pneumonia is a frequent complication of mechanical ventilation and an important factor in the prognosis of mortality. Endotracheal intubation short circuits the airway barrier defenses, compromising mucociliary clearance, resulting in epithelial cell peeling, leading to greater bacterial adhesion and tracheal colonization. In addition, it serves as a route by which microorganisms can enter the tracheobronchial tree.

A number of different laryngeal, pharyngeal and tracheal complications are caused by endotracheal tubes. These complications may occur at the moment of intubation (prolonged intubation attempt, right main stem bronchus intubation, arterial hypotension, airway damage), during the intubation period (mechanical malfunction of the endotracheal tube, leaking cuff, laryngeal ulceration), and after removal (stridor due to obstruction of the upper airways, hoarseness, difficulties with deglutition, stenosis of the trachea)

Sinusitis is a common cause of fever with no obvious focus and of bacteremia in patients on mechanical ventilation. The risk is related to the presence of tubes in the nasopharynx and the duration of ventilation, and can therefore, be minimized by NIV.

Reduced Discomfort

The pain resulting from the presence of the endotracheal tube in the oral cavity is the main source of discomfort among intubated patients. Furthermore, endotracheal intubation prevents the patient from speaking. Communication with relatives and health professionals is frustrating because of the inability to verbalize, which interferes with the ability to cooperate. The patient becomes agitated and is treated with sedatives, further compromising communication. The majority of patients with a facial or nasal mask tolerate them relatively well and present a gradual reduction in dyspnea.

Mechanism of Action

- Improvement in pulmonary mechanics and oxygenation NIV augments alveolar ventilation and allows oxygenation without raising the $PaCO_2$. The work of breathing equals the product of pressure change across the lung and volume of gas moved. During inspiration, most of the work is done to overcome elastic recoil of the thorax and lungs, and the resistance of the airways and non-elastic tissues.
- Partial unloading of respiratory muscles NIV reduces transdiaphragmatic pressure, pressure time index of respiratory muscles and diaphragmatic electromyographic activity. This leads to an increase in tidal volume, decrease in respiratory rate and increase in minute ventilation. Also overcomes the effect of intrinsic PEEP.
- Resetting of respiratory center ventilatory responses to $PaCO_2$ In patients with COPD, the ventilatory response to raised $PaCO_2$ is decreased especially during sleep. By maintaining lower nocturnal $PaCO_2$ during sleep by administering NIV, it is possible to reset the respiratory control center to become more responsive to an increased $PaCO_2$ by increasing the neural output to the diaphragm and other respiratory muscles. These patients are then able to maintain a more normal $PaCO_2$ throughout the daylight hours without the need for mechanical ventilation.

Timing of NIV

1. Different stages of ARF
2. Respiratory failure is defined as a failure to maintain adequate gas exchange and is characterized by abnormalities of arterial blood gas tensions.

   Type 1 failure is defined by a PaO_2 of <80 mm Hg with a normal or low $PaCO_2$.

   Type 2 failure is defined by a PaO_2 of 80 mm Hg kPa and a $PaCO_2$ of >60 mm Hg kPa.

   Type 2 is further divided into—acute, chronic, or acute-on-chronic.

How to Decide to Initiate?

- Diagnosis
  - What is the evidence?
  - Reversibility?
- Does the patient need ventilatory assistance?
- Does the patient have contraindications to NIV?

Respiratory Failure

- Hypoxemic (Type 1)
- Hypercapnic (Type 2)
  - NIV seems to work better for this.

Types

- PSV
  - Inspiratory pressure (IPAP)
- CPAP
  - Expiratory pressure (EPAP)
- Bilevel NPPV
  - Inspiratory and expiratory pressures
  - PSV + CPAP
  - BiPAP.

CPAP

- Same as PEEP (Used in spontaneous breathing patients)
- Most helpful in cardiogenic pulmonary edema
  - Decreases preload
  - Decreases after load, improves CO.
- Increases the FRC, decreases shunt and improves oxygenation.

  Although not a true ventilator mode because it does not actively assist inspiration, CPAP is used for certain forms of acute respiratory failure. By delivering a constant pressure during both inspiration and expiration, CPAP increases functional residual capacity and opens collapsed or underventilated alveoli, thus decreasing right to left intrapulmonary shunt and improving oxygenation. The increase in functional residual capacity may also improve lung compliance, decreasing the work of breathing.

CPAP may reduce the work of breathing in patients with COPD. A few uncontrolled trials have observed improved vital signs and gas exchange in patients with acute exacerbations of COPD treated with CPAP alone, suggesting that this modality may offer benefit to these patients.

Selection Criteria
Acute Respiratory Failure
At least two of the following criteria should be present:
- Respiratory distress with dyspnea
- Use of accessory muscles of respiration
- Abdominal paradox
- Respiratory rate >25/min
- ABG shows pH <7.35 or $PaCO_2$ >45 mm Hg or PaO_2/FiO_2 <200.

Chronic Respiratory Failure (Obstructive Lung Disease)
- Fatigue, hypersomnolence, dyspnea
- ABG shows pH <7.35, $PaCO_2$ >55 mm Hg, $PaCO_2$ 50–54 mm Hg
- Oxygen saturation <88% for >10% of monitoring time despite O_2 supplementation.

Thoracic Restrictive/Cerebral Hypoventilation Diseases
- Fatigue, morning headache, hypersomnolence, nightmares, enuresis, dyspnea
- ABG shows $PaCO_2$ >45 mm Hg
- Nocturnal SaO_2 <90% for more than 5 minutes.
    - COPD
        - Strongest evidence for use of NPPV
        - Intubation rate by up to 66%
        - Mortality, complications, hospital days
- Acute asthma
    - Arterial blood gas tensions should be considered in all individuals with breathlessness of sufficient severity to warrant admission to hospital. In certain subgroups of patients—for example, asthmatic patients with no features of a severe attack—oxygen saturation can be used as an initial screen, proceeding to arterial blood gas analysis in those with a SpO_2 of <92%. However, it is important to note that oximetry alone may provide false reassurance in patients on supplemental oxygen in whom oxygenation is well-maintained in the face of dangerous hypercapnia.
- Hypoxemic respiratory failure
    - Role of NPPV in nonhypercapnic respiratory failure is controversial
    - Studies support its use, but many studies include COPD patients
    - Evidence supports use of NPPV but evidence less compelling than COPD

- Cardiogenic pulmonary edema
  - CPAP
    - Evidence supports its use
  - Bilevel NPPV
    - Controversial
    - Need for intubation reduced
    - Possible ↑ cardiovascular events
    - Reserve for pulmonary edema + hypercapnia.

Indications for Acute NIV

- NIV may be undertaken as a therapeutic trial with a view to tracheal intubation if it fails, or as the ceiling of treatment in patients who are not candidates for intubation. A decision about tracheal intubation should be made before commencing NIV in every patient.
- NIV should be considered in patients with an acute exacerbation of COPD in whom a respiratory acidosis (pH <7.35, H^+ >45 nmol/L) persists despite maximum medical treatment on controlled oxygen therapy.
- Continuous positive airway pressure (CPAP) has been shown to be effective in patients with cardiogenic pulmonary edema who remain hypoxic despite maximal medical treatment. NIV should be reserved for patients in whom CPAP is unsuccessful.
- NIV is indicated in acute or acute-on-chronic hypercapnic respiratory failure due to chest wall deformity or neuromuscular disease.
- Both CPAP and NIV have been used successfully in patients with decompensated obstructive sleep apnea. Although no direct comparison is available, NIV (in the form of bi-level pressure support) should be used for these patients if a respiratory acidosis is present.
- CPAP should be used in patients with chest wall trauma who remain hypoxic despite adequate regional anesthesia and high flow oxygen. NIV should not be used routinely.
- In view of the risk of pneumothorax, patients with chest wall trauma who are treated with CPAP or NIV should be monitored on the ICU.
- Many patients with acute pneumonia and hypoxemia resistant to high flow oxygen will require intubation. In this context, trials of CPAP or NIV should only occur in HDU or ICU settings.
- CPAP improves oxygenation in patients with diffuse pneumonia who remain hypoxic despite maximum medical treatment. NIV can be used as an alternative to tracheal intubation if the patient becomes hypercapnic. In this context, patients who would be candidates for intubation if NIV fails, should only receive NIV in an ICU.
- NIV should not be used routinely in acute asthma.
- A trial of NIV may be undertaken in patients with a respiratory acidosis (pH <7.35, H^+ >45 nmol/L) secondary to an acute exacerbation of bronchiectasis, but excessive secretions are likely to limit its effectiveness and it should not be used routinely in bronchiectasis.

- NIV has been used in a variety of other conditions (such as acute respiratory distress syndrome, postoperative and post-transplantation respiratory failure) with reduced intubation rates, ICU stay and mortality. In this context, patients who would be considered for intubation if NIV fails should only receive NIV in ICU.
- NIV has been used successfully to wean patients from invasive ventilation, and should be used when conventional weaning strategies fail.

Strong (Level A) (Recommended)
- Acute hypercapnic RF—in COPD
- Cardiogenic pulmonary edema (CPAP)
- ARF in immunocompromized.

Intermediate (Level B)
- Asthma
- Community acquired pneumonia (COPD)
- Extubation failure (COPD)
- Hypoxemic respiratory failure
- Do-not-intubate patients
- Postoperative respiratory failure.

Do not intubate patients: Terminally ill patients. NIV is used in these patients, mainly to relieve symptoms like dyspnea, preserve patient autonomy and permit verbal communication with the family. However some would argue this is delaying the dying process and lead inappropriate resource utilization.

Weaker (Level C)
- Acute respiratory distress syndrome (ARDS)
- Community-acquired pneumonia (non-COPD)
- Cystic fibrosis
- Facilitation of weaning/extubation failure (non-COPD)
- Obstructive sleep apnea/obesity hypoventilation.

Contraindications
- Respiratory arrest/unstable cardiorespiratory status
- Uncooperative patients
- Unable to protect airway—impaired swallowing and cough
- Facial/esophageal or gastric surgery
- Craniofacial trauma/burns
- Anatomic lesions of upper airway.

Relative Contraindications
- Extreme anxiety
- Morbid obesity
- Copious secretions
- Need for continuous or nearly continuous ventilatory assistance.

Other Contraindications

- NIV should not be used in patients after recent facial or upper airway surgery, in the presence of facial abnormalities such as burns or trauma, if there is fixed obstruction of the upper airway, or if the patient is vomiting.
- Contraindications to NIV include recent upper gastrointestinal surgery, inability to protect the airway, copious respiratory secretions, life-threatening hypoxemia, severe comorbidity, confusion/agitation, or bowel obstruction. NIV can be used in the presence of these contraindications provided contingency plans for tracheal intubation have been made, or if a decision has been made not to proceed to invasive ventilation.
- Although NIV has been used successfully in the presence of a pneumothorax, in most patients with a pneumothorax an intercostal drain should be inserted before commencing NIV.

It is too late for NIV when the patient is:

- Apneic (arresting)
- Medically unstable (shock, acute MI or upper GI bleed)
- Agitated and uncooperative (but coma OK!)
- Unable to clear secretions
- Severely hypoxemic (PaO_2/FiO_2 <75)
- Multiorgan failure or nonreversible disease.

Interfaces (Figs 12.1 and 12.2)

Interfaces are devices that connect the ventilator tubing to the face allowing the entry of pressurized gas to the upper airway. Nasal, oronasal masks and mouthpieces are currently available. Masks are usually made from a non-irritant material such as silicon rubber. It should have minimal dead space and a soft inflatable cuff to provide a seal with the skin. Face masks and nasal masks are the most commonly used interfaces. Nasal masks are used most often in chronic respiratory failure while face masks are more useful in acute respiratory failure.

Ventilators

Ventilators can be conventional and NIV devices.

- Many different types of ventilator have been used successfully to provide NIV, local expertise will influence the choice of ventilator used.
- Bilevel pressure support ventilators are simpler to use, cheaper, and more flexible than other types of ventilator currently available; they have been used in the majority of NIV and are recommended when setting up an acute NIV service.
- Volume-controlled ventilators should be available in units wishing to provide a comprehensive acute NIV service.

While there are many ventilators designed specifically for NIV (bilevel), in principle any ventilator is capable of performing noninvasive ventilation. Conventional respirators separate the inspiratory and expiratory gas mixtures,

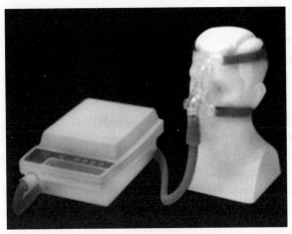

Fig. 12.1: Interface device

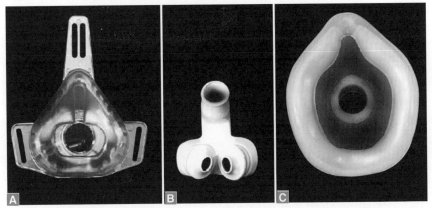

Figs 12.2A to C: (A) Nasal mask; (B) Nasal pillow; (C) Face mask

which prevents reinhalation and permits monitoring of inspiratory pressure and exhaled ventilation by minute, parameters on which the alarms are based. Ventilators of the bilevel type have only one circuit for gas and exhalation can be active (the ventilator opens an exhalation valve) or passive [expiratory positive airway pressure (EPAP) directs the expired air to leave via an exhaust valve]. They are cheaper, easier to use and portable, they have an input valve for oxygen and do not need humidification.

Modes

- Spontaneous
- Spontaneous/timed
- Pressure cycle
- Time

  – Patient

  – Patient/machine

  – Machine

  – Machine

Complications

- Aspiration: <5% (most dreaded)
  - Limit IPAP <20: 25 cm H_2O
  - NGT if above pressures needed
- Most common
  - Skin irritation
  - Eye irritation.

The most common complications of noninvasive ventilation are pressure necroses, especially around the bridge of the nose or chin.

"The most dreaded complication is aspiration.

System has fixed leak in circuit. Mask should not have air-tight seal maintain CPAP of at least 4–5 cm H_2O. Potential for rebreathing and $PaCO_2$ retention with bilevel NIV Single limb circuit NIV should not be used as a substitute for tracheal intubation and invasive ventilation when the latter is clearly more appropriate.

Initiation of Treatment

- Bilevel NIV
  - IPAP (PSV) = 8–12 cm H_2O
  - EPAP (CPAP or PEEP) = 3–5 cm H_2O
- Δ Ventilation = Δ IPAP
- Δ Oxygenation = Δ EPAP
- If no decrease in dyspnea or respiratory rate, then increased IPAP or PS 2–3 cm H_2O
  - Maximum IPAP = 20–25 cm H_2O
- If hypoxemia present, increase EPAP (or CPAP or PEEP) in 2–3 cm H_2O increments
  - Maximum EPAP = 15 cm H_2O.

What do you Monitor

- Clinical
- Labs.

Monitoring

- Clinical evaluation of the patient should include assessment of patient comfort, conscious level, chest wall motion, accessory muscle recruitment, coordination of respiratory effort with the ventilator, respiratory rate and heart rate. Patients receiving NIV should be reviewed regularly to assess their response to treatment and to optimize the ventilator settings.

- The need for arterial blood gas analysis will be governed by the patient's clinical progress but should be measured in most patients after 1–2 hours of NIV and after 4–6 hours if the earlier sample showed little improvement. If there has been no improvement in $PaCO_2$ and pH after this period, despite optimal ventilator settings, NIV should be discontinued and invasive ventilation considered.
- Oxygen saturation should be monitored continuously for at least 24 hours after commencing NIV and supplementary oxygen administered to maintain saturations between 85% and 90%.
- Breaks from NIV should be made for drugs, physiotherapy, meals, etc. Patients who show benefit from NIV in the first few hours should be ventilated for as much as possible during the first 24 hours, or until improving.
- All patients who have been treated with NIV should undergo spirometric testing and arterial blood gas analysis while breathing air before discharge.
- All patients with spinal cord lesions, neuromuscular disease, chest wall deformity, or morbid obesity.

Clinical Assessment

- Chest wall movement—respiratory effort
- Coordination between machine and patient
- Use of accessory muscles—work of breathing (WOB)
- Heart and respiratory rate
- Patient comfort
- Mental state
- Nasal bridge erosion and skin peeling
- Abdominal distention.

When to End NIV

- Patient is intolerant
- Patient deteriorates (intubate)
- Lack of improvement at 2 hours—persisting dyspnea, tachypnea, gas exchange derangement (intubate)
- Patient improves (weaning).

Weaning

- Progressive decrease in level of IPAP/EPAP
  - Once low level of NPPV tolerated
  - IPAP = 5 cm H_2O
  - EPAP = 5 cm H_2O
- Progressive time off NPPV
  - Similar to "T-piece" approach.

Humidification

Humidification is not normally necessary during NIV. Use of heated humidifiers or heat/moisture exchangers significantly alters the compliance and resistance of the circuit and, in particular, can impair the function of inspiratory and expiratory triggers.

Summary

NIV should be reserved for patients with appropriate reversible diagnoses. Use at the onset of ARF or to facilitate weaning or avoid extubation failure. Initiation is a "window of opportunity" that opens when vent assist is needed and closes with contraindications. Avoid delays in needed intubation when patient fails to respond to NIV in 2–3 hours. End when patient is intolerant, deteriorating (intubate) or improving (wean).

■ HIGH FLOW THERAPY

Humidified high flow airway respiratory support is a method of delivering a high minute volume of respiratory gas via special nasal cannula, tracheostomy tube kit. The respiratory gas is heated to near body temperature and humidified, usually to saturation vapor pressure. This form of respiratory support is generally referred to as high flow therapy (HFT). HFT is also referred to as transnasal insufflation.

This is achieved through the integration of heated humidification and a precise blend of air and oxygen delivered via an innovative nasal cannula or tracheostomy tube. A number of physiological effects have been described with HFT: pharyngeal dead space washout, reduction of nasopharyngeal resistance, a positive expiratory pressure effect, an alveolar recruitment, greater humidification, more comfort and better tolerance by the patient, better control of FiO_2 and mucociliary clearance.

With our own experience in the department of critical care medicine, this therapy is achieved with AIRVO 2 (Fisher and Paykel)
Humidifier with integrated flow generator, generates high flows of warmed and humidified respiratory gases—up to 60 liter/min of flow, delivered to you, the patient, through a variety of nasal, tracheostomy and mask interfaces.

How does HFT work?

HFT has a number of physiological effects that could be used to illustrate its benefits. Several studies have shown that HFNC generates a low level of positive airway pressure, improves oxygenation, increases the end-inspiratory lung volume, reduces airway resistance, increases functional residual capacity and flushes nasopharyngeal dead space, thus helping to manage breathing reduction in acute respiratory failure from all causes. It also better tolerated and more comfortable for the patient. Finally, pulmonary defense mechanisms are restored.

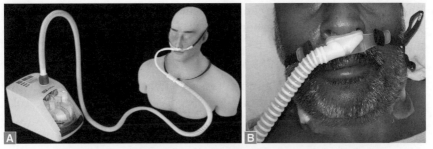

Figs 12.3A and B: Nasal high flow (*For color version, see Plate 3*)

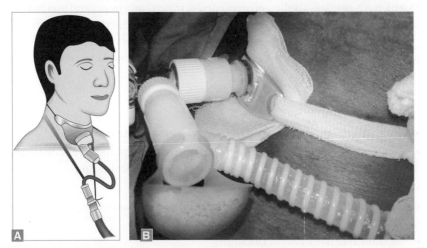

Figs 12.4A and B: High flow through tracheostomy tube (*For color version, see Plate 3*)

Physiological Effects of HFT

- Pharyngeal dead space washout
- Reduction of nasopharyngeal resistance
- Positive expiratory pressure (PEEP effect)
- Alveolar recruitment
- Humidification, great comfort and better tolerance
- Better control of FiO_2 and better mucociliary clearance
- Improved patient comfort and tolerance
- Greater therapy success than with face masks
- Improved lung volumes
- Improved respiratory rates.

Pharyngeal Dead Space Washout

The main effect of delivering high flow oxygen directly into the nasopharynx is to wash CO_2 and reduce CO_2 rebreathing. This allows the dead space to decrease and increases alveolar ventilation over minute ventilation ratio.

These properties have some clinical benefits for exercise tolerance, dyspnea reduction and better oxygenation.

Positive Expiratory Pressure (PEEP Effect)

Physiologically a positive airway pressure effect, generated by high flow oxygen, provides a certain level of pulmonary distending pressure and alveolar recruitment.

Alveolar Recruitment Effect

The high oxygen flows delivered may correct hypoxemia by several mechanisms and thus contribute to the alleviation of respiratory distress symptoms. The positive airway pressure effect provides a certain level of pulmonary distending pressure and alveolar recruitment, but it is unclear how their use affects lung volume.

Indications

- Pulmonary edema due to CHF, fluid overload, or near drowning
- Associated signs of CHF including edema of the legs, neck vein distention, and rales/wheezing on chest auscultation and examination
- Hypoxia—Pulse oximetry less than 90%
- Significant respiratory distress including use of accessory muscles and retractions
- Abdominal/paradoxical breathing
- Respiratory rate of >24 with signs and symptoms of respiratory distress.

■ CONTRAINDICATIONS

- Inability to follow commands (GCS 9-10)
- Hypoventilation requiring ventilator assistance
- Open stoma or tracheostomy
- Severe cardiorespiratory instability
- Systolic blood pressure <100 mm Hg
- Inability to maintain an open airway
- Unconsciousness
- Pneumothorax
- Facial trauma/burns
- Penetrating neck and chest trauma
- Recent facial surgery
- Recent gastric surgery
- Patient unable to tolerate mask
- Active vomiting.

HFT System Features

- Flow rates: 40–60 L/min
- Precise FiO_2 delivery: 21 to 80%
- Optimal humidity delivery
- Integrated oxygen mixing
- Inbuilt oxygen sensor
- No probes or external air supply required
- Simple controls.

Which may lead to:

- More effective treatment and reduced escalation of care
- Increased patient and caregiver satisfaction
- Reduced length of stay in ICU
- Reduced cost of care.

Normally with quiet breathing, the inspiratory flow rate of an adult usually exceeds 12 liters a minute, and can exceed 30 liters a minute for someone with mild respiratory distress. The typical upper limit of oxygen delivery via nasal cannula of six liters a minute does not meet the inspiratory flow rates of the average adult, and therefore, the oxygen is then diluted with room air during inspiration. Prior to the advent of HFT, when high flow was required for respiratory support, special face masks or intubation was required. With HFT, respiratory gas flow volume is delivered which meets or exceeds the patient's inspiratory flow rate, and is heated and humidified, allowing for comfortable delivery of respiratory support.

For HFT, a source of flow is usually with compressed air and oxygen. HFT requires the use of special nasal cannula or tracheostomy tube kit and tubing large enough to deliver flow rates of respiratory gas, up to 60 liters per minute in adults. The benefits of HFT are illustrated in Table 12.1.

Table 12.1: Benefits of HFT

Comfortable high flow delivery, reducing the likelihood of treatment failure	Less attendance time assisting uncomfortable patients
Can continue to eat, drink, talk and sleep	No need to change between multiple oxygen delivery devices and interfaces
A broad range of flows and oxygen concentrations can be delivered, providing both versatility and continuity of care as patients wean or their condition becomes more acute	Increased confidence in the actual fraction of inspired oxygen (FiO_2) being delivered to the patient
May displace the need for noninvasive or invasive ventilation through better patient tolerance	Easier oral care, maintaining the moisture in the oral mucosa
Improved respiratory efficiency	May be used to wean patients off noninvasive or invasive ventilation
Better secretion clearance, reducing the risk of respiratory infection	

Since the delivered flow rate of HFT can meet the inspiration flow rate, the delivered gases are not diluted by room air. The FiO_2 is controlled by the clinician, and can be set from 21% to 100% oxygen. High flow therapy reduces respiratory dead space and generates some positive airway pressure resulting from the expiratory resistance generated by continuous high flow gas delivery. Flow rates exceeding inspiratory demand may also provide positive pressure during inspiration. Heated humidification of the respiratory gas facilitates secretion clearance and decreases the development of bronchial hyper-response symptoms. Some patients requiring respiratory support for bronchospasm benefit using air delivered by HFT without additional oxygen. HFT is useful in the treatment of sleep apnea. During use of HFT, the patient can drink, and speak. Most patients find HFT more comfortable than using oxygen masks. As this is a noninvasive therapy, it avoids the risk of ventilator-associated pneumonia in situations where it can supplant the use of a ventilator.

■ BIBLIOGRAPHY

1. Brochard L. Noninvasive ventilation for acute respiratory failure. JAMA. 2002;288:932-35.
2. Gorini M, Ginanni R, Villella G, Tozzi D, Augustynen A, Corrado A. Non-invasive negative and positive pressure ventilation in the treatment of acute on chronic respiratory failure. Intensive Care Med. 2004;30(5):875-81.
3. Groves N, Tobin A. High flow nasal oxygen generates positive airway pressure in adult volunteers. Aust Crit Care. 2007;20:126-31.
4. International Consensus Conference in Intensive Care medicine: Noninvasive positive pressure ventilation in acute respiratory failure. Intensive Care Medicine. 2001;27:166-78.
5. Parke R, McGuinness S, Eccleston M. Nasal high-flow therapy delivers low level positive airway pressure. Br J Anaesth. 2009;103:886-90.
6. Rajesh C. Non-invasive mechanical ventilation—A practical guide. 1st ed. Feb. 2002. published for ISCCM (Delhi Chapter).
7. Ram FS, Picot J, Lightowler J, Wedzicha JA. Non-invasive positive pressure ventilation for treatment of respiratory failure due to exacerbations of chronic obstructive pulmonary disease. Cochrane Database Syst Rev. 2004;(1):CD004104.
8. Ricard JD. High flow nasal oxygen in acute respiratory failure. Minerva Anestesiol. 2012;78:836-41.
9. Riera J, Pérez P, Cortés J, Roca O, Masclans JR, Rello J. Effect of high flow nasal cannula and body position on end-expiratory lung volume. A cohort study using electrical impedance tomography. Respir Care. 2012.
10. Roca O, Riera J, Torres F, Masclans JR. High-flow oxygen therapy in acute respiratory failure. Respir Care. 2010;55:408-13.
11. Sztrymf B, Messika J, Bertrand F, Hurel D, Leon R, Dreyfuss D, et al. Beneficial effects of humidified high flow nasal oxygen in critical care patients: A prospective pilot study. Intensive Care Med. 2011;37:1780-6.
12. Ward JJ. High-Flow oxygen administration by nasal cannula for adult and perinatal patients. Respir Care. 2013;58:98-122.

PULMONARY REHABILITATION

◼ INTRODUCTION

The goals of rehabilitation are to reduce the symptoms, disability, and handicap and to improve functional independence in people with lung disease. The majority of patients considered for pulmonary rehabilitation programs will have chronic obstructive pulmonary disease.

The rehabilitation process incorporates a program of physical training, disease education, nutrition assessment and advice, and psychological, social, and behavioral intervention.

Rehabilitation is provided by a multiprofessional team, with involvement of the patient's family and attention to individual needs.

◼ WHO BENEFITS FROM PULMONARY REHABILITATION

In the past, pulmonary rehabilitation was used primarily for patients with COPD. However, it can also be helpful to people with other chronic lung conditions, such as:
- Interstitial diseases
- Cystic fibrosis
- Bronchiectasis
- Thoracic cage abnormalities
- Neuromuscular disorders.

Pulmonary rehabilitation can also be helpful to those who need lung transplants or other lung surgeries. Whether you have a chronic respiratory system disease or experiencing disabling symptoms, such as shortness of breath, cough, and/or mucus production, pulmonary rehabilitation can help. Even patients with severe disease can benefit.

Pulmonary rehabilitation is usually supervised and structured. This means that it will include:
- **Medical evaluation and management:** Evaluation of symptoms and current medical treatment ensure to get most out of the program. A medical evaluation also will pinpoint other concerns, such as heart problems, that might affect your ability to exercise.

- **Short-term and long-term goals:** After symptoms and other medical problems have been identified, short- and long-term goals are set that reflect specific needs. For instance, some people might want to be able to dress themselves every day while others might want to be able to walk 30 minutes every day. The ability to exercise and to perform daily tasks are determined before starting the program.
- **Therapy programs:** Which therapy programs you participate in, will depend on your needs and goals. For example, if you are a smoker, a smoking cessation program may be the most important short-term goal. (*See* below for specific therapy programs).

Evaluation of results: Each therapy program should be designed so that results can be measured. Measurable results may include easier breathing, the ability to exercise longer, and an improved quality of life.

All pulmonary rehabilitation programs generally include education of both patient and patient's family on how the program affects patient's COPD symptoms, the importance of the program to overall health, and how regular participation can help patient to meet the goals. Understanding COPD—how it progresses and is best treated—makes it easier to live with and manage the disease.

Support and encouragement from friends, family, and health professionals are crucial in helping patients to stick to the rehabilitation plan. Patient's health professional may recommend counseling for patient and patient's family. These groups can help patient and patient's family cope with COPD and its possible complications.

One of the greatest benefits of a pulmonary rehabilitation program is the opportunity to meet other highly motivated people with COPD and exchange information about living with COPD.

■ THERAPY PROGRAMS

Therapy programs are tailored to meet your specific needs. If you still smoke, stopping is the most important therapy program. Other therapy programs include exercise, breath training, and nutritional guidance.

Exercise

Regular exercise can improve how active you can be and can decrease your shortness of breath. If you stay active, you may develop fewer complications, have a better attitude about your life and the disease, and be less likely to be depressed. Exercise training for COPD often includes aerobic exercise, such as walking or using a stationary bike, and muscle-strengthening exercises for your arms and legs.

Always consult with your health professional before starting an exercise program. People with COPD may have heart problems, such as coronary artery disease (CAD) or high blood pressure, that may limit exercise options. You may need medical supervision when you start the program.

Lower Body Training

Lower body exercises like walking or riding a stationary bicycle will help strengthen your leg muscles and increase muscle tone and flexibility. These exercises will help you move about more easily, often for longer periods of time. They can also make certain tasks, like walking up stairs, easier to do.

Many patients find that as their technique improves, their motivation to continue with the exercise program increases as well. As a result, many patients report feeling better about themselves and their ability to control symptoms such as breathing difficulties.

Upper Body Training

Upper body training increases the strength and endurance of arm and shoulder muscles. Strengthening these muscles is important because they provide support to the ribcage and can improve breathing. These exercises can also help in tasks that require arm work such as carrying groceries, cooking dinner, lifting items, making the bed and vacuuming, taking a bath or shower, and combing hair. They can also decrease the amount of oxygen needed for these activities. This may be due to less worry about breathing difficulties and better coordination of the muscles involved in raising the arms.

Many patients with lung diseases are not in very good physical condition or have never exercised on a regular basis. Do not worry. Your pulmonary rehabilitation team will meet with you to assess your needs and will work with you to develop an exercise program designed specifically for you. They will advise you about which exercises will give you the best results, how often you should do them, for how long, and at what level. They will give you information on how to maintain your exercise abilities on a regular basis.

Ventilatory Muscle Training

Weakness of the respiratory muscles can contribute to breathing problems and make exercising difficult. For some patients, ventilatory muscle training (VMT) may improve respiratory muscle function, help reduce the severity of breathlessness, and improve the ability to exercise.

Research at this time does not support the use of VMT for everyone. However, it may be helpful for some patients with COPD who have respiratory muscle weakness and breathlessness. Your pulmonary rehabilitation team will let you know if you are a candidate for VMT.

Breath Training

If you have severe COPD, you may find that you take quick, small, shallow breaths. Breath training can help you take deeper breaths and reduce breathlessness. You must practice breath training regularly for you to do it well.

Three basic breath training methods are diaphragmatic breathing, pursed-lip breathing, and breathing while bending forward. They can be used to help you get through periods when you feel more short of breath.

- **Diaphragmatic breathing** helps your lungs expand so that they take in more air. (Your diaphragm is a muscle that helps draw air into your lungs as you breathe). Lie on your back or prop yourself up on several pillows. With one hand on your abdomen and the other on your chest, breathe in, pushing the abdomen outward as far as possible. You should be able to feel the hand on your abdomen moving out, while the hand on your chest should not move. When you breathe out, you should be able to feel the hand on your abdomen moving in. After you can do diaphragmatic breathing well-lying down, you can learn to do it sitting or standing. Many, but not all, people with COPD find this breathing method helpful. Diaphragmatic breathing should be practised for 20 minutes, 2 to 3 times a day.

- **Pursed-lip breathing** may help you breathe more air out so that your next breath can be deeper. In this type of breathing, you breathe in through the nose and out through the mouth while almost closing your lips. Breathe in for about 4 seconds and breathe out for 6 to 8 seconds. Pursed-lip breathing decreases shortness of breath and improves your ability to exercise.

- **Breathing while bending forward** at the waist may make it easier for you to breathe. Bending forward while breathing may decrease shortness of breath in those with severe COPD, both at rest and during exercise. This may be because bending forward allows the diaphragm to move more easily.

■ FLEXIBILITY AND STRETCHING

The flexibility and stretching exercises are suggestions only. Patients should only spend about 5 minutes within each class performing flexibility and stretching exercises as the emphasis within the class should be on endurance and strength training. The flexibility and stretching exercises could be incorporated into the home program. Trainers should prescribe and modify appropriate flexibility and stretching exercises according to individual needs.

Flexibility

Flexibility of the joints in the spine (particularly the thoracic spine) is important for people with respiratory disorders to enable thoracic mobility when breathing.

The exercises in the Table 13.1 are designed to move the joints through their range in order to improve or maintain flexibility.

Flexibility exercises are designed to move the joints through their range in order to improve or maintain flexibility. When prescribing flexibility exercises, the following points should be considered:

- Patients should perform two or three repetitions of each exercise using slow, smooth movements.

- Patients should only perform each exercise as far as they can without causing pain.

Stretching

The pectoral muscles may become shortened as a result of the forward lean position adopted by many patients with COPD when breathless, and therefore it is important to include stretches that aim to maintain the length of the pectoral muscles and in doing so, this may improve posture.

When prescribing stretching exercises, the following points should be considered:

- Ask the patient to hold each stretch for five to ten seconds.
- Ask the patient to perform two or three repetitions of each stretch.
- Patients should gradually lengthen the muscle to the point that feels as if they are stretching the muscle, but no pain is experienced.
- After this point is reached, the patient should be asked to 'hold it there'.
- Encourage the patient to gradually stretch a little further if they feel able to do so.
- Encourage patients to breathe while stretching, some patients hold their breath and others are unable to hold stretches for as long as 5 seconds due to breathlessness.
- The exercises in the Table 13.1 have been designed to help patients stretch muscles in their upper and lower limbs. Additional exercises include quadriceps stretching for individuals who report quads tightness or pain especially after cycle training.

Table 13.1: Flexibility and stretching exercises

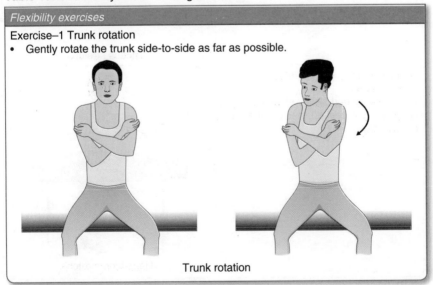

Flexibility exercises

Exercise–1 Trunk rotation
- Gently rotate the trunk side-to-side as far as possible.

Trunk rotation

Contd..

Contd..

Stretching exercises	
Exercise–1 Pectoralis stretch • Stand in the corner or in a doorway with your hands at shoulder level and your feet away from the corner or doorway. • Lean forward until a comfortable stretch is felt across the chest. • Take extra precaution if patient has shoulder pain.	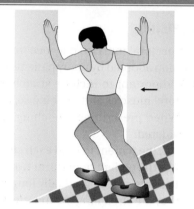 Pectoralis stretch
Exercise–2 Triceps stretch • Lift your arm so that your elbow is next to your ear. • Place your hand between your shoulder blades. • Gently push your elbow back with your other hand until you feel a stretch.	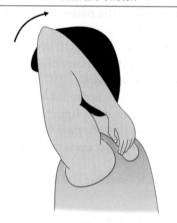 Triceps stretch
Exercise–3 Hamstring stretch Sit on the bed. Lean forward and slowly straighten your knee until you feel a stretch at the back of your thigh.	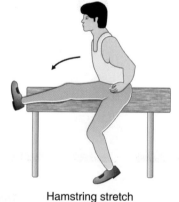 Hamstring stretch

■ BALANCE

Although there is no evidence suggesting that people with COPD have a higher prevalence of falls compared to a matched, healthy population, common risk factors for falls (such as reduced lower limb muscle strength, decreased daily physical activity and reduced standing balance capacity) are also associated with COPD. As a result, maintaining and enhancing balance is important especially for patients with a balance deficit or those with an increased risk of falls.

■ INSPIRATORY MUSCLE TRAINING

Inspiratory muscle training (IMT), performed in isolation using a threshold loading device or target-flow resistive device at loads equal to or greater than 30% of an individual's maximum inspiratory pressure generated against an occluded airway (PI_{max}) has been shown to increase inspiratory muscle strength and endurance and reduce dyspnea in patients with COPD. Training may also result in modest improvements in 6 minute walking distance and health-related quality of life. However, it remains unclear whether IMT combined with a program of whole-body exercise training confers additional benefits in dyspnea, exercise capacity or health-related quality of life in patients with COPD. At present, the evidence does not support the routine use of IMT as an essential component of pulmonary rehabilitation program.

■ HOME TRAINING

Patients should be encouraged to undertake a home exercise program concurrent with the supervised sessions of the pulmonary rehabilitation program. The home exercise program should be:

- Started within 1–2 weeks after commencing the supervised training program to allow any difficulties undertaking the home program to be discussed and resolved during the supervised period.
- Performed on 2 or 3 days per week (i.e. in addition to the 2 or 3 days that the patient is attending the supervised training program). In total, the patient should exercise 4 or 5 days per week.
- After the pulmonary rehabilitation program is completed, patients should be instructed to exercise a total of 4 or 5 days per week at home or in a local gymnasium. The home program may include attendance at a supervised maintenance exercise class, if available.

The home training program should consist of:
- Walking for 30 minutes at the same pace as in the supervised program.
- An exercise circuit that includes, where possible, identical exercises to the exercises that are completed during the supervised sessions.
- Progression of the exercises in the home program should occur at the same time that exercises are progressed during the supervised sessions.

The home training program should include the following advice to patients:

- Instructions not to exercise if unwell (e.g. flu, chest infection) or within 1–2 hours of a meal.
- Instructions to stop and rest in the event of the following symptoms: Excessive shortness of breath (much more than usual); chest, neck or arm pain of unknown origin in which case the patient should stop exercising immediately; excessive fatigue (much more than usual); dizziness, nausea, light-headedness; irregular heart beat or palpitations that are not usually experienced by the patient.

■ NUTRITIONAL GUIDANCE

Good nutrition is important to maintain your strength and health. Problems with muscle weakness and weight loss are frequent in COPD, and people with COPD who are profoundly underweight, especially those with emphysema, are at higher risk of death than are people with COPD who have a normal weight.

■ WHAT TO EXPECT AFTER TREATMENT

An ongoing pulmonary rehabilitation program can help you function better over the long-term. Each program should set short- and long-term goals to help you monitor change and success. This ensures that the program continues to meet your needs.

■ WHY IT IS DONE

Pulmonary rehabilitation is recommended for people who have respiratory disorders such as COPD. Most people who have COPD can benefit from pulmonary rehabilitation, especially people who use oxygen therapy and have often had to go to the emergency room or hospital. Therapy is not limited to people who have mild or moderate COPD.

■ HOW WELL IT WORKS

Pulmonary rehabilitation improves quality of life. A review of research reports that participating in pulmonary rehabilitation:

- Relieves shortness of breath and fatigue.
- Gives you more control over your condition.
- Results in greater improvement of quality of life than using other types of treatment, such as medication.
- Modestly improves how much you can exercise.

An effective pulmonary rehabilitation program should be at least 2 months long; the longer the program is, the more effective it is.

■ RISKS

There is little or no risk to these programs if they are well supervised.

■ WHAT TO THINK ABOUT

The success of pulmonary rehabilitation relies on the relationship between you and your team of health professionals. This team must work with you to achieve goals. It is vital that you take an active role in the program and understand the importance of regular participation.

Although this therapy can improve your daily life, it does not reverse the effects that COPD has had on the lungs or other organs such as the heart. It does not cure COPD. It trains the mind, muscles, and heart to get the most out of damaged lungs.

Pulmonary rehabilitation provides the opportunity to interact with health professionals specializing in lung disease and to exchange information with others about living with COPD.

■ BIBLIOGRAPHY

1. American Thoracic Society. Pulmonary rehabilitation-99. The official statement of the American Thoracic Society. Am J Respir Crit Care Med. 1999;159:1666-82.
2. Foster S, Thomas HM III. Pulmonary rehabilitation in lung diseases other than COPD. Am Rev Respir Dis. 1990;141:601.
3. Hodgkin JE, Farrell MJ, Gibson SR, Kenner RE, Kass I, Lampton LM, et al. American Thoracic Society. Medical Section of American Lung Association. Pulmonary rehabilitation. Am Rev Respir Dis. 1981;124:663-6.
4. Mahler DA, Wells CK. Evaluation of clinical methods for rating dyspnoea. Chest. 1998;93:580-6.
5. Reardon J, Awad E, Normandin E, Vale F, Clark B, ZuWallack RL. The effect of comprehensive outpatient pulmonary rehabilitation on dyspnoea. Chest. 1994; 105:1046-52.
6. Schwartz MI, King TE Jr, Chernaik RM. General principles and diagnostic approach to the interstitial lung diseases. In: Murray JF, Nadel JA, editors Textbook of Respiratory Medicine. Philadelphia: WB Saunders & Co.; 1994;2:1803-26.
7. Wijkstra PJ, Van Der Mark TW, Kraan J, Van Altena R, Koeter GH, Postma DS. Effects of home rehabilitation on physical performance in patients with COPD. Eur Respir J. 1996;9:104-10.

CHEST PHYSIOTHERAPY

■ INTRODUCTION

An integral part of respiratory therapy's recent advancement has been the adoption of chest physiotherapy techniques. The past few years have seen a great gain in the utilization of chest physiotherapy in large teaching centers. Most of this has been due to the availability of skilled therapists in aggressive respiratory care programs. A deterrent to widespread acceptance is that physical therapy and respiratory therapy are separate allied health fields. There is great reluctance on the part of some therapists to view these modalities as an integral part of respiratory therapy. Experience demonstrates that a team approach between respiratory therapy and physical therapy results in maximum patient benefit.

Therapists must have a basic knowledge of respiratory therapy to appreciate and understand the role that chest physiotherapy plays in bronchial hygiene and ventilation. On the other hand, respiratory therapists must be familiar with chest physiotherapy techniques and be qualified to deliver such therapy. It appears inevitable that the majority of hospital chest physical therapy treatments will be provided by respiratory therapists since the techniques are commonly used in conjunction with 'inhalation therapy' modalities and are required 24 hours a day. The role of the therapist must primarily be one of the supervision, teaching, and evaluation.

■ GOALS OF CHEST PHYSIOTHERAPY

Chest physiotherapy is a series of manipulative techniques designed to prevent pulmonary complications and improve function in acute and chronic pulmonary disease. From the viewpoint of respiratory therapy, it seems appropriate to classify the goals of chest physiotherapy:

- To prevent the accumulation and improve the mobilization of bronchial secretions.
- To improve the efficiency and distribution of ventilation.
- To improve cardiopulmonary reserve using exercise techniques to promote physical conditioning.

Chest physiotherapy techniques may be classified into three categories:
1. Techniques that promote bronchial hygiene.
2. Techniques that improve breathing efficiency.
3. Techniques that promote physical reconditioning.

Chest physiotherapy techniques may be applied therapeutically or prophylactically. Therapeutic use is the application of a specific technique to reverse a specific disease state. Prophylactic therapy is the application of a broad program to prevent the accumulation of secretion. The particular advantage of a prophylactic chest physiotherapy regimen is that it can be effectively carried out by a trained nursing staff as part of routine nursing care.

■ TECHNIQUES PROMOTING BRONCHIAL HYGIENE

Bronchial hygiene has been defined as the maintenance of clear airways and the removal of secretions from the tracheobronchial tree. The mucociliary complex and cough mechanism can be aided by techniques such as aerosol, Intermittent Positive Pressure Breathing (IPPB), and; (1) postural drainage; (2) percussion and vibration; and (3) coughing assistance.

Postural Drainage (Fig. 14.1)

Essential segmental anatomy of the lungs for purposes of postural drainage.

Also called bronchial drainage, this refers to the positions that make use of gravity to aid in the mucus clearance. In order to be effective, the head must be lower than the chest. This allows the mucus to flow toward the trachea, where it can be more easily coughed out. Different postures are useful for targeting different regions in the lungs. These six positions are to be used in a systematic manner, working from the upper to the lower lobes. There are a total of nine regions that can be drained in this manner. Achieving the correct positions can be done using a tilt table, a positional hospital bed, or pillows.

Postural drainage is most effective when combined with chest percussions and vibrations. This is called CPT. It has also been called 'clapping' or 'thumping.' In years past, the caregiver administering CPT did so by cupping his or her hand, and beating on patient's back in each of the regions of the lungs. Its effectiveness was almost solely determined by technique. Improper cupping of the hand produced only a slapping sensation, painful to both patient and caregiver. Also, as fatigue set in, the steady, rhythmic pounding would slow down and lose intensity.

The 'clapping method' of CPT, is no longer in widespread use for adults having CF. Certain aspects of postural drainage, however, are still useful for infants. Instead of clapping, however, the caregiver instead taps with two fingers on the different lung regions, while holding the child in the different postural drainage positions. In place of clapping, which as mentioned before was sometimes fatiguing, a motorized massage/percussion tool is used. Respiratory therapists in hospitals use a professional model, such as the GK3 postural drainage and percussion massagers.

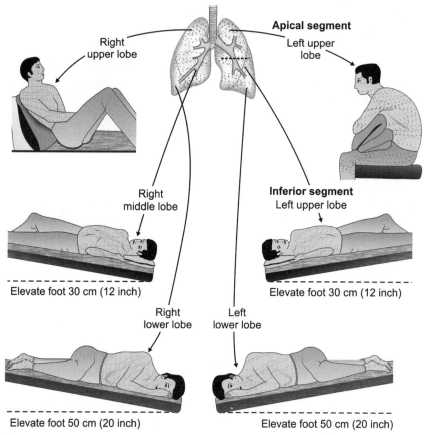

Fig. 14.1: Essential segmental anatomy of the lungs for purposes of postural drainage

The mucociliary escalator is greatly enhanced when aided by gravity, i.e. the mucus drainage of a lung segment is facilitated by body positions that allow mucus to flow in the direction of gravity. Obviously, postural drainage must be based upon a firm knowledge of tracheobronchial anatomy. Since branching of the tracheobronchial tree is variable and complex, practical postural drainage positions are best limited to areas of lung that commonly retain secretions.

Therapies involving positive expiratory pressure (PEP) are designed to keep the airways opened when the patient breathes out. There are a few different PEP devices, each having their own limitations and benefits. The way that PEP therapy works is that it keeps the lungs inflated with air. Basic science tells us that two things cannot occupy the same space. In people with cystic fibrosis, the mucus occupies precious space in the airways, preventing them from taking a full, deep breath.

The PEP devices are either stand-alone, or can be used with a nebulizer. All PEP devices work by having a one way valve that creates resistance when the patient breathes out against it. With PEP therapy, the pressure difference that occurs when a patient breathes out allows the lungs to fill with additional air, which in turn will push the mucus out as the lungs try to return to an equilibrant volume.

In simpler terms, PEP therapy functions very similarly to trying to get mustard out of a squeeze bottle. If you were to just squeeze the bottle without shaking it, you would only get a puff of air, and that little bit of watery mustard when you shake the bottle, you move the amount of air in the bottle to the bottom, which will force the mustard out when you squeeze.

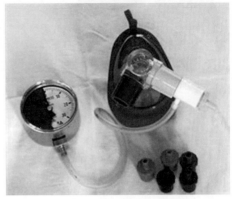

Fig. 14.2: PEP mask

PEP therapy is very effective when combined with postural drainage. However, the postural drainage positions, especially the ones in which a patient must lie face down, may make breathing against a PEP device too difficult. Some PEP therapies combine vibratory pressure, which helps loosen the mucus and dislodge it from the linings of the airways. The Acapella use a combination of vibrations and PEP to promote airway clearance.

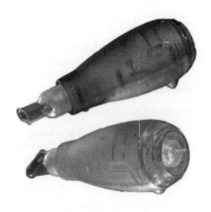

Fig. 14.3: Acapella

Below are some pictures of different types of PEP therapy:

1. Positive expiratory pressure (PEP) mask (Fig. 14.2)
2. Acapella (Fig. 14.3).

■ LUNG SEGMENTS (FIG. 14.4)

Divides the lungs into four quadrants for purposes of postural drainage. Each quadrant contains four 'drainage' segments. The lingual is considered a left middle lobe since the location and direction of the lingular segmental bronchus is a mirror image of the right middle lobe bronchus.

The upper lobes are composed of an apical, interior and posterior segment plus a middle lobe. Although there are far more precise clinical purposes, these four segments are the ones commonly involved in upper lobe disease.

The lower lobes have four segments: Apical, anterior basilar, posterior or basilar, and lateral basilar. The posterior basilar segment is the largest,

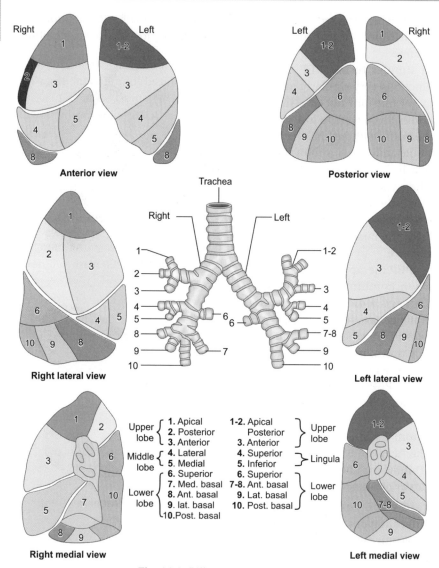

Fig. 14.4: Different lung segments

encompassing at least half of the posterior chest wall and resting directly in the diaphragm. Figure demonstrates that the apical and posterior basilar segmental bronchi do not have the advantage of gravity for drainage in the usual hospital bed positions. This is undoubtedly a major reason why these particular segments are most commonly involved in atelectasis and pneumonia.

Clinical indications

When normal bronchial hygiene mechanisms malfunction, the patient becomes a candidate for postural drainage therapy. Diseases often requiring postural drainage include, but are not limited to, bronchiectasis, cystic fibrosis, COPD, acute atelectasis, lung abscess, ventilator care, and pneumonia. Postural drainage is also often required for postoperative patients and patients who have been on prolonged bed rest. There is always potential for contamination of the opposite lung when secretions are mobilized in unilateral disease. A general rule of postural drainage therapy is that care must be taken to assure prophylactic drainage of the opposite (contralateral) lung following therapeutic drainage of the diseased side.

Lung abscess is a collection of purulent material (pus) within lung.

Precautions

There are several precautions, which must be considered when applying postural drainage. Position change may be a significant physiologic stress to the cardiovascular system, especially in critically ill patients. Further; a 'head-down' position may diminish venous return from the head and result in increased intracranial pressure. It is best to avoid head-down positions in postoperative neurosurgical patients and in patients with known intracranial disease.

Postural drainage positions must not place stress on 'healing' tissue, e.g. patients with recent spinal fusion or skin grafts. Postural drainage techniques must be weighed in terms of the potential benefit therapist's and physician's clinical evaluation!

Chest Percussion (Figs 14.5 and 14.6)

The technique of chest percussion is most often used in conjunction with postural drainage to loosen adherent bronchial secretions. The object is to have cupped-shaped hands 'clap' the chest wall, trapping air between the hand and the chest wall. This sudden compression of air produces an energy wave that is transmitted through the chest wall tissues to the lung tissue. This energy wave will theoretically loosen adherent mucus plugs and allow better mobilization of secretions via gravity and coughing techniques.

The procedure is performed by rhythmically and alternately striking the chest wall with the cupped hands, producing a loud clapping noise without pain, discomfort, or bruising. Bony prominences (clavicle, spine of the scapula, spinal column) and female breast tissue should be avoided. Chest percussion is an excellent adjunct to bronchial hygiene therapy and is usually performed in conjunction with postural drainage. Judgement must be exercised when a patient is fragile on 'brittle'. A skilled therapist can administer chest percussion to patients with brittle bones or fractured ribs; however, this takes great expertize and must not be done by the occasional therapist.

Hemorrhagic conditions, 'fragile' bones, bony metastases, and undrained empyema are contraindications to chest percussion. The procedure is usually avoided in patients with respectable tumors of the lung so that tumor spread is minimized prior to surgery.

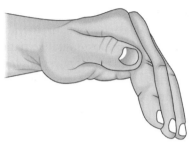

Fig. 14.5: Cup your hands when performing chest percussions

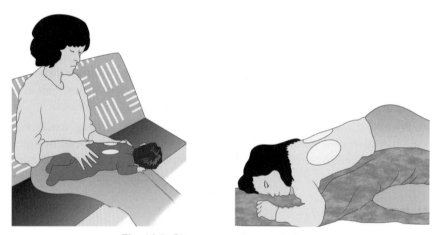

Fig. 14.6: Chest percussions techniques

Chest Vibration

Position hands as shown below when performing chest vibrations (Fig. 14.7).

Sequential positions for complete postural drainage:
1. Upper lobes, anterior segments
2. Upper lobe, posterior segment, right posterior bronchus
3. Upper lobe, posterior segment, right posterior bronchus
4. Right middle lobe
5. Left lingula
6. Lower lobes, apical segment
7. Lower lobes, anterior basal segment
8. Lower lobe, lateral basal segment
9. Lower lobes, posterial basal bronchus.

The technique of chest vibration is accomplished by placing the hands on the chest wall and producing a very rapid vibratory motion in the arms while gently compressing the chest wall. A skilled therapist can develop a vibratory frequency in excess of 200 per minute. This becomes an extremely effective means of mobilizing secretions toward the gravity-dependent major airways

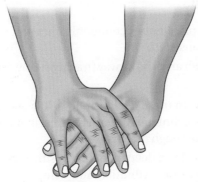

Fig. 14.7: Position of hands while performing chest vibration

in conjunction with postural drainage and following chest percussion. Chest vibration is performed during exhalation following a deep inspiration and is a very effective adjunct to IPPB therapy.

Cough Instruction

Cough instruction is a simple technique requiring a thorough understanding of the normal cough mechanism. The importance of a deep breath, the glottis, and the abdominal muscles must be appreciated. A patient receiving cough instruction must first be taught proper breathing techniques.

A simple technique is to have the patient take several deep breaths and then a maximum inspiration which he 'holds' for a count of 3. After mastering this maneuver, he is taught to forcefully contract his abdominal muscles on the count of 2 and expel the air by opening his glottis on the count of 3. Two coughs in succession may also be tried as an aid to mobilization of secretions.

Cough instruction is useful in conjunction with all respiratory therapy modalities and with postoperative abdominal and chest patients. A painful incision will limit the willingness of the patient to cough. It is helpful to have the patient 'cuddle' a pillow to his abdomen in a sitting position or for the therapist to support the incisional area with slight hand pressure. These maneuvers decrease the need to tighten abdominal muscles, the procedure that produces most of the pain.

In patients with spinal cord injury or disease, the abdominal musculature may be severely weakened. It is often helpful to apply an abdominal binder or hand pressure to provide support. Compressing the abdomen at the end of inspiration will help to increase intra-abdominal pressure and, therefore, increase the cough effectiveness.

Knowledge of the cough mechanism and the muscles of ventilation makes cough instruction an extremely simple and effective method of improving bronchial hygiene.

Cough Simulation

The respiratory care practitioner commonly encounters patients unable to cough effectively because of:

1. The placement of an artificial airway (tracheostomy or endotracheal tube).
2. Glottic disease.
3. Muscular inability: In these circumstances, it is effective to combine the bronchial hygiene techniques of chest physical therapy with IPPB therapy, thus simulating the cough mechanism.

The patient is provided a deep breath by positive pressure that is held for as long as reasonable. Chest vibration and compression is applied during this inspiratory pause. Exhalation is allowed to take place while the vibration and chest compression continue. This technique effectively produces a high-velocity airflow from the pulmonary tree, moving secretions to the trachea where they can be suctioned, coughed up, or swallowed. The positive pressure may be applied with a hand ventilator or an IPPB machine.

■ TECHNIQUES IMPROVING BREATHING EFFICIENCY

Few nurses are trained in the application of breathing techniques, and those with training have too little time to spend carrying them out. All respiratory therapy treatments necessitate proper breathing patterns and, therefore, all respiratory therapy practitioners must have an understanding of the techniques of breathing instruction and breathing retraining. Thorough understanding of the normal ventilatory cycle and the ventilatory muscles is mandatory.

Normal inspiration is accomplished primarily by contraction of the diaphragm. This results in an increased thoracic volume and a greater subatmospheric intrapleural pressure. This atmosphere-to-alveolar driving pressure results in gas movement towards alveoli. Recall that normal expiration is entirely passive, depending upon the elasticity of the chest wall and lung itself. With unlabored inspiration, one observes:

1. Abdomen rise because of the descension of the diaphragm.
2. Flaring out of the lower ribs.
3. A slight raising of the upper chest. During expiration, the abdomen moves in as the diaphragm rises and the lateral ribs return to the resting position.

A stressed inspiration includes use of the accessory muscles of ventilation, most commonly the scalenes, sternocleidomastoid, pectoralis major, and trapezius musles. These muscles act to elongate the bony thorax and exaggerate the increase in thoracic volume resulting from contraction of the diaphragm. Forced expiration is primarily accomplished by using abdominal musculature to increase intra-abdominal pressure. This forces the diaphragm upward.

These normal and forced ventilatory mechanisms are important to understand since it is the recognition of abnormal sequence or inefficient use of these mechanisms that allows the application of corrective measures. Such measures may greatly improve the patient's breathing mechanics. Any circumstance in which there is an abnormal breathing pattern is a circumstance where breathing retraining may be of dramatic aid. The abnormal breathing may be due to pain, apprehension and nervousness, surgery, bronchospasm, airway obstruction, restriction of the lungs and/ or chest wall, central nervous system disease, chronic lung disease, neuromuscular disorders, and countless others.

The tactile sense is most helpful in instructing a patient to assume a more appropriate breathing pattern. The therapist's hands are placed over the areas where muscular movement is desired and the patient is encouraged to concentrate on expanding the part of the chest under the hands. Proper diaphragmatic breathing instruction may be aided by placing the hand on the abdomen just beneath the xiphoid process and asking the patient to 'breathe in' against the hand. Proper diaphragm movement will cause the patient to feel his abdomen pushing away the hand. Relaxed shoulders and a slow, relaxed breathing pattern are essential to breathing instruction.

For segmental breathing instruction, the therapist's hand is placed on the chest area to be expanded. The patient is encouraged to breathe deeply and to preferentially 'send air' to that area of the chest where tactile stimulation is being applied by the therapist. On expiration, moderate compression is applied.

It is often helpful to have a patient with obstructive disease exhale through 'pursed lips'. A maneuver that increases resistance to exhalation at the month. This maneuver is believed to transmit an early expiratory back pressure to the bronchial tree. This back pressure is believed to prevent early collapse of small bronchioles and improve exhalation from alveoli.

CHEST PHYSIOTHERAPY POSITIONS FOR INFANTS AND CHILDREN

Below are the drainage positions for CPT. The white ovals show you where to percuss. During therapy, it is useful to have tissue or a basin handy to collect mucus. A glass of water may also be helpful for those who can cough better after their throat is wet.

Upper Lobes (Figs 14.8 and 14.9)

- Lean forward 30°. Percuss between the clavicle and the shoulder blade on each side of the chest.
- Lean back 30°. Percuss between the clavicle and the nipple on each side of the chest.

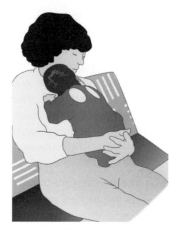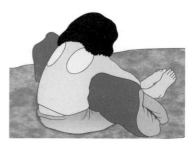

Fig. 14.8: Lean forward 30° position for upper lobe physiotherapy

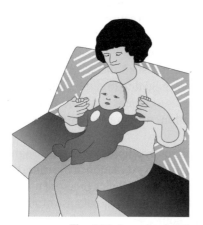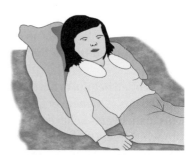

Fig. 14.9: Lean back 30° position for upper lobe physiotherapy

Lower Lobes (Figs 14.10 to 14.13)

The body should be positioned with the child's head down 30°and lying on the right side. Percuss on the left side below the underarm. Note: If your child has cystic fibrosis and is under the age of 5 years, you will not be tilting the chest area, but will keep the chest horizontal.

The body should be positioned with the child's head down 30°and lying on the left side. Percuss on the right side below the underarm. Note: If your child has cystic fibrosis and is under the age of 5 years, you will not be tilting the chest area, but will keep the chest horizontal.

The body should be positioned with the child's head down 30°and lying on the abdomen. Percuss between the lower edges of the rib cage and behind the underarm on each side of the spinal cord. Note: If your child has cystic fibrosis

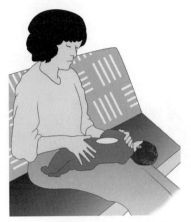
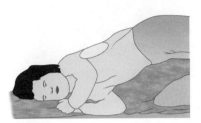

Fig. 14.10: Position for lower lobe physiotherapy, head down 30° and lying on the right side

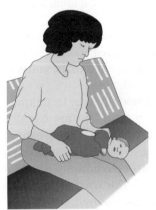

Horizontal

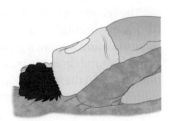

Head down 30°

Fig. 14.11: Head down 30° and lying the left side

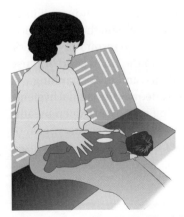
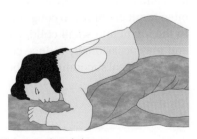

Fig. 14.12: Head down 30° and lying on the abdomen

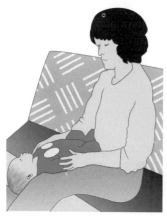 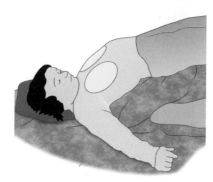

Fig. 14.13: Head down 30° and lying on the back

and is under the age of 5 years, you will not be tilting the chest area, but will keep the chest horizontal.

The body should be positioned with the child's head down 30°and lying on the back. Percuss on the front of the chest in the nipple area and just below. **Note:** If your child has cystic fibrosis and is under the age of 5 years, you will not be tilting the chest area, but will keep the chest horizontal.

The secret to the successful application of chest physiotherapy techniques in the small child is patience and understanding. Children are usually inquisitive and require a great deal of assurance that you are not going to hurt them. Postural drainage is easy to accomplish because the child is small and can be held in the lap and easily manipulated. Percussion is accomplished by simply tapping several fingers against the chest wall. This can be extremely effective and should not be accompanied by a 'slapping' sound, which may frighten the child. Above all, the therapist must be able to play 'a game' with the patient and to teach the family how to carry out the therapy in the chronically diseased child.

The most difficult modality of chest physical therapy to apply in pediatrics is coughing and breathing instruction. It is difficult to obtain the cooperation of a child who does not want to take a deep breath or is in respiratory distress. IPPB therapy is usually difficult and unrewarding in the small child because he is afraid of the mask and the machinery. Patience and understanding will often result in improved coughing technique and adequate bronchial hygiene. In the infant and small child, laughing and crying may assure deep breaths and may occasionally induce coughing like maneuvers. Nasopharyngeal or oropharyngeal suctioning may be necessary if secretions cannot be mobilized by other means.

INDEX

Page numbers followed by *f* refer to figure and *t* refer to table.

A

Abnormal breath sounds 45*t*
Acid-base disturbances
    mixed and complex 84*t*
    selected mixed and complex 84
Active exhalation 198*f*
Acute and chronic respiratory failure,
    distinctions between 111
Acute asthma 251
Acute lung injury 119
Acute respiratory acidosis
    1 for 10 rule for 84
    2 for 10 rule for 85
Acute respiratory distress syndrome (ARDS)
    137, 156
    ALI inclusion criteria 156
    ALI ventilator protocol 156
        exclusion 156
        scope 156
    recruitment maneuvers in 158
Acute ventilatory failure 70
    clinical findings 70
    physiologic consequences 70
    possible causes 70
    treatment 71
Adaptive support ventilation 127
Adjusting ventilation/oxygenation 138
Adult respiratory distress syndrome (ARDS)
    61, 64
    arterial blood gases 66
    clinical findings 66
    pathophysiology 64
    possible causes 66
    respiratory findings 66
    treatment 67
Air leak 208, 209*f*
Air trapping 197, 209*f*
Air trapping or auto-PEEP 196
Air, composition of 22
Airway management 212
    adjuncts to 213
Airway obstruction versus active exhalation
    195, 196*f*
Airway pressure release ventilation 126

Airway resistance
    conditions that increase 5*t*
    factors affecting 4
    normal 1
Airways, abnormalities of 109
Alveolar cells
    type I 1
    type II 1
Alveolar dead space 8, 14
Alveolar gas equation 14
Alveolar hypoventilation 93, 113
Alveolar macrophages 1
Alveolar overdistension 206, 207*f*
Alveolar recruitment effect 260
Alveolar shadows 48
Alveolar ventilation 9, 94
Alveolar ventilation and alveolar partial
    pressure for CO_2 95
Alveolar ventilation versus partial pressures 96*f*
Alveolar-arterial gradient 16
Alveoli
    abnormalities of 109
    cells types of 1
    expiration process 95*f*
    inspiration process 95*f*
    site of gas exchange 1
Anatomic dead space 8
Anxiety assessment findings 40
Aortic dissection 50
Apnea/low respiratory rate alarm 152
Arterial blood gas analysis 77
Arterial blood gases 54, 57, 78
Arterial blood pressure 161
    measurements, indications for 161
    physiology 162
    potential complications 164
    pulse pressure 164
Arterial catheter 161
Arterial lines, limitations of 162
Arterial pressure 22
Arterial pressure pulse 163
Arterial pulse pressure variation (PPV) 164
Arterial puncture 77
Arterial system
    pressure distribution in 163, 163*f*

Assist control (AC) 123
    advantages 124
    complications 124
    indication 123
Assisted versus controlled breath 199, 200*f*
Asthma 58
    arterial blood gases 59
    clinical findings 58
    possible causes 58
    respiratory findings 59
    treatment 59
Atelectasis 50
Atrial fibrillation 166
Automatic tube compensation 128
Auto-PEEP 150*f*

B

Barotrauma 126
Bellows lung 19
Bicarbonate buffer 35
BI-level positive airway pressure (BIPAP) 181
Blood pressure 22
Body plethysmography 25
Bougie 225, 226*f*
Breath sounds 45
    abnormal 45
    normal 45
Breathing 20
    control of 21
    efficiency, techniques improving 280
    gas exchange 21
    high work of 104
    mechanics 21
    through a tube 96
    type of 202, 202*f*
    work of 204, 205*f*
Bronchi, bronchial tree and lungs 20*f*
Bronchial carcinoma 48
Bronchial hygiene, techniques promoting 273
Bronchiectasis 48
Buffer systems 88

C

Capnography 173
    indications for use of 175
Carbon dioxide
    effects of 100
    elimination 14
    transport 35
Carbon monoxide 101
Cardiac function curve 165
Cardiac output 175
Cardiac tamponade 166

Cardiogenic pulmonary edema 252
Cardiopulmonary exercise testing 43
Cardiothoracic ratio 49
Carotid arteries 233
Central venous catheter 165
Chest MRI 72
Chest percussions 277, 278*f*
    techniques 278*f*
Chest physiotherapy 272
    goals of 272
    positions, for infants and children 281
Chest radiograph 135
Chest vibration 278
    position of hands 279*f*
Chest wall stiffness 7
Chest X-ray 46, 55, 57, 59*f*, 75
    increased opacity 60*f*, 62, 66*f*
    interpretation 47
Chronic bronchitis 53
    and emphysema 109, 110
    clinical findings 54
    possible causes 54
    respiratory findings 54
    structural changes 53
    treatment 54
Chronic lung disease (CLD) 131
Chronic obstructive pulmonary disease
    (COPD) 119
    ventilatory failure in 71
Chronic respiratory acidosis
    4 for 10 rule for 85
    5 for 10 rule for 85
Chronic respiratory failure (obstructive lung
    disease) 251
Circulation, ventilation, and perfusion 27
Closed loop control 127
Collateral ventilation 2
Combined oxygen and carbon dioxide
    transport 35
Combitube 225, 226*f*
Complications with PA catheters 170
Congestive heart failure 51
Consolidation 51
Continuous positive airway pressure (CPAP)
    119, 120, 181, 250
    advantages 120
    indications 120
Controlled mandatory ventilation (CMV) 121
    complication 121
    indications 121
Cor pulmonale 58
Coronary artery disease (CAD) 264
Coronary circulation 37
Correlation between X-rays 47
Cough instruction 279

Cough simulation 280
Cricoid cartilage 232
Cricothyroid membrane 233
Cricothyroidotomy 221, 231, 232
    absolute indication for 233
    anatomical landmarks 232
    definition 232
    equipment tray for 236*f*
    indications 233
    technique 232
Cuffed oropharyngeal airway (COPA) 224, 225*f*
CVP waveforms, pathological 166

D

Dead space
    factors affecting 96
    ventilation 8
Deep vein thrombosis (DVT) 97
Derived hemodynamic data 176
Diabetic ketoacidosis 88
Diaphragmatic breathing 266
Dicrotic notch 163
Difficult intubations 217
Difficult weaning, approach to 183
Diffusion capacity 15
    using CO 15
Diffusion rate 15
Dipalmitoyl phosphatidylcholine (DPPC) 7
Dyspnea
    classification of 45
    diagnostic approach to 41
Dyssynchrony 147

E

Echocardiogram 74
Elastance 12
Elastic forces 7
Electrocardiogram (ECG or EKG) 75
Emergency cricothyroidotomy
    advantages of 235
    disadvantages of 235
    dressing for 238*f*
Emphysema 55
    clinical findings 56
    complications of 57
    possible causes 56
    respiratory findings 56
    treatment 57
    types of 56
Endothelin receptor antagonists (ERAs) 75
Endotracheal tube 214
    function 215*f*
    process of inserting 214

Esophageal airway device 229
Esophageal gastric tube airway 230, 231*f*
Esophageal intubation 174*f*
Esophageal obturator airway (EOA) 229
    advantages of 229
    contraindications 229
Esophageal perforation 238
Esophagus 233
Ethylene glycol poisoning 88
Expected compensation 85*t*
Expiratory flow 146
    components of 194
    pattern 195*f*
Expiratory positive airway pressure (EPAP) 255
Expiratory reserve volume (ERV) 24, 25

F

Fetal hemoglobin 101
Fick principle 176
    definition 176
    oxygen extraction by 177*f*
Flail chest 67
    arterial blood gases 67
    clinical findings 67
    possible causes 67
    respiratory findings 67
    structural changes 67
    treatment 67
Flexibility and stretching exercises 267*f*
Flow and pressure plethysmographs 26
Flow patterns 193*f*
Flow versus time curve, basics of 192
Flow-related pulse wave, graphical displays
    of 172*f*
Flow-volume loop 208, 208*f*
    components of 208
    interpretation 192*f*
Forced vital capacity (FVC) 24
Frank-starling curve 165
FRC *See* Functional residual capacity (FRC)
Functional residual capacity (FRC) 24, 25
    and P-V loop 202, 203*f*

G

Gas exchange 22
    in humans and mammals 32
Gas exchange or respiration 30
Gas exchange/transport 30
Gas trapping 127
Gas velocity 12
Gaseous diffusion 34
    process of 33*f*
General cell metabolism 33

Griggs forceps (portex) technique 244
Guidewire insertion 243*f*
    through needle 243*f*

H

Head tilt/chin lift 212
Helical CT 72
Hemodynamic monitoring 161
Hemoglobin 43
Hepatic portal system of circulation 37
HFOV *See* high frequency oscillatory
    ventilation (HFOV)
High airway pressure 145
High anion gap acidosis 87
High flow therapy (HFT) 258
    benefits of 261*t*
    contraindications 260
    indications 260
    physiological effects of 259
    system features 261
High flow through tracheostomy tube 259*f*
High frequency jet ventilation 131
High frequency oscillatory ventilation (HFOV)
    131
    adverse effects 135
    basic principles 133
    contraindications 135
    initial settings 132
    physiology 133
    theory 133
High frequency ventilation 130
    disadvantages 131
    proposed advantages 130
High peep alarm 152
High pressure trigger, patient effort in 149*f*
High respiratory rate alarm 152
Higher peep/lower FiO$_2$ 158*t*
Hypercapnic/hypoxemic respiratory failure,
    type II 110
Hypercarbia, causes of 94
Hyperinflation (COPD) 51
Hyperventilation 174*f*
Hypoventilation 97, 103
Hypoxemia 92, 120
    causes of 97
    pathophysiology 113
    treatment 114
Hypoxemic respiratory failure 251
    type I 110
Hypoxia 102
    pulmonary vasoconstriction 28
    signs and symptoms of 103*t*

I

Ideal gas law 14
Inadequate inspiratory flow 149*f*, 202, 207, 207*f*
Increased airway resistance 206, 210, 210*f*
Increased anion gap metabolic acidosis 87
Increased WOB 206
Inflation pressure
    components of 200, 200*f*
Initial FiO$_2$ 138
Initial ventilator settings 137
Inspiratory capacity (IC) 24
Inspiratory flow 146
    components of 194
    pattern 194*f*
Inspiratory muscle training 269
Inspiratory plateau 140
    positioning 140
    prophylaxis 141
    sedation 141
Inspiratory reserve volume (IRV) 24
Intensive care units (ICUs) 178
Interface device 255*f*
Intermittent positive pressure breathing
    (IPPB) 273
Intra-alveolar pressure 2
Intrapleural pressure 2
Intrapulmonary shunting 113
Intrinsic PEEP 127
Intubation 214
    indications for 107
Intubation and ventilation, criteria for 106
Intubation device 215*f*
Iron lung 118*f*
Ischemia 88

J

Jaw thrust 212
Joints flexibility 266
Jugular veins 233

L

Lactic acidosis 88
Laminar resistance 13
Laminar versus turbulent flow 3
Laryngeal mask airway (LMA) 213, 214
    guide to use 214
Laryngeal tube 224, 225*f*
Low expired volume alarm 145
Low inspired oxygen partial pressure 93
Low PEEP alarm 152
Lower lobes 282
    physiotherapy 283*f*
Lower PEEP/higher FiO$_2$ 157*t*

Lung apex 29
Lung base 29
Lung compliance 6
　basis of 7
　conditions that decrease 8t
　decreased 184, 201, 205
Lung diseases 97, 102
Lung expansion 6
Lung fields, abnormalities in 48
Lung segments 275
Lung volumes 23
Lungs 2, 17, 27
　anatomy 19
Lungs and alveoli, anatomy of 18f

M

Macintosh pattern laryngoscope 216
Magill's forceps 217, 217f
Manual methods 212
Mean arterial pressure (MAP) 164
Mechanical breath 192, 193f, 199
Mechanical ventilation
　airway resistance 1
　indication for use 118
　monitoring 153
　spontaneous mode 119
Mechanical ventilator 116
Mechanical ventilatory support 178
Meconium aspiration syndrome (MAS) 132
Mediastinal carcinoma 49
Metabolic acid-base disorders, rules for 86
Metabolic acidosis 82
　analysis 86
　one and a half plus eight rule 86
Metabolic alkalosis 83
Methanol poisoning 88
Methemoglobinemia, effects of 101
Mini-wright peak flow meter 27f
Minute ventilation 9, 13, 94
Minute volume (MV) 180
Mouth-to-mask breathing 229

N

Nasal intubation 220
Nasal trumpet 223
Nasopharyngeal airway 223, 223f
Negative pressure ventilation 117
Neurally adjusted ventilatory assist (NAVA) 128, 129
NIV See Noninvasive ventilation (NIV)
Nodular shadowing 48
Noninvasive ventilation (NIV) 248
　acute, indications for 252

　advantages 248
　complications 256
　disadvantages 248
　humidification 258
　initiation of treatment 256
　interfaces 254
　mask 152
　mechanism of action 249
　modes 255
　reduced discomfort 249
　reduced incidence of complications 248
　selection criteria 251
　　acute respiratory failure 251
　summary 258
　timing of 250
　types 250
　ventilators 254
　when to end 257
Normal alveolus versus injured alveolus 65f
Normal anion gap 87
　metabolic acidosis 87
Normal capnography waveform 174f
Normal chest X-ray 47f
Normal CVP waveforms 166
Normal pulmonary artery pressures (PAP) 38
Nosocomial pneumonia. 126

O

Obstructed airway 233
Ohm's law 12
Oral intubation: a step-by-step guide 227
Oropharyngeal airway 222, 222f
　disadvantages 225
　history and usage 222
　indications and contraindications 223, 224
　insertion 222, 224
　key risks of use 223
Overperfusion and underperfusion 28
Oxygen transport 33
Oxygen uptake 14
Oxygenation criteria 180
Oxygenation status using PaO_2, interpretation of 102t
Oxyhemoglobin dissociation curve 99, 99f

P

PaO_2/FiO_2 ratio, calculations 180
Paraldehyde poisoning 88
Parameters 184
Partial lower airway obstruction 174f
Partial pressure (P) of gas, definition of 93
Patient-ventilator dyssynchrony 147
　causes of 147

Patient-ventilator system check 155
Peak expiratory flow rate (PEFR or PEF) 26
Peak flow meter 26
Peak inspiratory flow (PIFR) level 194
Peak inspiratory flow rate 140
Peak inspiratory pressure (PIP) 199
Peak pressure (high) 5
Pectoral muscles, stretching 267
PEEP *See* Positive end-expiratory pressure
    (PEEP)
Percutaneous dilatational tracheostomy
    (PDT) 240
Percutaneous tracheostomy 239
Persistent pulmonary hypertension of the
    newborn (PPHN) 132
Pharyngeal dead space washout 259
Phosphodiesterase-5 inhibitors (PDEI) 75
Physiological dead space 9, 14
    clinical conditions that increase 9*t*
Placement of the stethoscope, locations for 44
Plain tubes 221
Plateau pressure 5, 200
Pleural effusion 51
Pleurisy 2
Pneumonia 48, 59
    arterial blood gases 60
    clinical findings 60
    pathophysiology 60
    possible causes 60
    respiratory findings 60
    treatment 61
Pneumothorax 2, 49, 68
    clinical findings 69
    possible causes 69
    respiratory findings 69
    structural changes 68
    treatment 69
Point seven plus twenty rule, for a metabolic
    alkalosis 86
Positive end-expiratory pressure (PEEP) 6, 119,
    140, 199, 203
    complications associated with 120
Positive expiratory pressure (PEP) 260, 274
    mask 275*f*
Positive pressure ventilation 118
Postural drainage 273
    segmental anatomy of lungs for 274*f*
Pressure assist ventilation 123
Pressure controlled mechanism, process of
    122*f*
Pressure controlled ventilation 122
Pressure regulated volume control (PRVC) 125
Pressure support (PS) 181
    slow weaning protocol 188*f*
Pressure versus time curve 199*t*

Pressure-regulated volume control/volume
    support (PRVC/VS), slow weaning
    protocol 188*f*
Pressures within pulmonary circulation 37
Pressure-volume loop 202
    components of 202
    interpretation 191*f*
    lung compliance changes in 206*f*
    PEEP level on 204*f*
Pulmonary angiogram 73
Pulmonary arteriovenous malformation 71
Pulmonary artery catheters (PACs) 168, 169
    contraindications to 169
    physiology 169
    settings in 168
Pulmonary blood flow 36*f*
Pulmonary blood flow and metabolism 36
Pulmonary capillary occlusion pressure,
    limitations to 170
Pulmonary capillary wedge pressure (PCWP)
    38, 165, 169
Pulmonary edema 50, 61
    arterial blood gases 62
    clinical findings 62
    pathophysiology 61
    possible causes 61
    respiratory findings 62
    treatment 62
Pulmonary embolism 63
    arterial blood gases 64
    clinical findings 64
    pathophysiology 63
    possible causes 63
    treatment 64
Pulmonary embolus 96
Pulmonary function tests 56, 60, 67
Pulmonary hypertension 57, 73
    clinical findings 74
    diagnosis 74
    possible causes 74
Pulmonary insufficiency 40
Pulmonary measurements 180
Pulmonary rehabilitation 263
    balance 269
    breath training 265
    exercise 264
    flexibility and stretching 266
    home training 269
    lower body training 265
    nutritional guidance 270
    therapy programs 264
    upper body training 265
    ventilatory muscle training 265
    WHO benefits from 263
Pulmonary resistance 13

Pulmonary vascular resistance (PVR) 39, 176
Pulmonary vascular resistance index (PVRI) 176
Pulse oximetry 171
  reading of 171*f*
Pursed-lip breathing 266
P-V loop, components of 203*f*

R

Rapid sequence induction (RSI) 221
Rapid shallow breathing index (RSBI) 184
Rapid weaning 182
  success of 182
Registered pulmonary function technologists (RPFT) 25
Residual volume (RV) 24, 25
Respiratory acid-base disorders, rules for 84
Respiratory acidosis 81
Respiratory alkalosis 82
Respiratory breathing patterns 41
Respiratory care and surgery, preoperative evaluation 70
Respiratory diseases 52
Respiratory exchange ratio 12, 14
Respiratory failure 250
  classification of 110
  clinical manifestations 112
  diagnostic studies 112
Respiratory function 17
Respiratory muscle fatigue 184
Respiratory physiology 22
  equations 12
Respiratory pressures 13
Respiratory quotient (RQ) 11, 14
Respiratory rate 21
Respiratory system
  anatomy of 233*f*
  resistance 13
Restrictive and obstructive diseases, differentiation 25*t*
Reticular shadowing 48
Richmond agitation-sedation scale 185
Right arterial pressure (RAP) 165
Ring shadows and tram lines 48

S

Sarcoidosis 49
Scalar graphics, analysis of 192
Scalloping 149
Shunt equation 15, 16
Specific resistance 13
Spiral CT 43
Spontaneous breath 192, 192*f*, 198
Spontaneous breathing trial 185

Spontaneous respiratory rate (RR) 179
Sputum observation 46, 46*t*
Starling equation 15
Stroke volume index (SVI) 176
Subcutaneous emphysema 239
Surfactant, role of 8
Surgical tracheostomy 239
Synchronized intermittent mandatory ventilation (SIMV) 122, 124, 181
  interpretation 125*f*
  mandatory breath triggering mechanism 124
  PC with PS 125
  spontaneous breath triggering mechanism 125
Systemic circulation 37
Systemic vascular resistance (SVR) 176
Systemic vascular resistance index (SVRI) 176

T

Taylor dispersion 134
Terminal weaning 184
Thoracic gas volume (VTG) 25
Thoracic restrictive/cerebral hypoventilation diseases 251
Thoracic walls 2
Thyroid cartilage 232
Thyroid gland 233
Tidal volume (TV) 24
Tidal volume and inspiratory pressure limit 137
Tidal volume/inspiratory time 146
Total lung capacity (TLC) 24
Trachea 232
  examination of 45
Tracheoesophageal fistula 238
Tracheostomy 239
  advantages 246
  contraindications 246
  disadvantages/complications 246
    delayed 247
    immediate 246
    late 247
  indications 246
  insertion techniques 240
  preparation 245
  procedure 245
  technique 241
Tracheotomy 221
Transairway pressure 200
Tricuspid regurgitation 166
Tube
  insertion over guidewire 244*f*
  maintenance 220
  position of 221
  types of 221

Tuberculosis 48
Turbulent resistance 13

U

Uncuffed tubes 221
Upper lobe physiotherapy 282*f*
Uremia 88

V

Variable and waveform control 141
Veins 27
Ventilation and oxygenation, effects on 5
Ventilation
    definition of 94
    goals 142
    indications for 107
    pathophysiology 106
    respiratory failure 107
Ventilation/perfusion lung scan 30, 75
Ventilation-perfusion mismatch (V/Q) 15, 104, 113
    defects 105
Ventilation-perfusion ratio 10
    alveolar gases 10
    decreased 11
    end-capillary gases 11
    increased 11
Ventilation-perfusion relationships 9
Ventilator dependence, reversible causes of 183

Ventilator graphics 190
    general concepts 190
Ventilator settings 127
Ventilator settings and alarms 144
Ventilator-induced lung injury, pathogenesis of 131
Ventilatory criteria 179
Ventilatory failure 106
Ventilatory muscle training (VMT) 265
Ventricular septal rupture (VSR) versus acute mitral regurgitation 168
Vital capacity (VC) 20, 23, 24
    and spontaneous tidal volume (VT) 179
Volume targeted ventilation 205, 205*f*
Volume versus time 93*f*
    curve, basics of 197
    scalar 197*f*

W

Wean screen 183
Weaning 178, 257
    criteria 179
    failure 178
        causes of 183
        signs of 179*t*
    method of 181
procedure 186
    protocol, for medical respiratory intensive care unit 184*t*
    success 178